AF800165

Septal Surgery Challenges in Rhinoplasty

Springer Nature More Media App

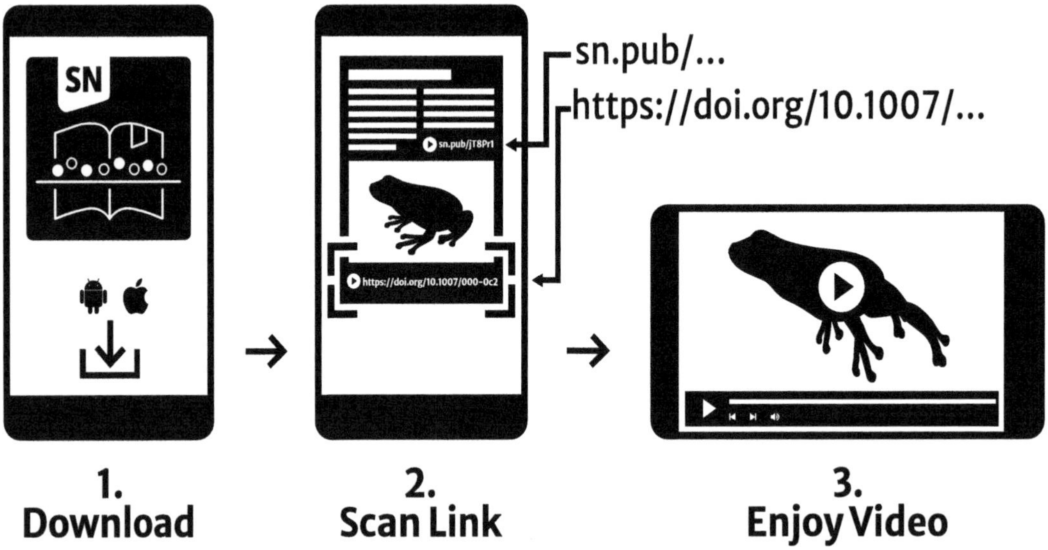

Support: customerservice@springernature.com

Fazıl Apaydın

Septal Surgery Challenges in Rhinoplasty

Springer

Fazıl Apaydın
Department of Otorhinolaryngology
Ege University
Izmir, Türkiye

This work contains media enhancements, which are displayed with a "play" icon. Material in the print book can be viewed on a mobile device by downloading the Springer Nature "More Media" app available in the major app stores. The media enhancements in the online version of the work can be accessed directly by authorized users.

ISBN 978-3-031-74733-5 ISBN 978-3-031-74734-2 (eBook)
https://doi.org/10.1007/978-3-031-74734-2

© The Editor(s) (if applicable) and The Author(s), under exclusive license to Springer Nature Switzerland AG 2025

This work is subject to copyright. All rights are solely and exclusively licensed by the Publisher, whether the whole or part of the material is concerned, specifically the rights of translation, reprinting, reuse of illustrations, recitation, broadcasting, reproduction on microfilms or in any other physical way, and transmission or information storage and retrieval, electronic adaptation, computer software, or by similar or dissimilar methodology now known or hereafter developed.
The use of general descriptive names, registered names, trademarks, service marks, etc. in this publication does not imply, even in the absence of a specific statement, that such names are exempt from the relevant protective laws and regulations and therefore free for general use.
The publisher, the authors and the editors are safe to assume that the advice and information in this book are believed to be true and accurate at the date of publication. Neither the publisher nor the authors or the editors give a warranty, expressed or implied, with respect to the material contained herein or for any errors or omissions that may have been made. The publisher remains neutral with regard to jurisdictional claims in published maps and institutional affiliations.

This Springer imprint is published by the registered company Springer Nature Switzerland AG
The registered company address is: Gewerbestrasse 11, 6330 Cham, Switzerland

If disposing of this product, please recycle the paper.

Preface

As a surgeon performing rhinoplasty for 32 years and septal surgery for 38 years, I found that nasal septal deformities could cause special difficulties for the surgeon. In my practice, inadequate correction is the most common reason for revision rhinoplasty. I already had a very special interest in this part of the nose during rhinoplasty, and I wanted to share my vast experience with my colleagues in this book. If my colleagues find some of the information in this book helpful, it will be a great pleasure for me.

When I joined the Department of Otorhinolaryngology at Ege University in 1987, as a first-year resident, one of the first operations I assisted and later performed was submucous resection of the nasal septum. It was performed under local anesthesia through Killian incision at that time. The traditional packing involved inserting gauze strips. The removal of these packs was later performed in 20 min, which was a very painful procedure for the patient. I started assisting with rhinoplasties during my residency years. In my department, traditional Joseph techniques were applied without touching the tip.

The only operation I learned and performed during my residency years was submucous resection of the nasal septum. When I went to Tübingen for a research project in 1993, I had a chance to observe the Cottle type of maxilla-premaxilla approach to the nasal septum. Since then, I have learned how to handle caudal septal deviations.

In 1992, I had the opportunity to start rhinoplasty during my military service. In 1999, when my chairman asked me to choose a subspecialty, I chose facial plastic surgery. When I visited Chicago to learn more from Dr. Eugene Tardy and Dr. Dean Toriumi, I learned the details of endonasal and external rhinoplasty and subtotal septal reconstruction. Since that time, because of working in a tertiary referral center, I have had the chance to operate on all difficult cases and crooked noses, which became a kind of challenging passion for me.

When I started organizing meetings and lecturing on rhinoplasty and septoplasty after 2000, I had a chance to listen and learn techniques and tricks from masters in rhinoplasty. I had a chance to learn about extracorporeal septoplasty from Prof. Gubisch during these meetings. After trying this method in some cases, I realized that it was very difficult and unpredictable for me. I chose to master splinting techniques and subtotal reconstruction techniques without removing the entire cartilaginous septum. However, in revision rhinoplasty, the situation is different from that in primary rhinoplasty. In these challenging cases, I learned to use the ear and rib cartilages effectively.

During my rhinoplasty journey, I learned a lot from my teachers, colleagues, and students. However, my best teachers were always my patients. I learned more about rhinoplasty and challenging cases of septal surgery after video recording, taking pictures, using Gunter diagrams, keeping records in Rhinobase, and consistent follow-up for as long as possible.

I have been a keen history reader during my life. Therefore, I dedicated the first chapter to the history of septal procedures. I am absolutely fascinated by reading the numerous articles on historical developments of septal surgery and rhinoplasty. I was very much amazed when I read the original article by Killian because it was almost the same operation that I had learned to perform during my residency. I also found that during the recent 150 years, the advances in septorhinoplasty realized by our forefathers followed each other step by step. I also found that unfortunately, some of this valuable information was neglected and seemed to be forgotten when passing it on to newer generations. Therefore, I highly recommend my colleagues to learn more about the history and previously written articles thoroughly if they would like to learn more details and techniques of our previous masters.

In Chap. 2, a brief description of surgical anatomy was given to remind my colleagues about some important details that can be helpful during surgery.

Physiology of the nose is the third chapter in this book. Unfortunately, some surgeons tend to forget the importance of the physiology of the nose, which is of utmost importance for functional rhinoplasty. The surgeon must have a clear understanding of the physiology of the nose to enlighten the patients about the reaction of the nose to surgery.

I must admit that I am shocked when I see some rhinoplasty surgeons performing surgery without a detailed examination of the nose. As far as I understand, this is because rhinoplasty is performed by ENT surgeons, plastic surgeons, and more recently by maxillofacial surgeons. Among these three specialties, the examination of the nose is a standard procedure only for ENT surgeons during their residencies. Therefore, plastic surgeons and maxillofacial surgeons who are interested in rhinoplasty should rotate in ENT departments to learn more about surgical anatomy, physiology, and examination of the nose. This is one of the reasons why Chaps. 2–4 are added to this book.

I have been claiming for decades that septal surgery must be accepted as a major surgery and not a minor procedure. The surgeon should definitely come up with an operative plan before surgery after identifying the real problems that patients encounter. In Chap. 5, it is recommended how it can be done systematically.

There is no universally accepted classification of septal deviations. In Chap. 6, some widely used classifications and my own classification are presented.

In Chap. 7, the incisions used for septal surgery alone or together with rhinoplasty are presented. I wanted to share my thoughts and experience on each of these incisions with my colleagues.

The traditional surgical methods for septal surgery must be mastered by all rhinoplasty surgeons. There is no shortcut in this matter. Surprisingly, I heard from a famous rhinoplasty surgeon a year ago that "I do not believe in septal surgery. If you rotate the nose, the function becomes good without touching the septum." Please simply disregard these kinds of wrong statements and read Chap. 8 to revive traditional septoplasty methods and hear about my thoughts and experience.

One of the most difficult challenges in rhinoplasty is the presence of caudal septal deflections. Because this is the part just under the nasal tip and this part of the nose is most prone to trauma and is also the most flexible part of the nose. In Chap. 9, the methods used to correct these deformities are described by some case examples.

In Chap. 10, solutions to correct the dorsal deviations of the nose are reported. The preferred methods are given by some case examples.

In Chap. 11, a more complicated but less often discussed problem is the focus: dorso-caudal deviations of the nasal septum. Rhinoplasty surgeons tend to speak about caudal or dorsal deviations, but not on combined deviations. In this chapter, the solutions for this particular situation are reported by presenting some concepts that I have popularized in recent years.

In Chap. 12, the focus is on deviations of the bony septum. This part of the nasal septum is usually neglected during surgery and is simply resected. In this chapter, the fundamentals of bone recycling are covered.

Dorsum preservation has been revitalized within the last decade with growing interest. Regardless of the technique used, the nasal septum is always at the epicenter of these interventions. This issue is addressed in Chap. 13.

The surgical management of nasal septal perforations is discussed in Chap. 14. It is always a big challenge for the surgeon to close septal perforations. You can find different techniques to close septal perforations in this chapter.

In Chap. 15, different techniques for the management of the nasal valve are detailed. Although the nasal septum can be a reason for nasal valve stenosis, the upper lateral cartilages and external valves can play a role as well.

When there is severe septal deviation in the nose, enlargement of the inferior and middle turbinates is very common. The surgical techniques that can be used in these situations are considered in Chap. 16.

Should packing and splinting be used at the end of septorhinoplasty? You can find the answer to this important question in Chap. 17.

Every surgeon creates their own algorithm for postoperative follow-up and care after septal surgery. In Chap. 18, I want to share my own thoughts with my colleagues, thinking that it can be helpful to them.

It is the dream of every resident in training and surgeon to have a useful model to practice the different steps of rhinoplasty and septal surgery. I find lamb head as a very useful model for this aim, and I share the details of its use in Chap. 19.

This book reflects my experience of three decades on the challenges in septal surgery during rhinoplasty. I hope that my colleagues will find it useful and adapt some of these techniques in their surgical armamentarium.

I consider myself a blessed person in many ways. I am very grateful to my teachers in elementary school, high school and my professors at the university. Prof. Dr. Orhan Cura and Prof. Dr. Ovunc Gunhan from Ege University were two pillars in my ENT education and training, and in my academic life. Prof. Dr. Eugene Tardy, Prof. Dr. Dean Toriumi, and Prof. Dr. Regan Thomas introduced me to the fascinating world of facial plastic surgery. There are numerous Professors, colleagues, friends, fellows, and residents who helped me and guided me during this journey. I am also very grateful to Mr. Tony Bull, who accepted me as a member of the European Academy of Facial Plastic Surgery. I happened to serve this Academy, my friends, and colleagues until now with great passion and enthusiasm. I am also grateful to my friends and colleagues in Türkiye, where I had the opportunity to share my passion for learning and teaching. I have been working with them in ENT and Facial Plastic Surgery societies in Turkey for decades.

I would like to express my gratitude to Merve Evren, PhD, who worked with me on the illustrations for 18 months with great effort. With her skillful touch, this book became more colorful and descriptive.

I was born in Izmir, and all my education occurred in Izmir. I still live in Izmir. My family and many of my friends live in Izmir. My father, my mother, and my two brothers were always my main inspirations during my childhood. However, the best luck of my life was meeting my wife, Sebnem Apaydin, while I was a university student. She is always the main person supporting me by all means. I would like to thank her from the bottom of my heart through this book. If you work so hard in your life, you can never be a great father, but my daughter Ipek is always the joy of my life.

I hope that this book will be helpful to my friends and colleagues.

Izmir, Turkey Fazıl Apaydın
2024

Contents

1 History of Nasal Septal Surgery

1.1 Introduction

The first submucous septal resection was published by Heylen in 1847 [1]. Linhart performed submucous surgery on a deviated anterior septum in 1862 [2].

Adams employed force to induce a septal fracture using forceps with flat, parallel blades in 1885. He used a steel-screw compressor to support the septum for 2–3 days, which was subsequently replaced with ivory plugs to maintain support [3].

Ingals classified septal deviations, and in the case of anterior cartilaginous septal deviations, he recommended a vertical incision in the mucosa and removal of a small triangular piece of cartilage from the deviated portion. He also recommended a horizontal incision of the mucosa and removal of the bone with a saw to remove bony crests or spurs [4].

In 1892, Hajek described a modification in which the incision was made just at the anterior edge of the cartilage, and the caudal septal cartilage was resected along with the anterior nasal spine [5].

Krieg reported his technique in 1886, which involved resecting the mucous membrane entirely on one side and then resecting a large piece of the cartilaginous septum while leaving an L-strut framework in place, termed the "window operation" (Fenster operation). He allowed the defect to heal through granulation [6]. Boenninghaus refined Krieg's technique in 1889, adding the resection of the vomer and perpendicular plate to the deviated cartilage and even reported resection of the entire cartilage without complications [7].

Until 1896, the Bosworth operation was the most common procedure in the United States for managing septal deviations. This involved using a small intranasal saw to remove the obstructing spur with its mucosa on the convex side, plus the underlying cartilage and bone, while preserving the mucosa on the concave side [8].

In 1896, Watson [9] presented a technique that began with one or more beveled incisions on the convex side of the deviation, which could be linear, hockey stick-shaped, or T-shaped in design. After elevating the perichondrium, some obstructive cartilage was resected. The remaining cartilage was then pushed toward the concave side of the septum to obtain the benefit of the beveled incision and the position of the bony septum, both of which could help maintain the position of the septum in the midline, often using pins, nasal packing, or hollow metal tubes (Fig. 1.1).

Gleason [10] published his technique in 1896. It consisted of inserting a Bosworth saw into the obstructed nasal passage and cutting transversely until it penetrated the cartilage or bone. Then, the direction of the sawing was changed to a vertical position in order not to harm the contralateral mucosa while cutting. A U-shaped incision was made through the septum, wide enough to expose the entire deviated area of the septum. The deflected parts of the septal cartilage and bony septum were removed. The beveled cut surface of

© The Author(s), under exclusive license to Springer Nature Switzerland AG 2025

F. Apaydın, *Septal Surgery Challenges in Rhinoplasty*,
https://doi.org/10.1007/978-3-031-74734-2_1

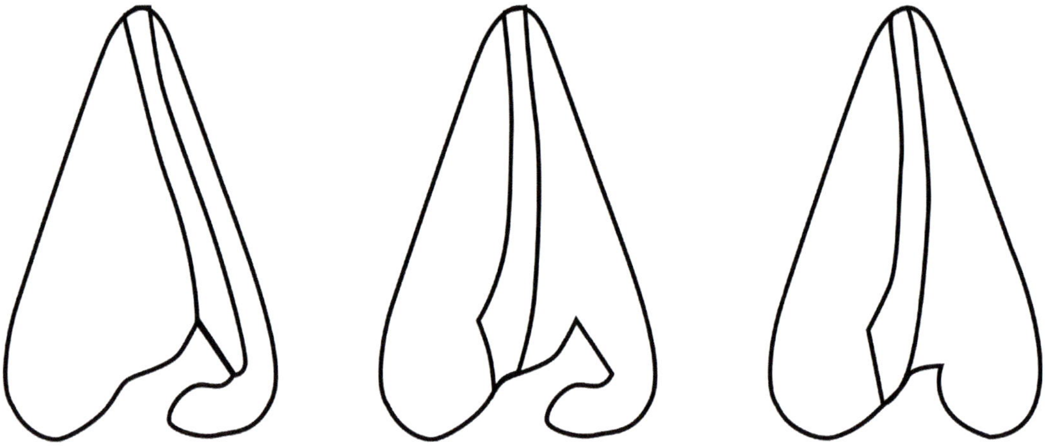

Fig. 1.1 Watson resected some obstructive cartilage and spur, then pushed the septum toward the concave side to position it in the midline by obtaining the benefit of the beveled incision and the position of the bony septum

the septum was pushed to the midline, jumping over the lower bony septum, which helped the septal cartilage maintain its midline position. The techniques of Watson and Gleason shared many technical similarities, which sparked significant debate at the time.

Asch noted that previous methods did not yield satisfactory results and proposed a different approach in 1896. He pointed out that the vital point to attain was to destroy the resiliency of the cartilage. He transected the nasal septum with scissors and then manipulated it digitally to fracture it severely, aiming to disrupt cartilage memory and prevent recurrence of the deviation, followed by using hollow tubular splints to keep the nose open [11].

Freer presented the "Submucous resection" method in 1902. He used an L-shaped incision to gain access to the nasal septum while leaving the caudal septum intact. He emphasized the importance of leaving an L-shaped cartilaginous strut of 6–8 mm to maintain nasal support and prevent common deformities such as columellar retraction and supratip depression [12].

Killian reported some difficulties following the techniques of Krieg and Boenninghaus, such as occasional granulations and a longer need for tampons during the healing process. He decided to leave the mucosa in place and observed that healing was much faster and better. He presented his technique in 1899 during a German meeting and named his procedure "Submucous window resection of nasal septum." In his technique, the oblique incision started from below, which was 5 mm away from the caudal septum, moving obliquely to stay 10 mm away from the caudal septum at the upper end (Fig. 1.2). His idea was to leave a piece of the caudal septum to support the outer nose. He elevated bilateral subperichondrial flaps, used Hartman nasal forceps to resect the septal cartilage like opening a window on the septal cartilage, and used a chisel and hammer to

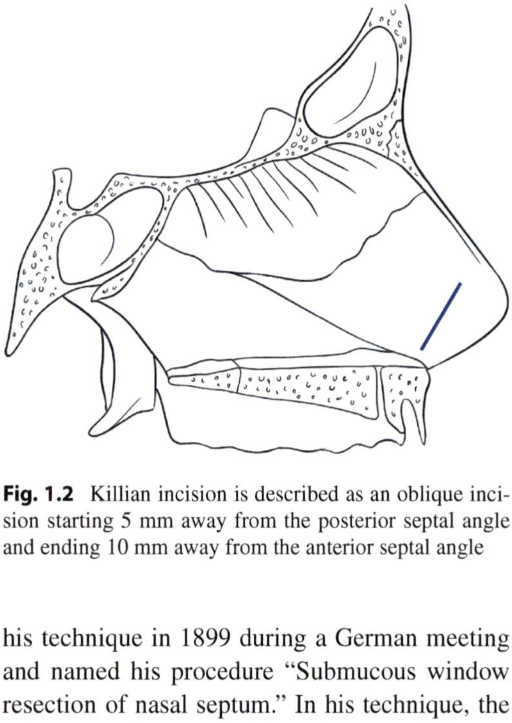

Fig. 1.2 Killian incision is described as an oblique incision starting 5 mm away from the posterior septal angle and ending 10 mm away from the anterior septal angle

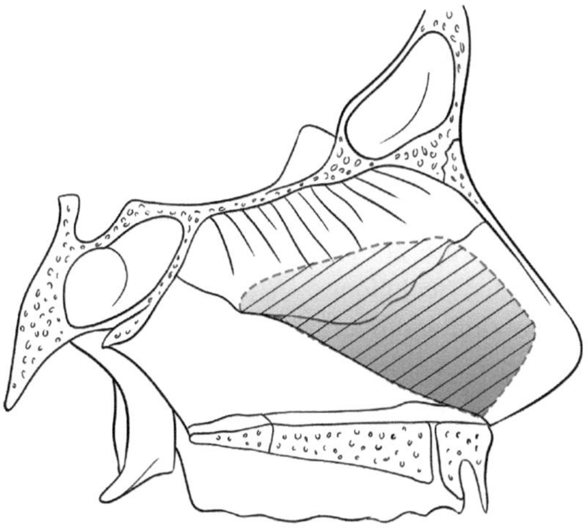

Fig. 1.3 The nasal septal cartilage is removed by leaving a portion of the superior and caudal part of the septum

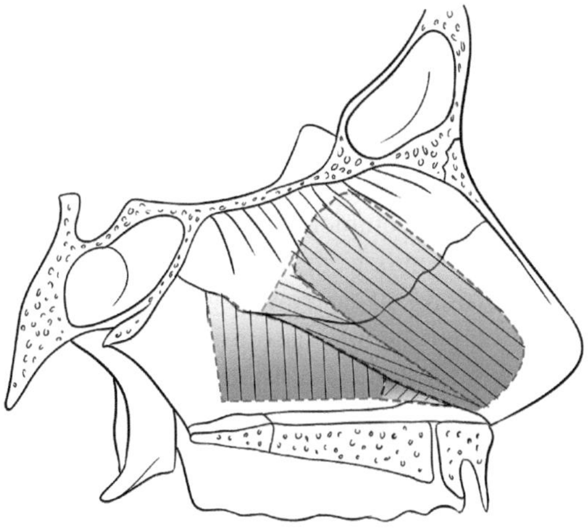

Fig. 1.4 Killian used a chisel and hammer to resect the bone of the ethmoid plate and vomer in addition to resecting the cartilage

resect the bone of the ethmoid plate and vomer (Figs. 1.3 and 1.4). He reported that the use of nasal speculums of his own design, available in different lengths, helped him see clearly through a narrow incision. He published all the details of his meticulous work in 1905 [13].

Although submucous resection was a revolutionary method that dominated other methods at the beginning of the twentieth century, its use was limited to deviations of the caudal septum. Metzenbaum was the first to report a technique for correcting deviations of the caudal septum in 1929, emphasizing the significance of this structure in supporting the nasal tip and its role in esthetic and functional outcomes [14]. Therefore, if the displaced cartilage was removed, the tip would drop, it would come closer to the upper lip, a retracted columella would be seen, and the difficulty in breathing could remain. If the caudal septum was replaced, the columella would stiffen, the soft tissues of the nasal tip would be supported, the depressed nasal tip would be raised, the patency of the nostrils would be restored, and the nasal tip would develop normally in children. He also insisted that a fractured or dislocated caudal septum had to be reset at the time of the injury regardless of the patient's age. In his technique, it was first necessary to diagnose the problematic portions of the nasal septum. The incision was made along the caudal margin of the septum. The mucosa of the contralateral side was detached until the angle of deflection was reached. One or two narrow strips of cartilage parallel to the incision could be removed or cross-hatched to straighten the caudal septum and replaced in a groove at the anterior nasal spine and into a pocket opened retrogradely in the columella (Fig. 1.5). He used the analogy of a door to explain his technique, which was later called the "swinging door" technique [14].

Peer [15] developed a technique for cases where replacement of the dislocated caudal septum was not possible because of severe distortion. After an incision over the caudal margin of the septal cartilage, the nasal septum was exposed through bilateral dissection of the mucous membrane. The distorted lower segment was completely resected, a large piece of cartilage was removed from the remaining nasal septum using a Bellanger swivel knife, and the anterior portions of the ethmoid and vomer were also resected. A caudal septal replacement graft was carved and placed in a pocket opened in the columella, extending from the nasal spine to the dorsal septum (Fig. 1.6).

Seltzer described a reconstructive technique for the nasal septum in crooked noses in 1944. It started with exposure of the crooked lower half of the nose through intercartilaginous and transfix-

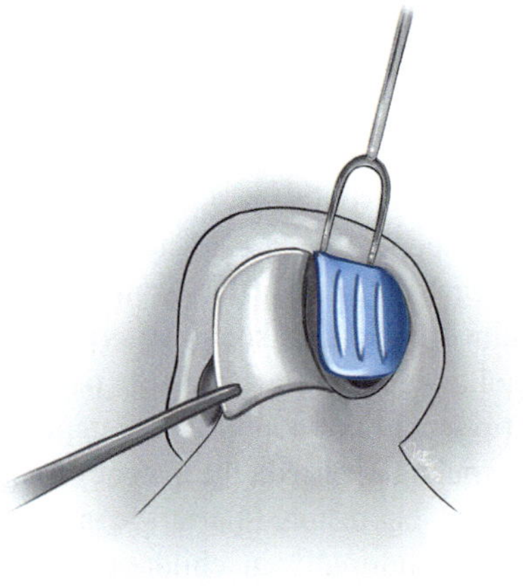

Fig. 1.5 Metzenbaum reported the technique of "swinging door" for correcting deviations of the caudal septum. After exposing and identifying the angle of deflection, one or two narrow strips of cartilage parallel to the incision were removed to straighten the caudal septum

ion incisions. After a narrow strip from the septum was removed from the deflected septum at the vertical plane, the displaced lower end of the septal cartilage was brought back into the midline (Fig. 1.7). The crucial part of this technique was to keep the mucoperichondrium on the opposite side intact. The caudal margin of the nasal septum was sutured to the columella [16]. Similar techniques were published by Salinger in the same year [17] and by Steffensen a few years later [18] (Fig. 1.8).

Galloway extensively resected the nasal septal cartilage to eliminate septal deviation. After opening a bed in the columella, he passed two pilot sutures from the columella and inserted the septal cartilage between the mucoperichondrial flaps. The pilot sutures were then used to engage the septal cartilage into the columellar bed, where it was fixed by two mattress sutures passing through the full thickness of the columella and graft. The pilot sutures were withdrawn after they met the surgeon's needs [19].

Fomon published a paper in 1946 to challenge the notion that maintenance of the profile projection of the nasal pyramid was mainly dependent on support by the septum. He reported that the upper lateral cartilages maintain the profile projection of the nose without the aid of the septum [20]. He also liked using Galloway's technique without the fear of saddling the dorsum because the reinserted cartilage could overcome cicatricial contracture.

King and Ashley reported a new technique, as they were not satisfied with the previously presented techniques. After one-sided hemitransfixion and intercartilaginous incisions, the mucoperichondrial flaps were elevated on both sides, and almost the entire septal cartilage was resected in one piece. Bony deviations were corrected. The cartilage was then carefully trimmed, straightened, and placed back in its bed, transfixed into the columella with mattress sutures [21].

Maliniac classified septal deformities associated with external malformation of the nose as follows: (1) septal deflection with oversized hump deformity, (2) crushed septal fracture with depressed external deformity, and (3) septal deflection with external lateral deviation. He reported that the axis of the external nose could not be completely straightened until all secondary bends were released either by vertical excisions of narrow segments along its entire height or by crisscrossing when curvatures were less marked [22]. He described the use of dorsal and columellar grafts in crushed deformities.

Cottle criticized the Killian incision and gave two reasons for switching to a more caudal incision: (1) If the incision is in the mucosa, the resultant scar can prevent normal ciliary activity; (2) A large flap to cover replaced bone and cartilage has been sectioned. He also showed that the cartilage and bone could be inserted between the mucous membranes like a mosaic to prevent scar formation and cicatricial contracture [23].

Goldman commented on the inadequacies of the three popular techniques described by Killian, Metzenbaum, and Fomon. He published a new technique for the correction of septal deviation in 1956. The mucoperichondrium was elevated bilaterally after the transfixion incision. The deviated caudal septum was converted into two vertical sections. The remaining septum was then displaced to the midline by fracturing or resect-

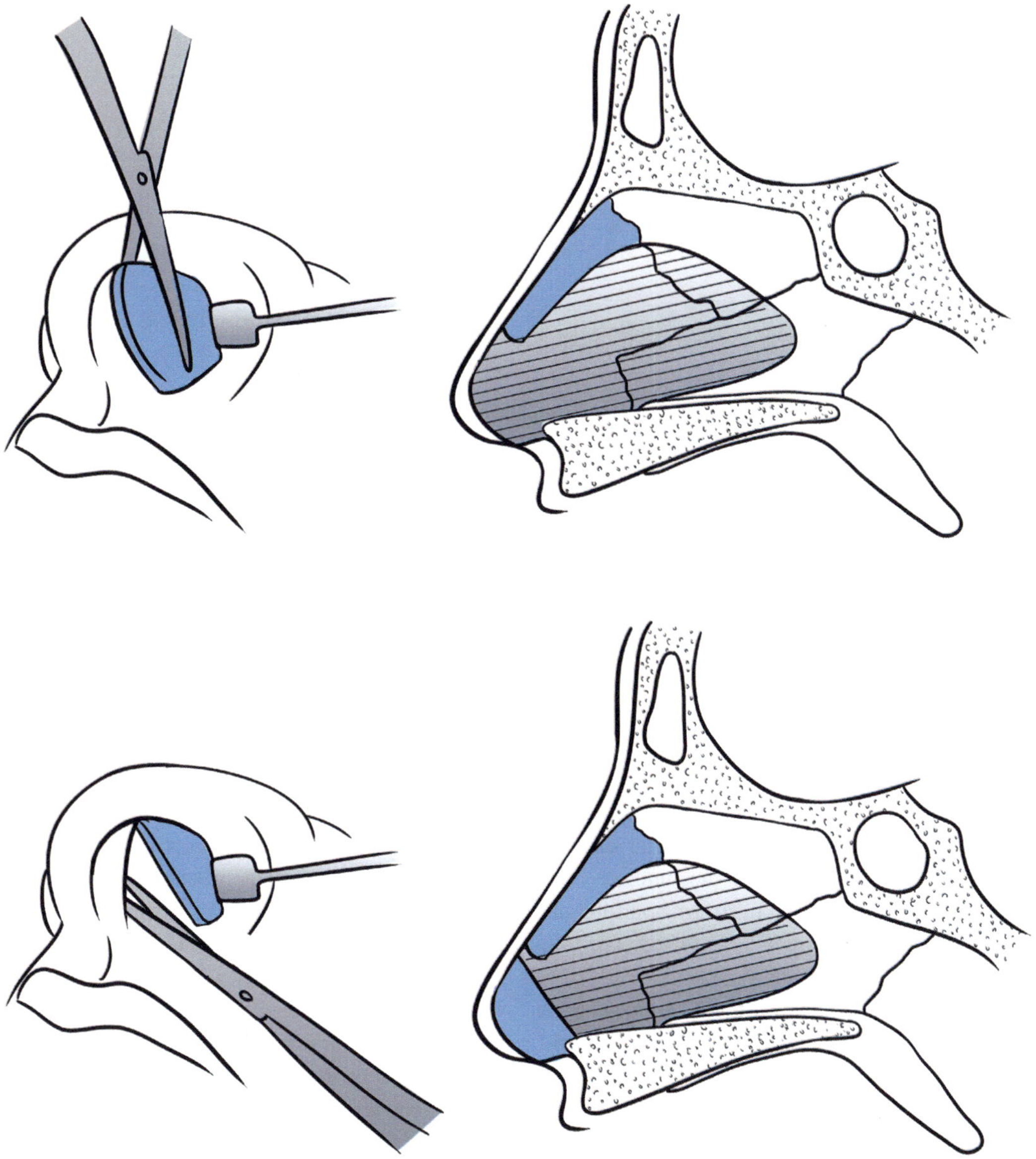

Fig. 1.6 Peer developed a technique for resecting the distorted lower segment of the nasal septum. Then a large piece of cartilage was removed from the remaining nasal septum, and the anterior portions of the ethmoid and vomer were also resected. A caudal septal replacement graft was carved and placed in a pocket opened in the columella, extending from the nasal spine to the dorsal septum

ing the osseous region. If there was overlapping or angulation of the cartilaginous and bony septum, a limited resection was performed. If the anterior nasal spine was at the midline, it could be brought back to the midline by fracturing. If the anterior nasal spine was too wide, it was completely or partly removed. He claimed that his technique could prevent saddling, tip drooping, septal flaccidity, columellar retraction, and vulnerability to trauma [24].

Cottle et al. published "the maxilla-premaxilla approach to extensive nasal septum surgery" in 1958. In this technique, a right-handed surgeon started the operation with a right hemitransfixion incision, exposing the caudal septum and opening a left anterior tunnel by dissecting the muco-

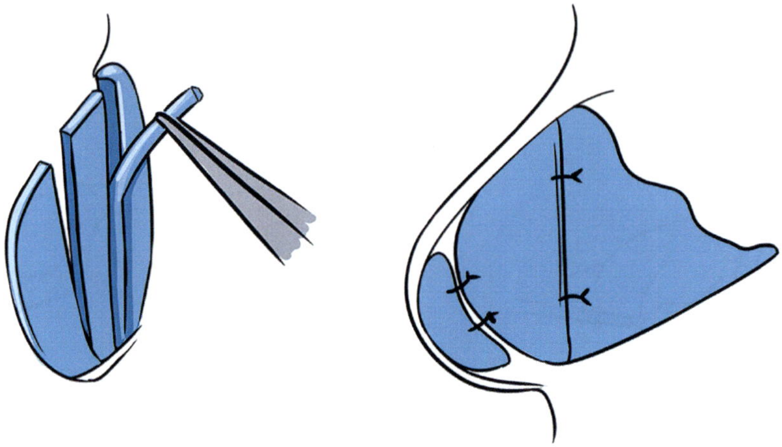

Fig. 1.7 Seltzer exposed the crooked lower half of the nose through intercartilaginous and transfixion incisions. After a narrow strip from the septum was removed from the deflected septum at the vertical plane, the displaced lower end of the septal cartilage was brought back into the midline. The crucial part of this technique was to keep the mucoperichondrium on the opposite side intact

perichondrium from the nasal septum on the left side, where the right-sided mucosa was attached to the nasal septum. When the posterior area was reached, the mucosa was separated further by bringing the elevator from behind forward and interiorly, which was frequently quite easy. In very severely injured noses, the anterior nasal spine, lower portion of the pyriform aperture, and floor of the nasal airway were exposed. The inferior tunnels were then dissected bilaterally. The cartilage was severed from the bone base as far back as the perpendicular plate of the ethmoid, and the right inferior tunnel was then entered. The left anterior and inferior tunnels were combined by careful dissection. The premaxillary bones were inspected and modified if needed. The posterior portion of the septal cartilage separated from the perpendicular plate of the ethmoid while remaining attached in its entirety to the right mucosal flap [25].

In 1986, Rees reported on 25 patients with severe internal and external deviation of the nose, where the entire bony and cartilaginous septum was removed while preserving the mucoperichondrial and mucoperiosteal flaps. The distorted cartilage was carefully trimmed to obtain one or more straight pieces of cartilage. These pieces were sutured to each other and inserted between the mucoperichondrial flaps to support the lower nose and midvault. The flaps were then sutured to hold the implants in place. He reported good esthetic and functional improvement in all cases [26]. Gubisch popularized and improved this technique first with the endonasal approach and then with the external approach [27, 28]. Jugo used this technique in children, using an external approach, with good results [29].

Endoscopic septoplasty was initially described by Lanza [30] and then by Stammberger [31] in 1991. The primary indication was isolated septal deviation in primary or secondary cases. The advantages were reduced morbidity and postoperative swelling because of the limited dissection area, improved visualization, and it served as an effective teaching tool. In fact, a similar technique was described by Maliniac in 1948 using a headlight [22]. Advances in the use of an endoscope during septal surgery or rhinoplasty have revolutionized nasal surgery. Surgeons can feel more comfortable in addressing the problems of the posterior part of the nose, the lower and middle turbinates, and the management of septal perforations and sinuses [32].

Toriumi published subtotal reconstruction of the nasal septum in 1994 with successful results. He reported that his technique was the first site-

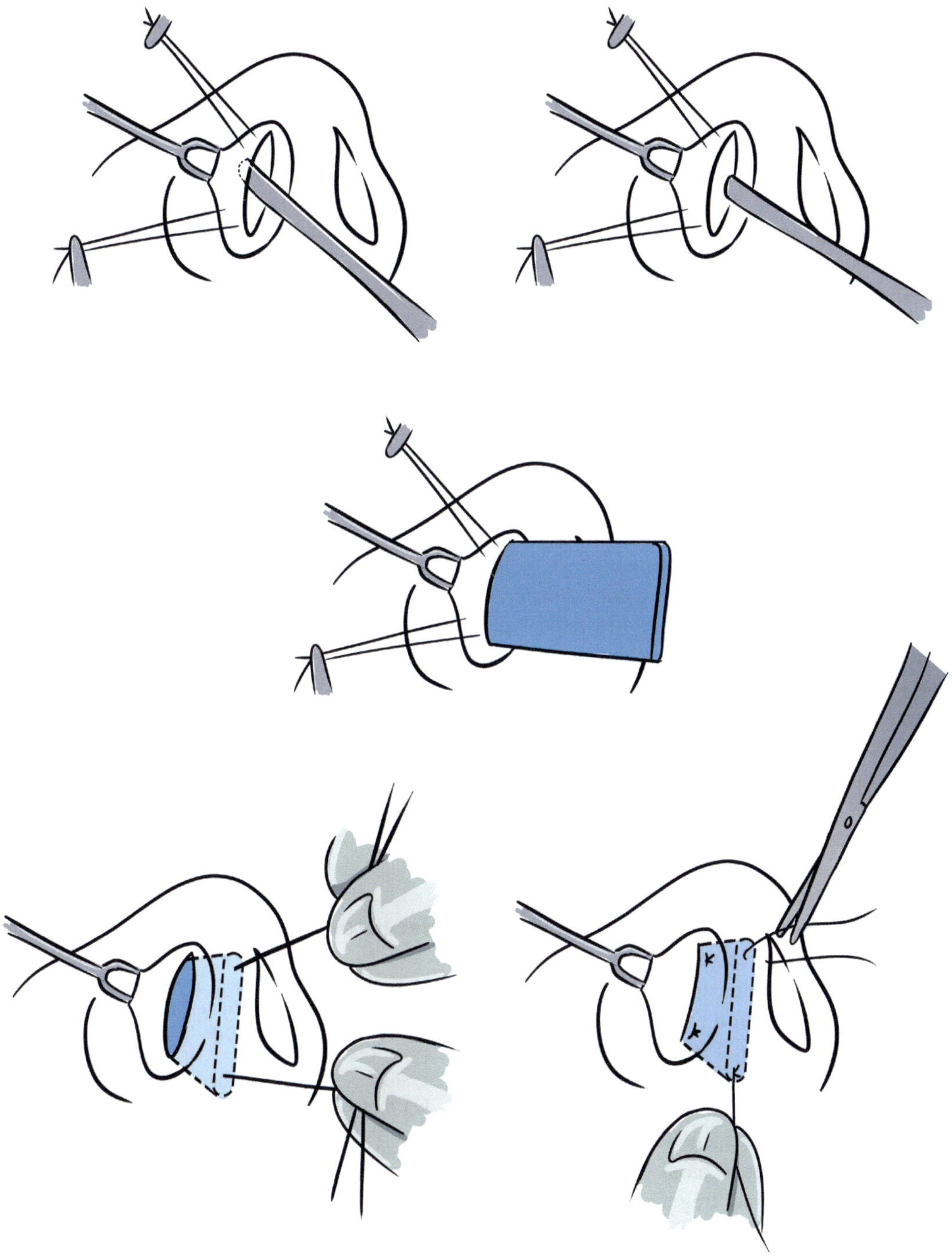

Fig. 1.8 Galloway resected most of the nasal septal cartilage to eliminate septal deviation. He prepared a big cartilaginous graft, opened a bed in the columella, passed two pilot sutures from the columella, and inserted the septal cartilage between the mucoperichondrial flaps. The pilot sutures were then used to engage the septal cartilage into the columellar bed, where it was fixed by two mattress sutures passing through the full thickness of the columella and graft

specific technique with an external approach that emphasizes the reconstitution of structural support. In 12 cases of severely crooked noses, he resected most of the septal cartilage in one piece by leaving 5 mm of cartilage at the key area and anterior nasal spine. A flat piece of cartilage was sculpted from the posteroinferior portion of the septal cartilage. This cartilage was then sutured to the remaining cartilages at the key area and anterior nasal spine. If there was no remnant at the anterior nasal spine, the caudal portion of the graft was sutured to the anterior nasal spine. If the dorsal segment had residual deflection, a unilateral spreader graft was used to create symmetry [33].

Byrd et al. reported different techniques for correcting crooked noses in 1998. After leaving 8–10 mm of the L-strut framework in place, the caudal strut was trimmed and sutured back to the anterior nasal spine to remove excess cartilage. A horizontal control suture of the Mustardé type was suggested for straightening dorsal, caudal, and anterior angle deformities. In this study, one-sided spreader-extension grafts and contralateral batten grafts for the caudal strut were also reported [34]. Rohrich et al. suggested weakening the dorsal strut with partial cuts and supporting it bilaterally with spreader grafts. They also reported the use of batten grafts for the caudal strut after cross-hatching [35]. Thus, the era of leaving the L-strut in place and using a splinting method began. Foda reported the use of bony batten grafts to straighten the dorsal and caudal deformities of the L-strut [36].

Boenisch published a study using polydioxanone foil in conjunction with septal cartilage in 2000. She performed almost the same operation as Rees; in other words, she removed almost all of the badly deviated nasal septal cartilage, divided it into straighter fragments, sutured them on PDS foil, and reinserted them as free grafts in 71 patients and 5 rabbits. She reported that no inflammatory foreign body reaction had occurred, and cartilage regeneration was observed [37]. The PDS foil was completely absorbed in 25 weeks. This technique brought a lot of excitement to septal surgery and was very well accepted by many prominent surgeons. However, its popularity started to fade out throughout the years because of septal cartilage loss, prolonged edema, and inflammation [38].

Toriumi extensively used rib cartilage to obtain splinting spreader grafts and caudal septal replacement grafts to reconstruct the nasal septum in crooked noses and/or revision rhinoplasties [39]. He used the Gibson and Davis principle of balanced cross-section to sculpt the grafts and eliminate warping [40]. Tastan et al. published an oblique split technique for sculpting rib cartilage [41]. This technique, which I am also fond of, enabled surgeons to obtain more grafts, thinner and better-sculpted grafts for nasal septal reconstruction [42].

I am always thrilled to read about the history of surgical procedures. While preparing this chapter, I had the opportunity to learn small details of many procedures that were accepted as the state-of-the-art of that day. The techniques we are currently using are the result of the cumulative efforts of some of the pioneers presented in this chapter. As a rhinoplasty student and surgeon who is trying to get better and serve my patients better every day, I would like to express my gratitude to all the surgeons who did monumental work to perfect functional and esthetic surgery of the nose.

References

1. Heylen P. Déviation et longueur trop considérable du cartilage de la cloison du nez; resection d'une partie du cartilage; disparition de la difformité. Gaz Med Paris. 1847;12:810.
2. Linhart W. Compendium der chirurgischen Operationslehre. 2nd ed. Wien: Braunmueller; 1862.
3. Adams W. On the treatment of the broken nose by forcible straightening and mechanical retentive apparatus. BMJ. 1875;2:421–2.
4. Ingals EF. Deflections of the septum narium. Trans Am Laryngol Assoc. 1882;4:61–9.
5. Hajek M. Laryngo-rhinologische mitteilungen: operation der septumdeviationen [Laryngology rhinology cures: operation of the deviated septum]. Internationale Klinische Rundschau. 1974;6:1419–1423.
6. Krieg P. Beitrage zur resection der cartilage quadrangularis narium zur heilung der skoliosis septi [Contributions of resection of the quadrangular cartilage to cure scoliosis of the septum]. Berliner Klinische Wochenschrift. 1889. pp. 699–700.

7. Boenninghaus G. Bemerkungen zum aufsatze loewes: zur chirurgie der nasenscheidewand. Monatsschr Ohrenh. 1900;34:287.
8. Bosworth FH. Treatment of nasal stenosis due to deflective septa with or without thickening of the convex side. Laryngoscope. 1899;6:337–9.
9. Watson AW. The operation for deviation of the nasal septum. N Y Med J. 1896;1–6
10. Gleason EB. A new operation for the correction of deflections of the nasal septum. Laryngoscope. 1896;1:265–9.
11. Asch MJ. Treatment of nasal stenosis due to deflective septa with or without thickening of the convex side. Laryngoscope. 1899;6:340–3.
12. Freer OT. The corrections of deflections of the nasal septum with a minimum of traumatism. JAMA. 1902;38:636–42.
13. Killian G. The submucous window resection of the nasal septum. Ann Otol Rhinol Laryngol. 1905;14:384.
14. Metzenbaum M. Replacement of the lower end of the dislocated septal cartilage versus submucous resection of the dislocated end of the septal cartilage. Arch Otolaryngol. 1929;9:282–92.
15. Peer LA. An operation to repair lateral displacement of the lower border of the septal cartilage. Arch Otolaryngol. 1937;25:475–7.
16. Seltzer AP. The nasal septum: plastic repair of the deviated septum associated with a deformed tip. Arch Otolaryngol. 1944;40:433.
17. Salinger S. Traumatic deformities of the nasal septum. Ann Otol Rhinol Laryngol. 1944;53:274.
18. Steffensen WH. Reconstruction of the nasal septum. Plast Reconstr Surg (1946). 1947;2(1):66–71.
19. Galloway T. Plastic repair of the deflected nasalseptum. Arch Otolaryngol. 1946;44:141.
20. Fomon S, Syracuse VR, Bolotow N, Pullen M. Plastic repair of the deflected nasal septum. Arch Otolaryngol. 1946;44:141–56.
21. King ED, Ashley FL. The correction of the internally and externally deviated nose. Plast Reconstr Surg (1946). 1952;10(2):116–20.
22. Maliniac JW. Role of the septum in rhinoplasty. Arch Otolaryngol. 1948;48(2):189–201.
23. Cottle MH, Loring RM. Surgery of the nasal septum—new operative procedures and indications. Ann Otol Rhinol Laryngol. 1948;57:705–13.
24. Goldman IB. New technique in surgery of the deviated nasal septum. Arch Otolaryngol. 1956;64:183–9.
25. Cottle MH, Loring RM, Fischer GG, Gaynon IE. The "maxilla-premaxilla" approach to extensive nasal septum surgery. AMA Arch Otolaryngol. 1958;68:301–13.
26. Rees TD. Surgical correction of the severely deviated nose by extramucosal excision of the osseocartilaginous septum and replacement as a free graft. Plast Reconstr Surg. 1986;78(3):320–30.
27. Gubisch W. Das schwierige septum. HNO. 1988;36:286–9.
28. Gubisch W. Extracorporeal septoplasty for the markedly deviated septum. Arch Facial Plast Surg. 2005;7(04):218–26.
29. Jugo S. Total septal reconstruction through decortication (external) approach in children. Arch Otolaryngol Head Neck Surg. 1987;13:173–86.
30. Lanza DC, Kennedy DW, Zinreich SJ. Nasal endoscopy and its surgical applications. In: Lee KJ, editor. Essential otolaryngology: head and neck surgery. 5th ed. New York: Medical Examination; 1991. p. 373–87.
31. Stammberger H. Special problems. In: Hawke M, editor. Functional endoscopic sinus surgery: the Messerklinger technique. Philadelphia: BC Decker; 1991. p. 432–3.
32. Hwang PH, McLaughlin RB, Lanza DC, Kennedy DW. Endoscopic septoplasty: indications, technique, and results. Otolaryngol Head Neck Surg. 1999;120(5):678–82.
33. Toriumi DM. Subtotal reconstruction of the nasal septum: a preliminary report. Laryngoscope. 1994;104(7):906–13.
34. Byrd HS, Salomon J, Flood J. Correction of the crooked nose. Plast Reconstr Surg. 1998;102(6):2148–57.
35. Rohrich RJ, Gunter JP, Deuber MA, Adams WP Jr. The deviated nose: optimizing results using a simplified classification and algorithmic approach. Plast Reconstr Surg. 2002;110(6):1509–23.
36. Foda HM. The role of septal surgery in management of the deviated nose. Plast Reconstr Surg. 2005;115(2):406–15.
37. Boenisch M, Mink A. Clinical and histological results of septoplasty with a resorbable implant. Arch Otolaryngol Head Neck Surg. 2000;126(11):1373–7.
38. Wang LL, Frankel AS, Friedman O. Complications of polydioxanone foil use in nasal surgery: a case series. Facial Plast Surg. 2018;34(3):312–7.
39. Toriumi DM. Subtotal septal reconstruction: an update. Facial Plast Surg. 2013;29(6):492–501.
40. Gibson T, Davis WB. The distortion of autogenous cartilage grafts: its cause and prevention. Br J Plast Surg. 1958;10:257.
41. Taştan E, Yücel ÖT, Aydin E, Aydoğan F, Beriat K, Ulusoy MG. The oblique split method: a novel technique for carving costal cartilage grafts. JAMA Facial Plast Surg. 2013;15(3):198–203.
42. Apaydin F. Oblique split technique: a game changer in costal cartilage sculpting. Plast Aesthet Res. 2019;6:9.

2 Surgical Anatomy of the Nasal Septum

2.1 Introduction

The nasal septum is located in the middle of the nasal cavity and divides it into two passages. It is also the middle wall of the nasal pyramid. The nasal cavity is surrounded by mucosa, except at the entrance. Under the mucosa, the nasal septum comprises the cartilaginous and bony septum. In front of the caudal septum, there is a structure called the membranous septum, which does not have any solid structure.

2.2 Growth of the Nasal Septum

The nasal septum is solely composed of cartilage from the columella to the sphenoid in a newborn baby. The vomer is in the form of vomeral wings as a thin layer of bone on each side of the basal rim of the cartilaginous septum [1]. Two zones of thicker cartilage have been described in newborns: the sphenospinal and sphenodorsal zones. The first is the lower, thicker zone extending from the sphenoid to the anterior nasal spine, and the latter extending from the sphenoid to the nasal dorsum [2]. The cartilage between these two zones is the thinnest. The caudal portion of the septum is also thinner. This pattern of cartilaginous thickness does not change in later years [3] (Fig. 2.1).

A controversial topic among surgeons is the timing of rhinoplasty and septal surgery. I was taught not to touch the nose until the age of 18 since my residency years. The nasal septal cartilage is believed to be a key growth center that contributes to nasofacial skeletal development, especially the development of the midface. There are different studies in the literature that give different ages for the maturation of nasofacial growth. In one study, it was reported that it would stop at the age of 13 years for girls and 15 years for boys [4]. It was found to be 16 in girls and 18 in boys in another study [5]. In my region, it was found to be 12 years of age in girls and 15 years in boys [6]. Although some surgeons are comfortable operating on children at a relatively early age [7, 8], I am still reluctant to start rhinoplasty earlier than 15 years in girls and 16 years in boys unless there is a prominent nasal obstruction causing marked discomfort.

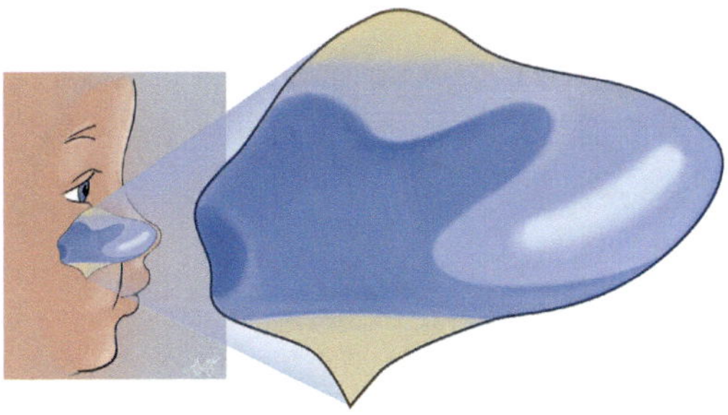

Fig. 2.1 The nasal septum is entirely composed of cartilage in newborn babies. The sphenospinal and sphenodorsal zones are two zones of thicker cartilage. The cartilage between these two zones is the thinnest. The caudal portion of the septum is also thinner

© The Author(s), under exclusive license to Springer Nature Switzerland AG 2025

F. Apaydın, *Septal Surgery Challenges in Rhinoplasty*,
https://doi.org/10.1007/978-3-031-74734-2_2

2.3 Cartilaginous Septum (Quadrangular Cartilage)

The septal cartilage is rectangular, which is why it is also called quadrangular cartilage. It sits at the top of the maxillary crest and vomer. The caudal margin is connected by fibrous tissue to the membranous septum and inferiorly to the medial crura. Superiorly, it continues with the upper lateral cartilages, and the uppermost portion goes below the nasal bones. The posterior margin is attached to the ethmoid lamina with a strong joint (Fig. 2.2).

The caudal septum makes the anterior septal angle superiorly, the middle septal angle, and the posterior septal angle inferiorly. Approximately 5 mm behind the posterior septal angle, the septal cartilage is attached to the anterior nasal spine by strong soft tissue attachments [9] (Fig. 2.3).

The septum cartilage in white adults averages 3–4 mm in thickness [10]. As mentioned above, it has different thicker zones, the sphenodorsal and sphenospinal zones, and thinner zones. In 1892, Zuckerkandl described a thicker zone and named it “processes laterales ventrales” [11]. The inferior border of the quadrangular cartilage sitting on the maxillary crest shows lateral extensions of approximately 2–4 mm on each side, forming a cartilage 4–8 mm thick. Similar lateral extensions of the cartilage are frequently observed in the dorsally attached upper lateral cartilages. Cottle suggested referring to them as the “processus laterales dorsales” [10] (Fig. 2.4). These thicker portions act as excellent graft sources during rhinoplasty. In addition, shaving a 1–2 mm cartilaginous hump, especially close to the keystone area, does not pose a problem in terms of maintaining the brow-tip esthetic lines and preserving the valve area. This is a critical detail I had missed for years. I was always trying to use spreader grafts in such cases; however, this small detail eliminated the use of spreader grafts in each case after hump removal.

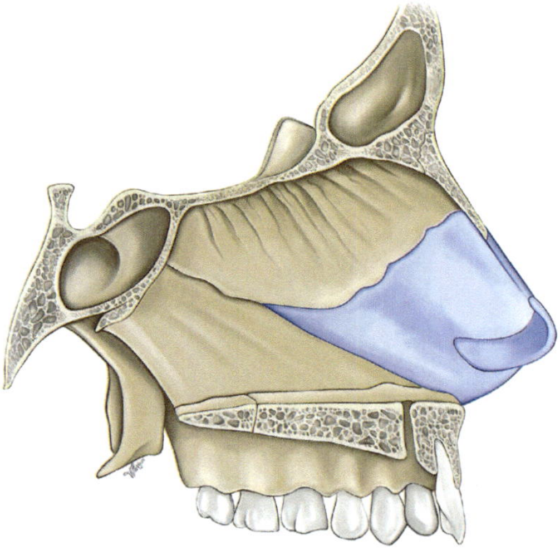

Fig. 2.2 The septal cartilage is rectangular and sits at the top of the maxillary crest and vomer. Superiorly, it continues with the upper lateral cartilages, and the uppermost portion goes below the nasal bones. The posterior margin is attached to the ethmoid lamina with a strong joint

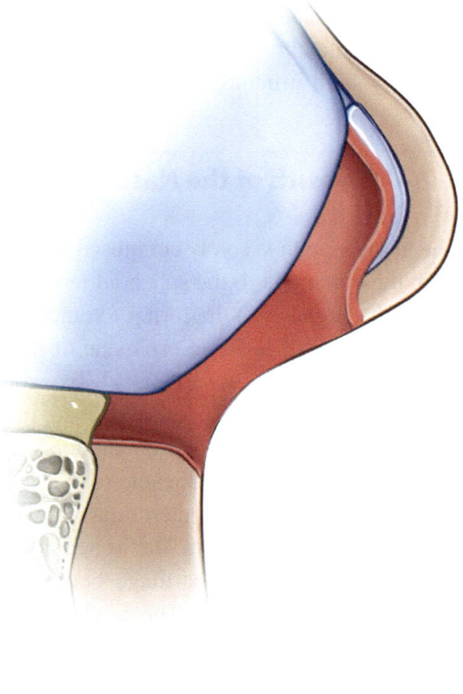

Fig. 2.3 The caudal septum makes the anterior septal angle superiorly, the middle septal angle, and the posterior septal angle inferiorly. It is connected to the membranous septum anteriorly. Approximately 5 mm behind the posterior septal angle, the septal cartilage is attached to the anterior nasal spine with strong soft tissue

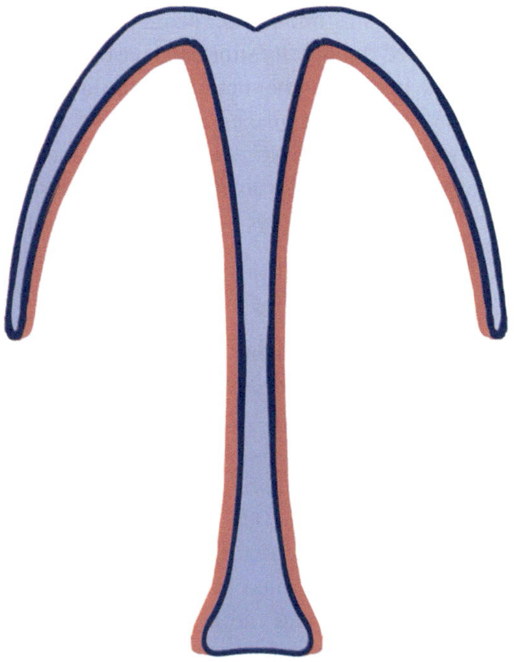

Fig. 2.4 The superior border of the quadrangular cartilage is thicker and shows extensions laterally of approximately 2–4 mm on each side to form a cartilage 4–8 mm thick. This thicker part is attached to the upper lateral cartilages and is coined as processus laterales dorsalis by Cottle

2.4 Premaxilla and Anterior Nasal Spine (ANS)

It was shown in the last century that the premaxilla has its own bony center [12]. The anterior nasal spine projects from the anterior surface of the premaxilla and has two alar wings. These wings are approximately 12 mm long and 6 mm high [12] (Fig. 2.5). The incisive canal is located just behind these wings and is also the start of the junction of the vomer in adults. ANS is important for maintaining the shape of the lip, subnasale, columella, and position of the alveolus. Therefore, it is not a good idea to resect it completely because the support for these structures will be gone. The septal cartilage forms a pseudoarthrosis with the premaxilla, supported by ligaments, paraseptal cartilages, perichondrium, and soft tissues [12] (Fig. 2.6). Paraseptal cartilages are thin bars of cartilage lying lateral to the septum and reaching the vomer. This robust connection between the premaxilla and septal cartilage should be preserved as it is unless there is a prominent deviation or a Cottle-type septal mobilization is performed [10].

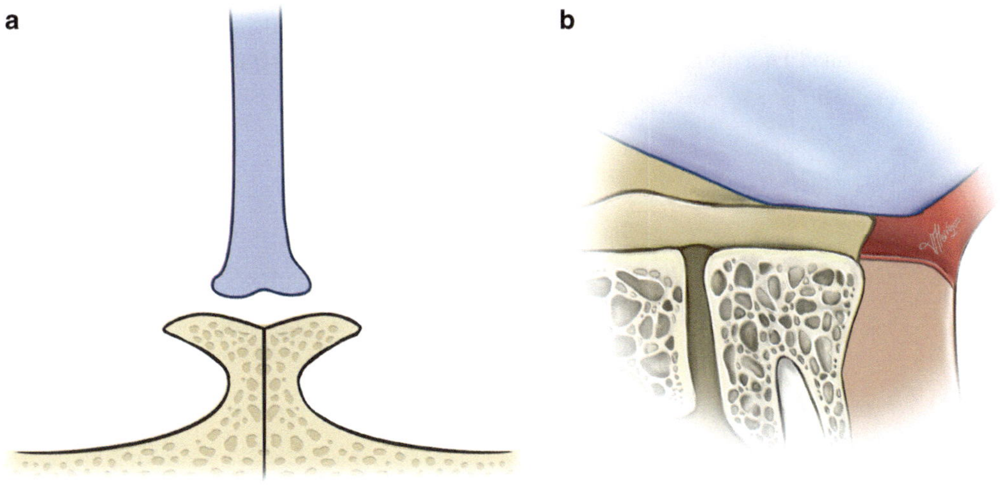

Fig. 2.5 The anterior nasal spine projects from the anterior surface of the premaxilla and has two alar wings (**a**). These wings are approximately 12 mm long and 6 mm high. The incisive canal is located just behind these wings and is also the start of the junction of the vomer in adults (**b**)

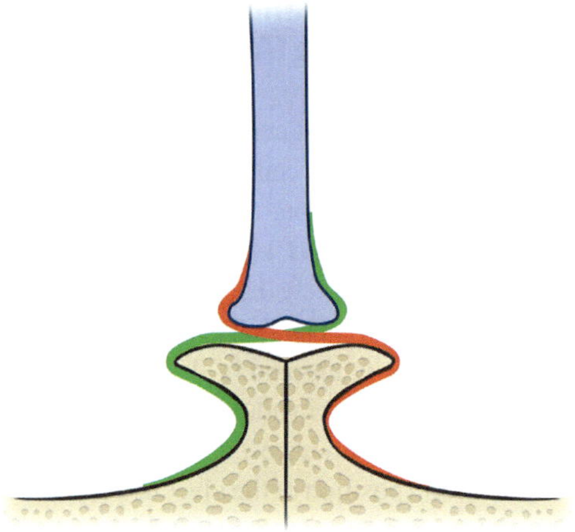

Fig. 2.6 The septal cartilage forms a pseudoarthrosis with the premaxilla, supported by ligaments, paraseptal cartilages, perichondrium, and soft tissues

2.5 Are the Quadrangular and Upper Lateral Cartilages Separate Anatomic Structures?

Until 1955, it was thought that the septal cartilage and upper lateral cartilage were separate anatomical structures. In 1955, Straatsma et al. proposed that ULCs might be continuous with the septal cartilage [13]. This concept was investigated and confirmed later using more modern methods such as micro-MRI studies [14]. As an experienced rhinoplasty surgeon, I have been cutting this junction of the septal cartilage and nasal septum to resect the cartilaginous hump. Therefore, during surgery, I had a chance to observe that the septal cartilage and the upper lateral cartilages are one anatomical structure (Fig. 2.4).

2.6 Perpendicular Plate of the Ethmoid Bone

It is a thin bone and part of the ethmoid extending anteriorly to the nasal bones and nasal spine of the frontal bone, downwards to the quadrangular cartilage, and backwards to the vomer and sphenoid bone. Its upper portion is connected to the lamina cribrosa, which is part of the anterior skull base [12]. Therefore, manipulation with the perpendicular plate must be very gentle in order not to create a problem at the skull base. A very important anatomical detail, especially for dorsum preservation, is that it extends to the middle of the nasal bones in 49% of cases and to the lower third of the nasal bones in 38% [11] (Fig. 2.7). In recent years, this junction has become crucial for successful dorsum preservation surgery. The thick inferior border of the perpendicular plate is attached to the nasal septal cartilage.

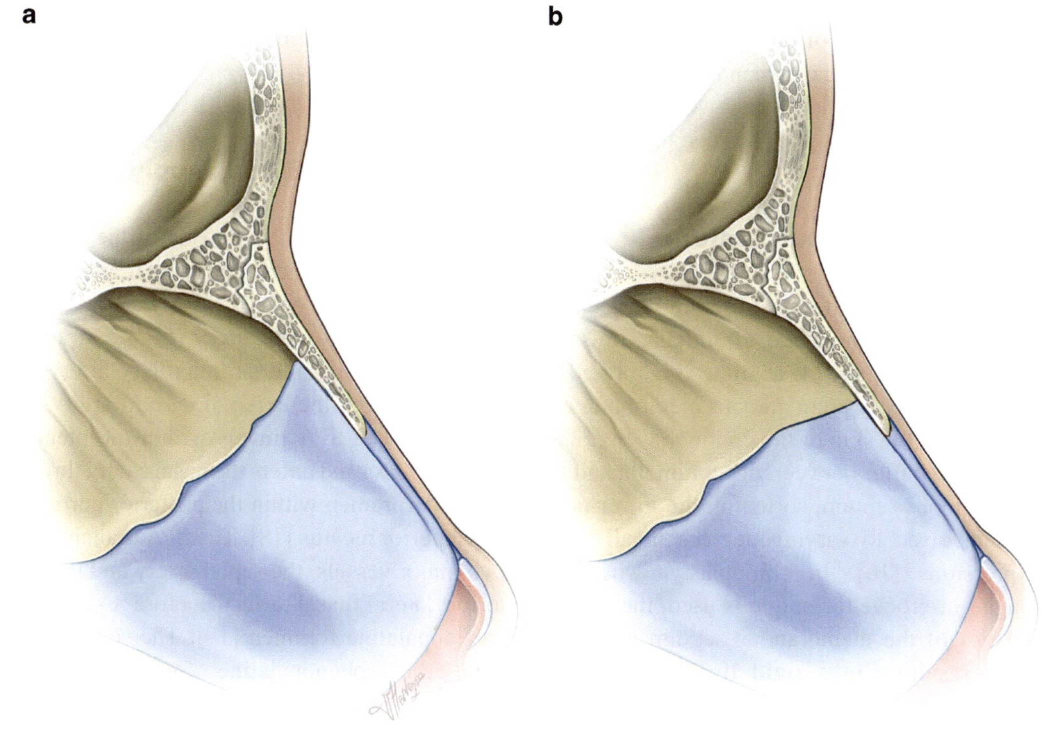

Fig. 2.7 The septal cartilage extends to the middle of the nasal bones in 49% of cases (**a**) and to the lower third of the nasal bones in 38% (**b**)

2.7 Vomer

The vomer is found in the posteroinferior portion of the nasal septum. It is thin, flat, and almost trapezoidal in shape [12]. It has two surfaces and four borders. The nasopalatine groove runs obliquely downward and forward on the lateral surfaces, lodging the nasopalatine nerve and vessels (Fig. 2.8). The superior border is the thickest border and is connected to the rostrum of the sphenoid, the medial pterygoid plates of the sphenoid behind, and the sphenoidal processes of the palatine bones in front [15].

The inferior border articulates with the crest formed by the maxilla and palatine bones. The anterior border is the longest and slopes downward and forward. Its upper half is fused with the perpendicular plate of the ethmoid, and its lower half is grooved for the inferior margin of the septal cartilage of the nose. The posterior border is free, concave, and separates the choanae. It is thick and bifid above and thin below. It is a bilaminar bone that can be part of a one-sided spur, which is very often seen in the human nose. The inferior border articulates with the median

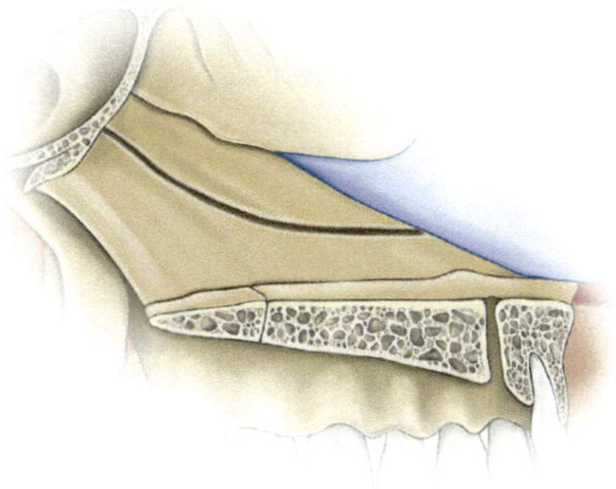

Fig. 2.8 The nasopalatine groove runs obliquely downward and forward on the lateral surfaces, lodging the nasopalatine nerve and vessels

nasal crests of the maxilla and palatine bones. The anterior border of the vomer is the longest and articulates with the perpendicular plate of the ethmoid bone superiorly and with the inferior margin of the nasal septal cartilage inferiorly.

2.8 Membranous Septum

It is the portion of the nasal septum between the cartilaginous septum and columella. It is the most flexible part of the septum. It is formed by the union of the septum mucous membranes and blends with the skin of the columella (Fig. 2.3). It acts as a buffer between the columella and the cartilaginous septum, softening the lower nose. It is involved to varying degrees in all facial expressions [16]. In rhinoplasty, when the tongue-in-groove technique is used, the characteristics of the membranous septum are sacrificed, resulting in a rigid tip. This situation seems reasonable to many surgeons because tip projection and rotation can be adjusted and preserved after surgery.

2.9 Arterial Blood Supply

The major arteries of the inside of the nose are the anterior and posterior ethmoidal arteries and the sphenopalatine artery (Fig. 2.9).

The sphenopalatine artery (SPA) is a terminal branch of the internal maxillary artery that originates from the external carotid artery system [17]. The SPA travels within the pterygopalatine fossa and enters the nasal cavity through the SPA foramen within the posterior portion of the superior meatus [18]. The SPA branches into two major vessels, the septal artery and the posterior lateral nasal artery, before exiting the sphenopalatine foramen [19]. The septal artery exits the sphenopalatine foramen, courses

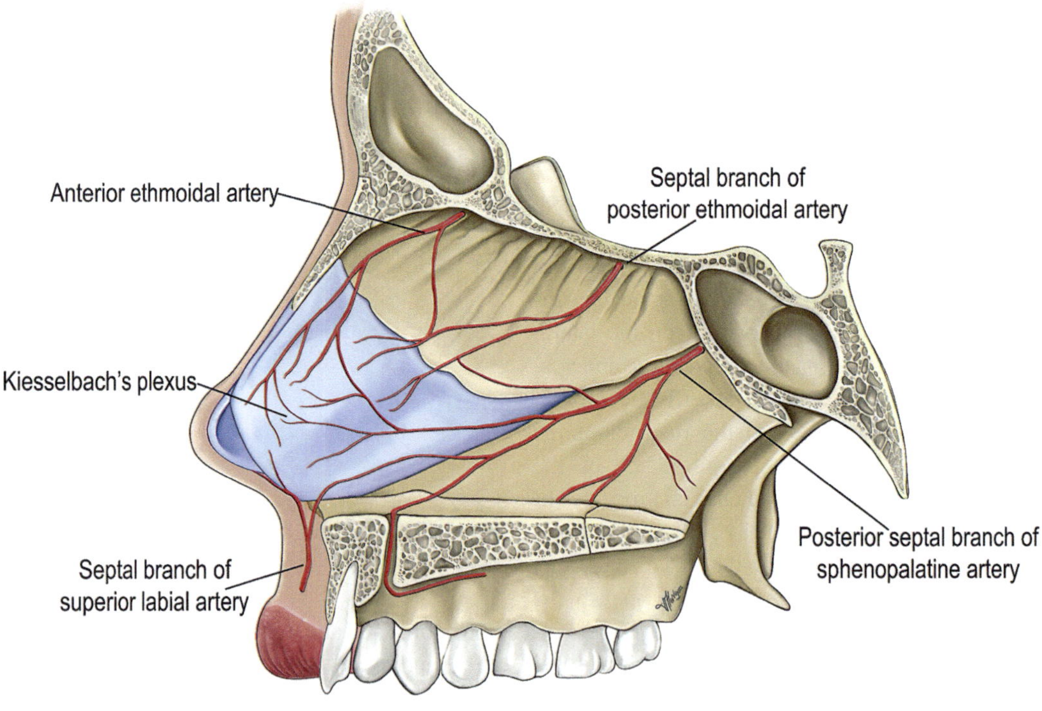

Fig. 2.9 The major arteries of the inside of the nose are the anterior and posterior ethmoidal arteries and the sphenopalatine artery

through the anteroinferior wall of the sphenoid sinus, and distributes on the nasal septum. The posterior lateral nasal artery exits the sphenopalatine foramen, courses downward anteriorly to the posterior end of the middle turbinate along the lateral nasal wall, and runs inferiorly on the perpendicular plate of the palatine bone, giving off branches to the inferior and middle turbinate [20].

In most cases, the septal artery is divided into the upper, middle, and lower branches. The lower branch is usually the largest and runs downward and forward toward the incisive foramen to anastomose with the termination of the greater palatine artery. The middle branch runs anteriorly to the anterior septum. The upper branch is variably present and is the smallest in caliber [21].

2.9.1 Anterior Ethmoid Artery (AEA)

The ethmoidal arteries arise from the ophthalmic artery. Both enter the nasal cavity from the orbit through the ethmoidal foramina and lamina papyracea. The arteries run along the ethmoid roof from lateral to medial, reaching the lateral lamella of the cribriform plate. The AEA supplies the anterior superior part of the septum (anterior septal branch) and the anterior ethmoidal cells, the frontal sinus, and the middle turbinate (anterior lateral nasal branches) [22].

2.9.2 Posterior Ethmoidal Artery

It is smaller than the AEA and passes through the posterior ethmoidal canal. It supplies the posterior ethmoidal cells and nasal branches that descend into the nasal cavity through apertures in the cribriform plate, anastomosing with branches of the sphenopalatine.

Kiesselbach's plexus is formed by the anterior and posterior ethmoidal arteries, the superior labial artery, the greater palatine artery, and the posterior septal branch of the SPA [21].

2.9.3 Veins

Veins arise from the dense venous network of the nasal mucosa and accompany the arteries. The main drainage from the nasal septum runs backward, accompanied by the sphenopalatine artery. They pass through the pterygopalatine foramen into the pharyngeal plexus and, via the ethmoid branches, into the cavernous sinus (Fig. 2.10). The ethmoidal arteries are usually accompanied by veins that anastomose with the veins of the dura mater of the anterior cranial fossa and with the superior sagittal sinus through the foramen caecum [12].

The submucosa of the interior of the nose comprises well-developed venous plexi, which are particularly prominent on the inferior nasal concha, inferior meatus, and posterior part of the septum. They function like erectile tissue [23].

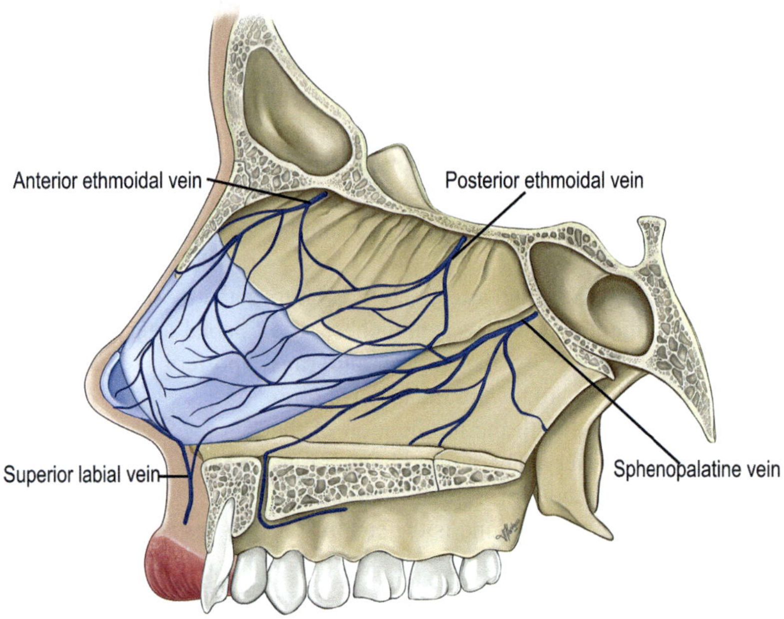

Fig. 2.10 Veins arise from the dense venous network of the nasal mucosa and accompany the arteries. The main drainage route passes through the pterygopalatine foramen into the pharyngeal plexus and via the ethmoid branches into the cavernous sinus

2.10 Innervation of the Nasal Cavity

The nasal cavity is innervated by three groups of nerves: the olfactory nerve, the ophthalmic (V1) nerve, and the maxillary nerve (V2). The ophthalmic nerve is the first branch of the trigeminal nerve and carries only sensory fibers. It gives rise to the frontal nerve, lacrimal nerve, and nasociliary nerve. The nasociliary nerve gives rise to the posterior and anterior ethmoid nerves inside the nose. The anterior ethmoid nerve has an external, lateral internal, and medial internal nasal branch [12, 23, 24] (Fig. 2.11).

The pterygopalatine ganglion is found in the pterygopalatine fossa and is created by the maxillary nerve, which is the second branch of the trigeminal nerve. The branches of the pterygopalatine ganglion carry parasympathetic, sympathetic, and general sensory fibers. They pass through the sphenopalatine foramen inside the nose and produce six branches (Fig. 2.12). The nasopalatine nerve is the uppermost branch and innervates the septum, superior nasal concha, and superior lateral wall. It runs in an anteroinferior direction toward the incisive canal through the nasopalatine groove of the vomer. Its end branch penetrates the canal and supplies the superior gingiva. The nasopalatine nerve also supplies part of the vestibule and anastomoses with the nasal rami of the anterior superior alveolar branch of the infraorbital nerve. The posterior superior lateral nasal nerve innervates the middle and superior nasal conchae, the posterior aspect of the nasal septum, and the posterior ethmoidal air cells. The posterior inferior lateral nasal nerve, in fact, comes off the greater palatine nerve and supplies the medial and inferior nasal meatuses, along with the inferior nasal concha. The greater palatine nerve innervates the hard palate. The lesser palatine nerve innervates the soft palate, uvula, and tonsil. The pharyngeal nerve exits the pterygopalatine fossa via the palatovaginal canal and is responsible for innervating the mucosa and glands of the nasopharynx [12, 23, 24].

Rhinoplasty surgeons tend to look at the nose in terms of the bony-cartilaginous framework because that is the part that they are dealing with

Fig. 2.11 Innervation of the nasal septum

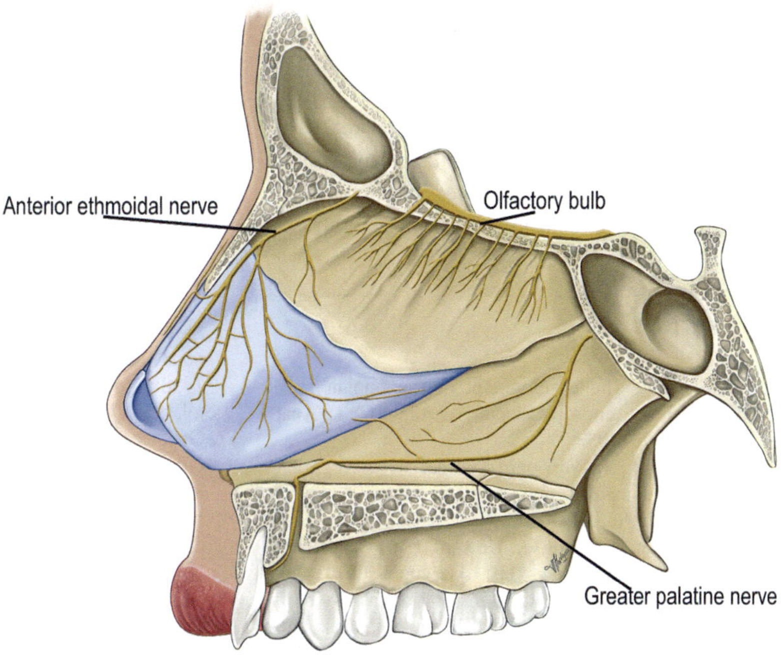

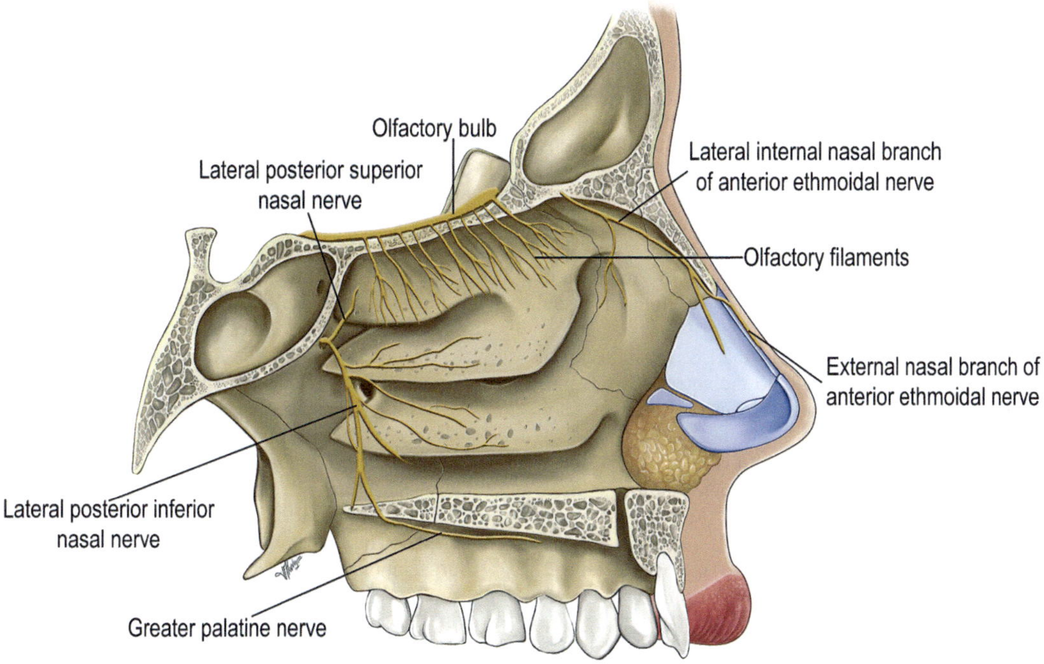

Fig. 2.12 Innervation of the lateral nasal wall. The nasal cavity is innervated by the branches of the ophthalmic and maxillary nerves

during surgery. However, in addition to the bony-cartilaginous framework, a surgeon should have a clear understanding of the arteries, veins, and nerves of the nasal cavity, so that in case of emergencies, necessary cautions can be taken. The student of rhinoplasty never graduates and should always repeat and refresh her/his knowledge about the surgical anatomy of the nasal cavity.

References

1. Fawcett M. The development of the human maxilla, vomer and paraseptal cartilages. J Anat. 1911;45:378–405.
2. Van Loosen J, Verwoerd-Verhoef HL, Verwoerd CDA. The nasal septal cartilage in the newborn. Rhinology. 1988;26:161–5.
3. Van Loosen J, Yiang J, Howard CV, Van Zanten GA, Verwoerd-Verhoef HL, Verwoerd CDA, Van Velzen D. Nasal cartilage maturation assessed by automated computer-assisted image analysis. Adv Otorhinolaryngol. 1997;51:51–60.
4. Huizing EH. Septum surgery in children: indications, surgical technique and long-term results. Rhinology. 1979;17:91–100.
5. Meng HP, Goorhuis J, Kapila S, Nanda RS. Growth changes in the nasal profile from 7 to 18 years of age. Am J Orthod Dentofacial Orthop. 1988;94:317–26.
6. Akgüner M, Barutçu A, Karaca C. Adolescent growth patterns of the bony cartilaginous framework of the nose: a cephalometric study. Ann Plast Surg. 1998;41:66–9.
7. Tasca I, Compadretti GC. Nasal growth after pediatric septoplasty at long-term follow-up. Am J Rhinol Allergy. 2011;25:e7–12.
8. Menger DJ, Tabink I, Nolst Trenité GJ. Treatment of septal hematomas and abscesses in children. Facial Plast Surg. 2007;23:239–43.
9. Goh S, Karamchandani D, Anari S. Relationship of the posterior septal angle to the anterior nasal spine in the Caucasian nasal septum. J Laryngol Otol. 2019;133:224–6.
10. Cottle MH, Loring RM, Fischer GG, Gaynon IE. The maxilla-premaxilla approach to extensive nasal septum surgery. AMA Arch Otolaryngol. 1958;68:301–13.
11. Zuckerkandl E. Geruchsorgan, Anatomische Hefte, 2. Abt. 1895, Wiesbaden, vol 5. 1896. pp. 131–145.
12. Lang J. Clinical anatomy of the nose, nasal cavity and paranasal sinuses. Stuttgart: Thieme; 1989.
13. Straatsma BR, Straatsma CR. The anatomical relationship of the lateral nasalcartilage to the nasal bone and the cartilaginous nasal septum. Plast Reconstr Surg. 1951;8:443–55.
14. Varoquier M, Rumeau C, Vuissoz PA, Perez M, Hossu G, Jankowski R. Do the upper lateral nasal cartilages exist? The concept of septolateral cartilages. Eur Ann Otorhinolaryngol Head Neck Dis. 2021;138:77–81.
15. Gray H. Anatomy of the human body. 1918. Reference > Anatomy of the human body > II. Osteology > 5b. 7. The Vomer. https://www.bartleby.com/107/43.html.
16. Stovin JS. The importance of the membranous nasal septum. AMA Arch Otolaryngol. 1958;67(5):540–1. https://doi.org/10.1001/archotol.1958.00730010554006. PMID: 13520023.
17. Gras-Cabrerizo JR, García-Garrigós E, Montserrat-Gili JR, Gras-Albert JR, Mirapeix-Lucas R, Massegur-Solench H, Quer-Agusti M. Anatomical correlation between nasal vascularisation and the design of the endonasal pedicle flaps. Indian J Otolaryngol Head Neck Surg. 2018;70(1):167–73.
18. Tanoue S, Kiyosue H, Mori H, Hori Y, Okahara M, Sagara Y. Maxillary artery: functional and imaging anatomy for safe and effective transcatheter treatment. Radiographics. 2013;33:e209–24.
19. El-Shaarawy EAA, Hassan SS. The sphenopalatine foramen in man: anatomical, radiological and endoscopic study. Folia Morphol (Warsz). 2018;77(2):345–55.
20. Eordogh M, Grimm A, Gawish I, Patonay L, Reisch R, Briner HR, Baksa G. Anatomy of the sphenopalatine artery and its implications for transnasal neurosurgery. Rhinology. 2018;56:82–8.
21. Chiu T, Dunn JS. An anatomical study of the arteries of the anterior nasal septum. Otolaryngol Head Neck Surg. 2006;134:33–6.
22. Lund VJ, Stammberger H, Fokkens WJ, Beale T, Bernal-Sprekelsen M, Eloy P, Georgalas C, Gerstenberger C, Hellings P, Herman P, Hosemann WG, Jankowski R, Jones N, Jorissen M, Leunig A, Onerci M, Rimmer J, Rombaux P, Simmen D, Tomazic PV, Tschabitscherr M, Welge-Luessen A. European position paper on the anatomical terminology of the internal nose and paranasal sinuses. Rhinol Suppl. 2014;24:1–34.
23. Oneal RM, Beil RJ. Surgical anatomy of the nose. Clin Plast Surg. 2010;37:191–211.
24. Lane AP. Nasal anatomy and physiology. Facial Plast Surg Clin North Am. 2004;12:387–95, v.

Physiology of the Nose

3

3.1 Introduction

As rhinoplasty surgeons, we are all used to thinking that the nose is mainly a cosmesis organ. In fact, it has many different important functions and roles in respiration, humidification, and heating of inspired air, olfaction, defense, and speech production [1].

"Nasal mucosa is the organ of the nose," a statement that I heard from Eugene Kern four decades ago. I still cannot agree more as I become more experienced working in the nose. The mucosa is mainly composed of respiratory epithelium, which is pseudostratified ciliated columnar epithelium composed of six cell types (Fig. 3.1). Goblet cells produce mucinogens and contain secretory granules. When mucinogen becomes hydrated, it becomes mucin. Once mucin is mixed with other materials in a watery environment, it is known as mucus. Ciliated columnar cells, like goblet cells, constitute approximately 30% of the total respiratory epithelial cell population. The cilia of these cells move mucus and its trapped particulate matter toward the nasopharynx for elimination, a process called mucociliary clearance, which is vital for a healthy nose [2]. Therefore, interventions in the nose can be very harmful to the mucosa and mucociliary clearance. More surgeries in the nose mean more dryness inside the nose because of damaged mucosa and mucociliary activity.

The major function of the nose is respiration. In a normal nose, air is directed to the middle meatus after passing through the nostril and valve area during inspiration. It follows a curved tract that stays parallel to the turbinates at the middle meatus and then downslopes toward the nasopharynx as a laminar flow [3]. In droopy tips, the inspired air can be directed to the upper meatus. When the rotation is increased just before surgery to show the effect of rotation, the patient can understand that increasing the rotation of a droopy tip is not only a cosmetic maneuver but also a functional one, increasing the amount of air passing through the middle meatus. During expiration, airflow is mainly through the inferior nasal meatus (Fig. 3.2).

The nasal valve area is approximately 1.5 cm from the nostril entrance in adults and is formed by the nasal septum, caudal margin of the upper lateral cartilages, head of the inferior turbinate, and floor of the nasal cavity. It is the narrowest portion of the entire respiratory tract. Its surface area is 50–70 mm^2. It is accepted as a major regulator of nasal airflow. The speed of airflow passing through the nasal valve area is six times more than that through the rest of the nose [3, 4]. The condition of the anatomic structures composing the valve area is important for healthy respiration (Fig. 3.3). According to my experience, this area is the most critical part in functional rhinoplasty, and most problems are caused by the deviation of the nasal septum in this area. This area is also the

© The Author(s), under exclusive license to Springer Nature Switzerland AG 2025

F. Apaydın, *Septal Surgery Challenges in Rhinoplasty*,
https://doi.org/10.1007/978-3-031-74734-2_3

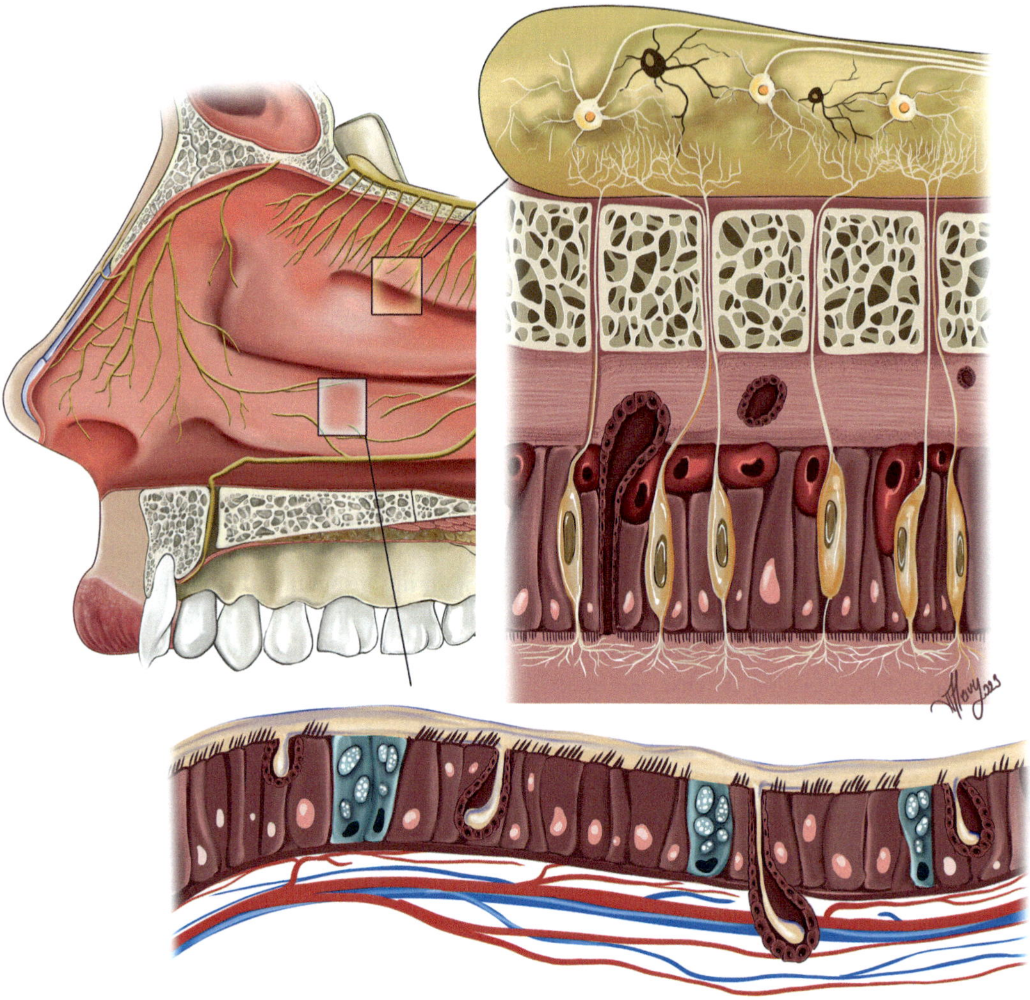

Fig. 3.1 The mucosa is mainly composed of respiratory epithelium, which is a pseudostratified ciliated columnar epithelium. It has Goblet cells (green) producing mucinogens and containing secretory granules. Ciliated columnar cells are responsible for mucociliary clearance. The olfactory region is in the attic and is composed of olfactory receptor neurons and their cilia, sustentacular cells, and basal cells

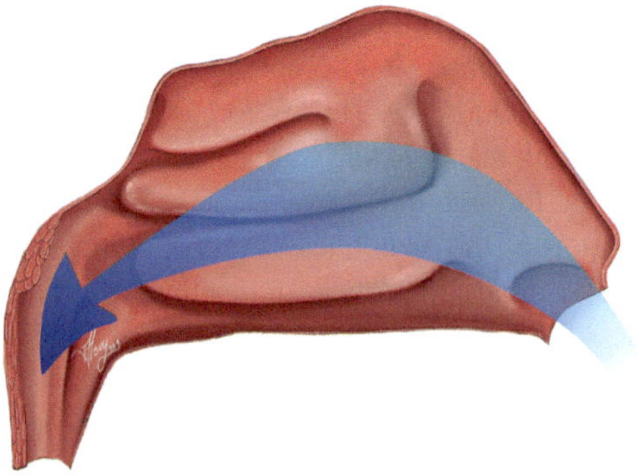

Fig. 3.2 The air passing through the nose follows a curved tract

victim of the requests of patients seeking the smallest nose.

The physical mechanism underlying the nasal cycle is an asymmetry in blood flow leading to engorgement of erectile tissue in the anterior part of the nasal septum and inferior turbinate. This reciprocal cycle changes every 3–5 h (Fig. 3.4). The total nasal resistance and airflow do not change [5]. Sometimes the nasal cycle is explored by patients, and they ask you to change it and create a condition in which both nasal passages receive the same amount of air all the time. Therefore, I usually need to explain the nasal

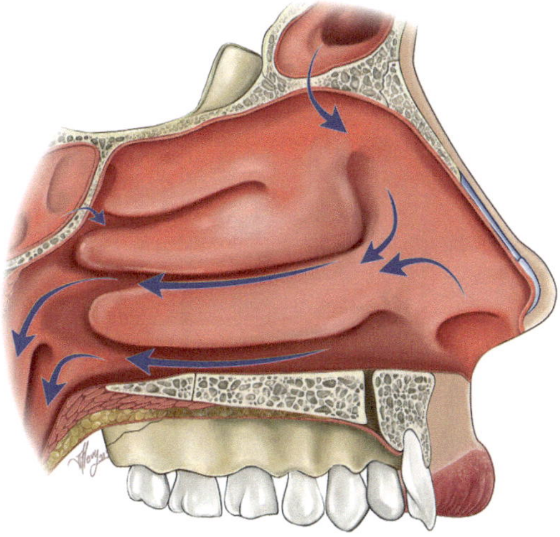

Fig. 3.3 During expiration, airflow can follow many tracts, but it mainly goes through the inferior nasal meatus

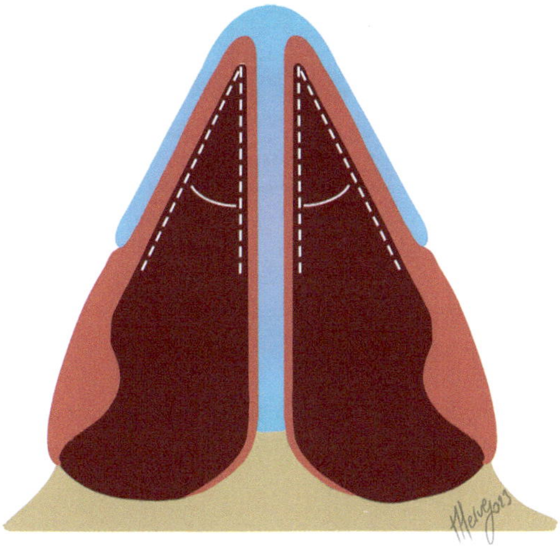

Fig. 3.4 The nasal valve area is formed by the nasal septum, the caudal margin of the upper lateral cartilages, the head of the inferior turbinate, and the floor of the nasal cavity. The internal nasal valve angle is 10–15°

cycle to most of my patients before surgery. Many patients tell us that they are addicted to vasoconstrictive nose sprays. I always explain to them how these sprays can interfere with this nasal cycle and can result in rhinitis medicamentosa when used for a long time. However, interestingly, I have seen many patients who were addicted to these sprays for years, and the mucosa did look quite healthy. Therefore, it should be kept in mind that not all patients who are addicted to vasoconstrictive sprays end up with rhinitis medicamentosa.

Olfaction is a feeling that we all neglect until we lose it during a common cold or similar upper respiratory tract infection. I always tell my patients that the animals find their food, partner, friend, and what to do by olfaction. I also tell them that humans have lost their sensitivity to olfaction as they have become more civilized. The olfactory region is located in the attic of the nasal airway and is usually not affected by surgery. However, the application of packing and splinting and edema caused by surgery can result in temporary loss or weakening of olfaction. Patients must be informed about this situation before surgery (Fig. 3.1).

One of the important tasks of the mucosa is to heat and humidify the inspired air. The internal valve area is the most effective part of the nasal cavity for this task. It was revealed that an air temperature of about 31–34 °C and a relative humidity of approximately 90–95% after inspiration could be observed within the nasopharynx [3].

Mucociliary transport is the migration of the superficial viscous layer covering the mucosa. Its speed is 0.5–2.0 cm/min in the dorsal direction by the to-and-fro movements of the cilia. A normal ciliary beat consists of an effective and a recovery stroke. During the effective stroke, the cilium is stretched and reaches the gel layer, with its tip pushing the upper viscous layer of mucus. During the recovery stroke, the cilium curves and bends backward to its rest phase [1].

The nose provides mechanical, humoral, and cellular defenses to protect the airways. In addition, the nasal cavity is an important resonator during speech. However, these two characteristics of the nose will not be detailed in this chapter (Figs. 3.5 and 3.6).

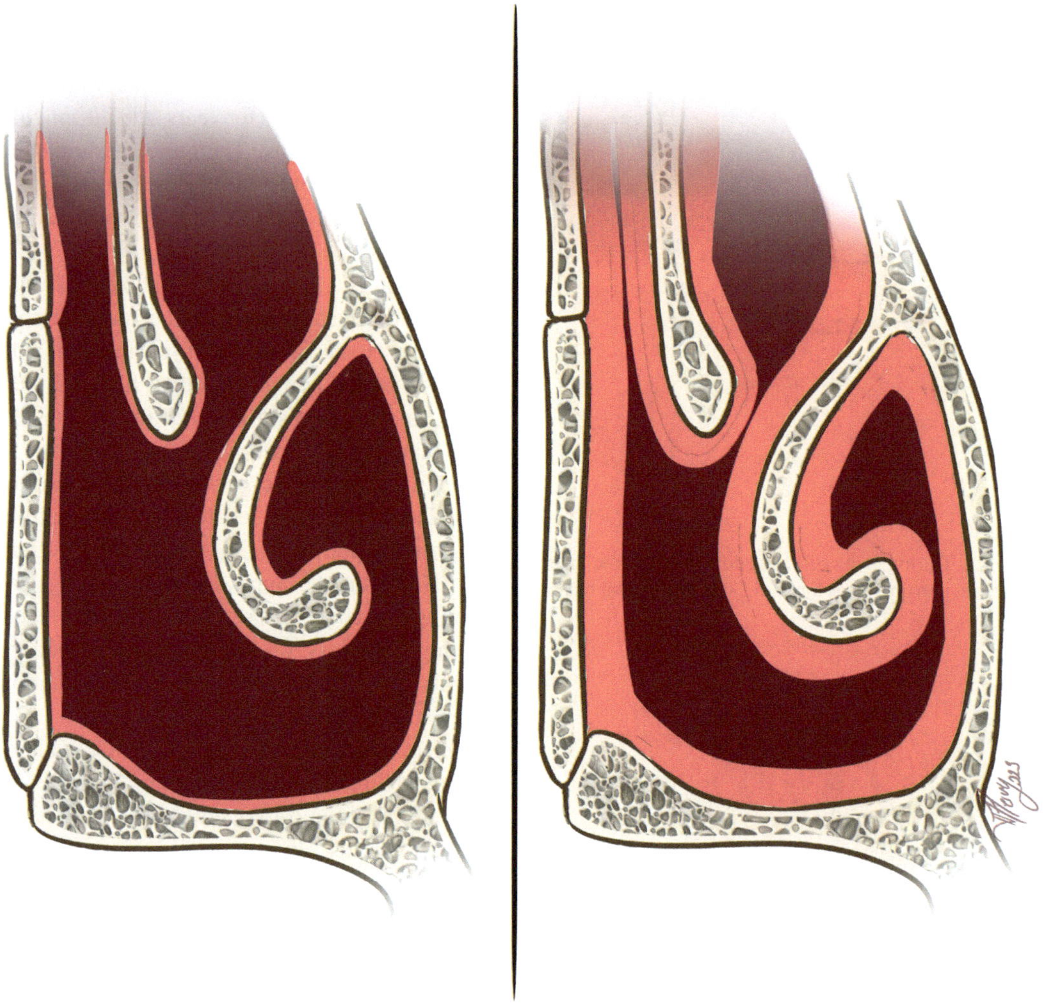

Fig. 3.5 The nasal cycle is an asymmetry in blood flow, leading to engorgement of erectile tissue in the anterior part of the nasal septum and the inferior turbinate. The size of the inferior turbinates changes every 3–5 h

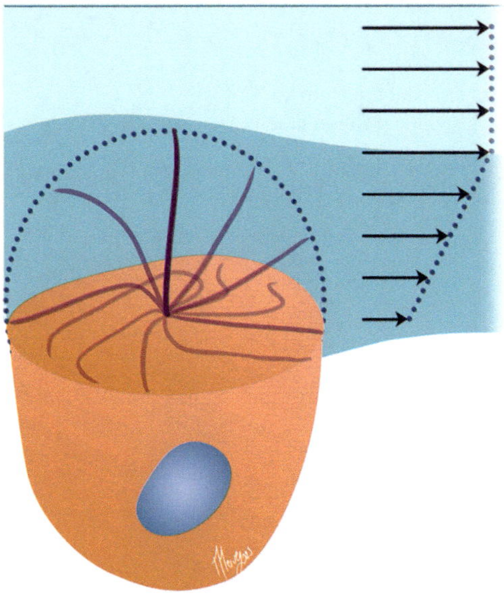

Fig. 3.6 The mucociliary transport moves toward the nasopharynx by the to-and-fro movements of the cilia. A normal ciliary beat consists of an effective and a recovery stroke. During the effective stroke, the cilium is stretched and reaches the gel layer with its tip, pushing the upper viscous layer of mucus. During the recovery stroke, the cilium curves and bends backward to its rest phase

References

1. Cole P. Physiology of the nose and paranasal sinuses. Clin Rev Allergy Immunol. 1998;16(1–2):25–54.
2. Gartner LP. Respiratory system. In: Textbook of histology. Elsevier; 2021.
3. Huizing book.
4. Kasperbauer JL, Kern EB. Nasal valve physiology. Implications in nasal surgery. Otolaryngol Clin North Am. 1987;20:699–719.
5. Kahana-Zweig R, Geva-Sagiv M, Weissbrod A, Secundo L, Soroker N, Sobel N. Measuring and characterizing the human nasal cycle. PLoS One. 2016;11:e0162918.

4 Examination of the Nose

4.1 Introduction

The examination of the nose begins with careful history taking. Each individual consultation starts by asking the patient what the complaints are. When directly asked, the patients tend to mention only the major problems, usually neglecting the minor ones. Therefore, the surgeon should find a way to systematize history taking.

In recent years, validated patient-reported outcome measures (PROMs) and similar questionnaires have become very popular for identifying the functional, esthetic, and psychological conditions of patients. Nasal obstruction symptoms evaluation (NOSE) scale [1], rhinoplasty outcomes evaluation (ROE) [2], Utrecht questionnaire [3], FACE-Q [4], standardized cosmesis and health outcomes survey (SCHNOS) [5], and body dysmorphic disorder questionnaire (BDDQ) [6] were all developed by different researchers. Having tried almost all of them, I have ended up using SCHNOS, which is also validated for Turkish [7] and BDDQ. However, I still find these PROMs very basic, and it is very easy to miss details, including the side, duration, consistency, and severity of some of the complaints. I developed my own questionnaire with some additional questions (Table 4.1). This questionnaire is provided to the patient before consultation. After looking at the details in this questionnaire filled out by the patient, it is relatively easy to have a certain opinion about the patient. I also like using this questionnaire to detail some of the answers given by the patient and for reflective listening. In fact, in 1999, when developing Rhinobase, a very detailed module was added, including all possible complaints and details about that complaint (Table 4.2; Fig. 4.1).

One of the most difficult factors to diagnose is the degree of nasal obstruction. The most widespread method is to simply ask the patient. I have developed a very simple method of asking two questions and detailing them as follows:

1. How often does your mouth open during the day? How long: 20%, 50%, 80%, or 100%?
2. How often does your mouth open during sleep? Never, sometimes, or always?

The patient is then asked about their medical history. A history of facial trauma, hypertension, diabetes mellitus, asthma, cardiac disease, peripheral vascular disease, renal disease, gastrointestinal and hepatic disease, neurological disease, psychiatric disorder, skin disorder, connective tissue disorder, and allergy are all asked. The same diseases are questioned in the family history.

It must not be forgotten to ask if the patient has undergone any kind of surgery around the

© The Author(s), under exclusive license to Springer Nature Switzerland AG 2025

F. Apaydın, *Septal Surgery Challenges in Rhinoplasty*,
https://doi.org/10.1007/978-3-031-74734-2_4

Table 4.1 The questionnaire that I have been using includes the standardized cosmesis and health outcomes survey (SCHNOS), the body dysmorphic disorder questionnaire (BDDQ), and some additional questions that I find important

NOSE Surgery (Rhinoplasty) Questionnaire						
(This questionnaire is prepared to evaluate your situation better and also to guide your doctor)						
Name Surname:____________________ Date: / /						
Age: Height: Weight: Cellphone: E-mail:						
Over the past **month**, how much of a **problem** was the following:						
	No problem					Extreme problem
1. Having a blocked or obstructed nose	0	1	2	3	4	5
2. Getting air through my nose during exercise	0	1	2	3	4	5
3. Having a congested nose	0	1	2	3	4	5
4. Breathing through my nose during sleep	0	1	2	3	4	5
5. Decreased mood and self-esteem due to my nose	0	1	2	3	4	5
6. The shape of my nasal tip	0	1	2	3	4	5
7. The straightness of my nose	0	1	2	3	4	5
8. The shape of my nose from the side	0	1	2	3	4	5
9. How well my nose suits my face	0	1	2	3	4	5
10. The overall symmetry of my nose	0	1	2	3	4	5
11. Have you ever had nose surgery before? (Please write the type of surgery, date, and place)						
12. Have you ever had facial trauma before? If so, when?						
[ ] Yes [ ] No , ________________						
13. Are you worried about your appearance in any way?						
[ ] Yes [ ] No						
14. Does these concerns preoccupy you? That is, do you think about it a lot and do you wish you could worry about it less?						
[ ] Yes [ ] No						
15. Did these concerns cause you a lot of distress, torment, or pain?						
[ ] No [ ] Mild [ ] Moderate [ ] Severe [ ] Extreme disabling						
16. Did these concerns cause you impairment in social, occupational, or other important areas of functioning?						
[ ] No [ ] Mild [ ] Moderate [ ] Severe [ ] Extreme disabling						
17. Did these concerns often significantly interfere with your social life?						
[ ] No [ ] Mild [ ] Moderate [ ] Severe [ ] Extreme disabling						
18. Did these concerns often significantly interfere with your schoolwork, job, or ability to function in your role?						
[ ] No [ ] Mild [ ] Moderate [ ] Severe [ ] Extreme disabling						
19. Are there things you avoid because of these concerns?						
[ ] Yes [ ] No						
20. Why now?						
21. Please write your three most important expectations from this nose surgery						
(a)						
(b)						
(c)						

nose. The patient could have previously undergone septoplasty, rhinoplasty, reduction of nasal bone fracture, sinus surgery, turbinate surgery, or any other surgery. If any of these procedures are reported, the time of these procedures must be noted as well. If the patient is seeking another surgery, there may be a need to obtain ear or rib cartilage.

The patient is asked if she is taking any medications regularly or if she has any drug allergies. The use of tobacco, alcohol, and any other drugs should be noted.

Table 4.2 The complete list of complaints regarding the nose

Complaint	Side	Duration	Consistency	Severity
[ ] Nasal obstruction	( ) R; ( ) L; ( ) B	( ) D, W, M, Y	A, O, S, R	1, 2, 3, 4
[ ] Deviated nose				
[ ] Tip drop				
[ ] Dorsal hump				
[ ] Wide osseocartilaginous vault				
[ ] Septal perforation				
[ ] Infected implant				
[ ] Facial pain/pressure				
[ ] Headache				
[ ] Postnasal drainage				
[ ] Snoring				
[ ] Epistaxis				
[ ] Exercise intolerance				
[ ] Rhinorrhea				
[ ] Crusting				
[ ] Dryness				
[ ] Allergy				
[ ] Smell disorder				
[ ] Tumor				
[ ] Other: ________________				
	R: Right	D: Days	A: Always	1: Mild
	L: Left	W: Weeks	O: Often	2: Moderate
	B: bilateral	M: Months	S: Sometimes	3: Marked
		Y: Years	R: Rarely	4: Severe

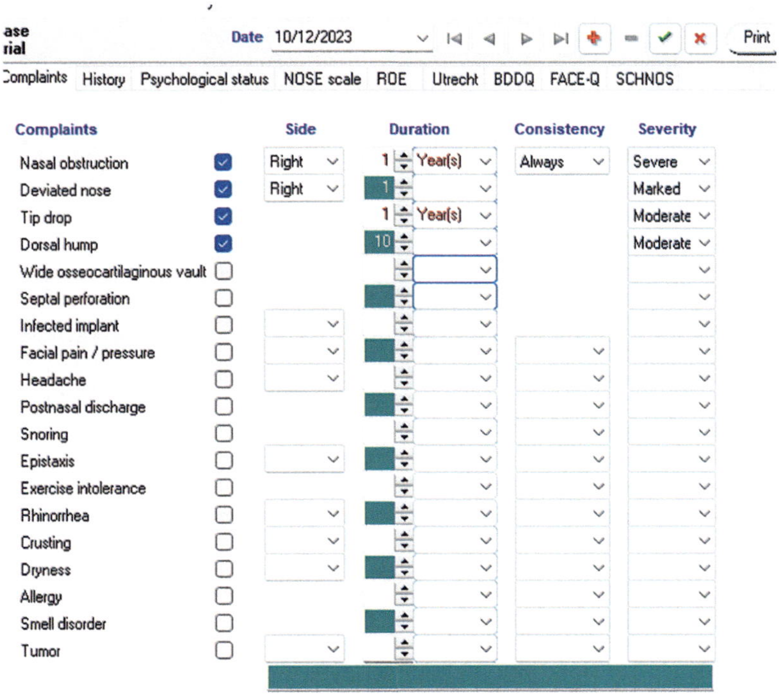

Fig. 4.1 In Rhinobase, a very detailed module is found, including possible complaints and their details

4.2 Inspection

Inspection of the nose starts while listening to the patient. This is the best time to obtain an opinion on the dynamic situation of the nose and its relationship with the other facial structures during speaking, smiling, and laughing. It is important to look at the nose from different perspectives. A systematic analysis of the nose from the frontal, lateral, and basal views is essential to reveal the deformities using an esthetic eye (Tables 4.3, 4.4 and 4.5). On the frontal view, the position of the nasal axis is noted to determine whether it is straight or deviated. The width of the nose can also provide a clue about the situation of the nasal septum. In the lateral view, the existence of a tension nose or saddle nose changes the surgeon's operative plan. The basal view is also crucial for detecting subluxations and deviations (Fig. 4.2).

The patient is asked to breathe quietly and then with effort to reveal any external or internal valve collapse (Fig. 4.3). The patient is asked to talk and smile to see if there is any tip ptosis upon animation. Tip ptosis can be minimal, moderate, or severe, which can affect the surgical plan.

Table 4.3 This is a list to realize a systematic analysis of the nose on the frontal view. The rhinoplasty surgeon should follow a certain discipline in facial analysis in order not to miss any detail

Esthetic analysis frontal view				
	1	2	3	4
Face shape	Oval	Round	Square	Diamond/pear
6/8	Proportional	Disproportional		
Horizontal thirds	Proportional	Disproportional		
Vertical fifths	Proportional	Disproportional		
Left Brow-tip line	Smooth	Irregular		
Right Brow-tip line	Smooth	Irregular		
Skin thickness	Thin	Moderate	Thick	
Sebaceous gland	Sparse	Moderate	Rich	
Skin discoloration	None	Present		
Scar	None	Present		
Deviation	Bony vault	Tip	Cartilaginous vault	
Radix	Normal	Wide	Narrow	
Bony vault	Normal	Wide	Narrow	
Cartilaginous vault	Normal	Wide	Narrow	
Tip	Normal	Wide	Narrow	
Alar axis	Divergent	Straight	Convergent	
Alar size	Normal	Wide	Narrow	
Alar flare	Normal	Excessive	Decreased	
Infratip lobule	Normal	Prominent	Recessed	
Chin width	Normal	Wide	Narrow	
Supraalar pinching	Absent	Present		
Tip bifidity	Absent	Present		
Parenthesis deformity	Absent	Present		
Unitip deformity	Absent	Present		
Bulbosity	Absent	Present		
Cephalically oriented lateral crura	Absent	Present		

Table 4.4 In the lateral view, instead of fixing on the problems, it is better to make a thorough analysis by using this checklist

Esthetic analysis lateral view			
Facial contour	Straight	Convex	Concave
Forehead	Flat	Protruding	Sloping
Occlusion	Orthognathic	Retrognathic	Prognathic
Midface	Normal	Retrognathic	Prognathic
Lower face	Normal	Retrognathic	Prognathic
Radix	Normal	Shallow	Deep
Nasal starting point	Normal	High	Low
Dorsum	Normal	Hump	Saddle
Nasal length	Normal	Short	Long
Nasal bones	Normal	Short	Long
Upper lateral cartilage	Normal	Short	Long
Supratip	Normal	Depressed	Prominent
Anterior septal angle	Normal	Overdeveloped	Underdeveloped
Tip projection	Normal	Underprojected	Overprojected
Tip rotation	Normal	Underrotated	Overrotated
Columella	Normal	Hanging	Retracted
Double break	Favorable	Accentuated	Poorly defined
Alar rim	Normal	Hanging	Retracted
Alar -facial relationship	Normal	Hooded	Recessed
Nasolabial angle	Normal	Acute	Obtuse
Upper lip orientation	Normal	Retro-inclination	Forward-inclination
Upper lip length	Normal	Short	Long
Nasal spine	Normal	Short	Long
Mentolabial sulcus	Deep	Normal	Shallow
Chin	Normal	Recessive	Prominent
Submental region	Normal	Moderate fat deposit	Marked fat deposit

Table 4.5 The basal view tells the surgeon a lot of information if the surgeon is intended to decipher them

Esthetic analysis basal view				
Shape	Triangular	Trapezoidal	Boxy	Irregular
Deviation	Absent	Right	Left	
Lobule	Normal	Wide	Narrow	
Columella/Lobule ratio	Normal	Increased	Decreased	
Columella	Normal	Short	Long	
Caudal septal position	Midline	Subluxation to the left	Subluxation to the right	
Medial crural footplate flare	Normal	Wide	Narrow	
Columellar width	Normal	Wide	Narrow	
Columella scar	Absent	Inverted-V	Stairstep	Straight
Nostril sill width	Normal	Short	Long	
Nostril floor Width	Normal	Depressed	Prominent	
Alar flare	Normal	Excessive	Narrow	
Alar width	Normal	Excessive	Narrow	
Angle of divergence	Normal	Wide	Narrow	
Alarbase-nostril floor	Cheek junction	Columellar junction	Labial junction	
Nostril configuration	Pear shaped	Round Oval	Slit-like	Asymmetric
Nostril size	Normal	Large	Small	Infantile

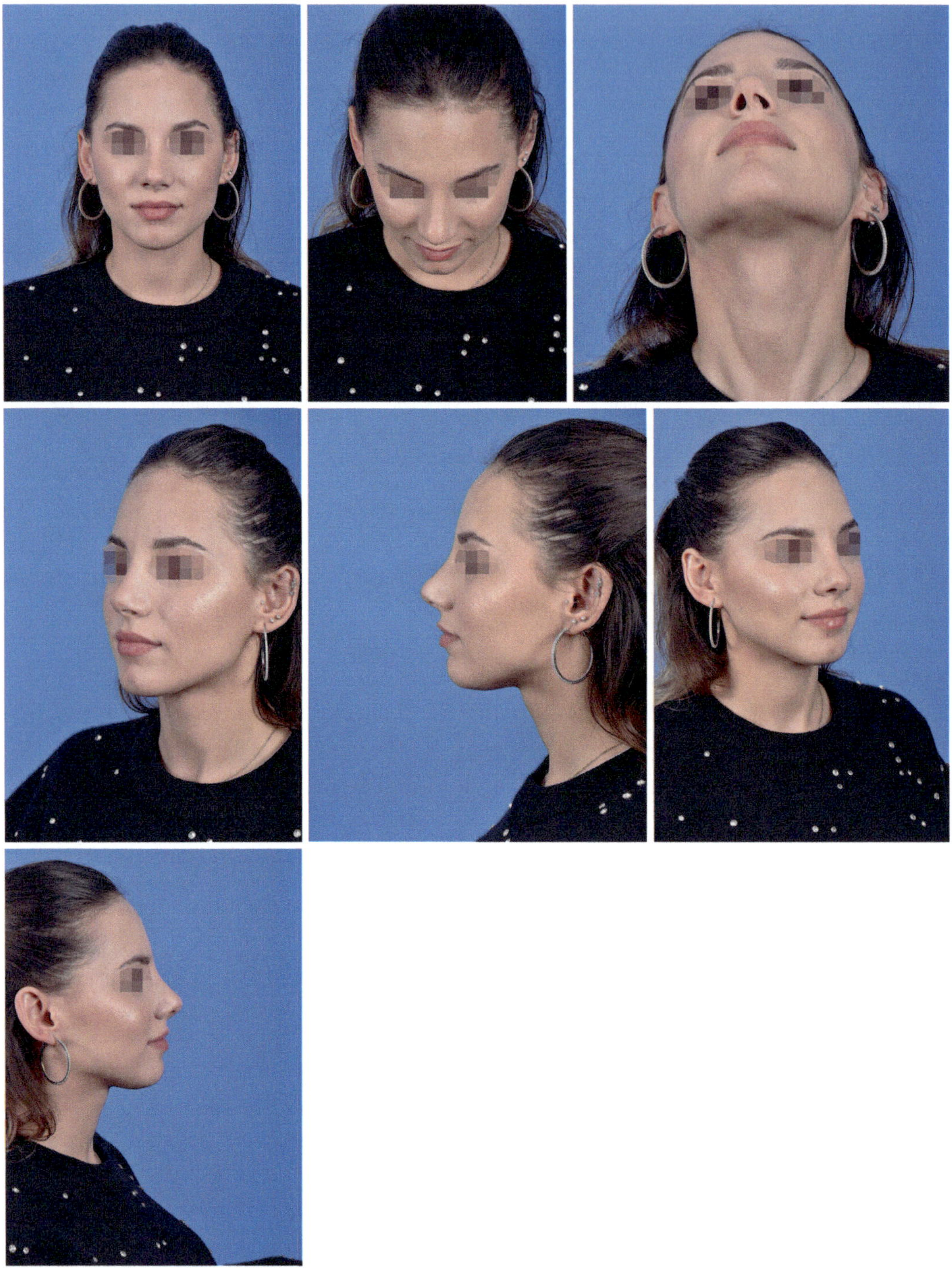

Fig. 4.2 Frontal, sky, semi-obliques, obliques, laterals, and basal views are all essential to reveal the deformities using an esthetic eye. In this case, the patient has a linear crooked nose to the right and a subluxation to the right

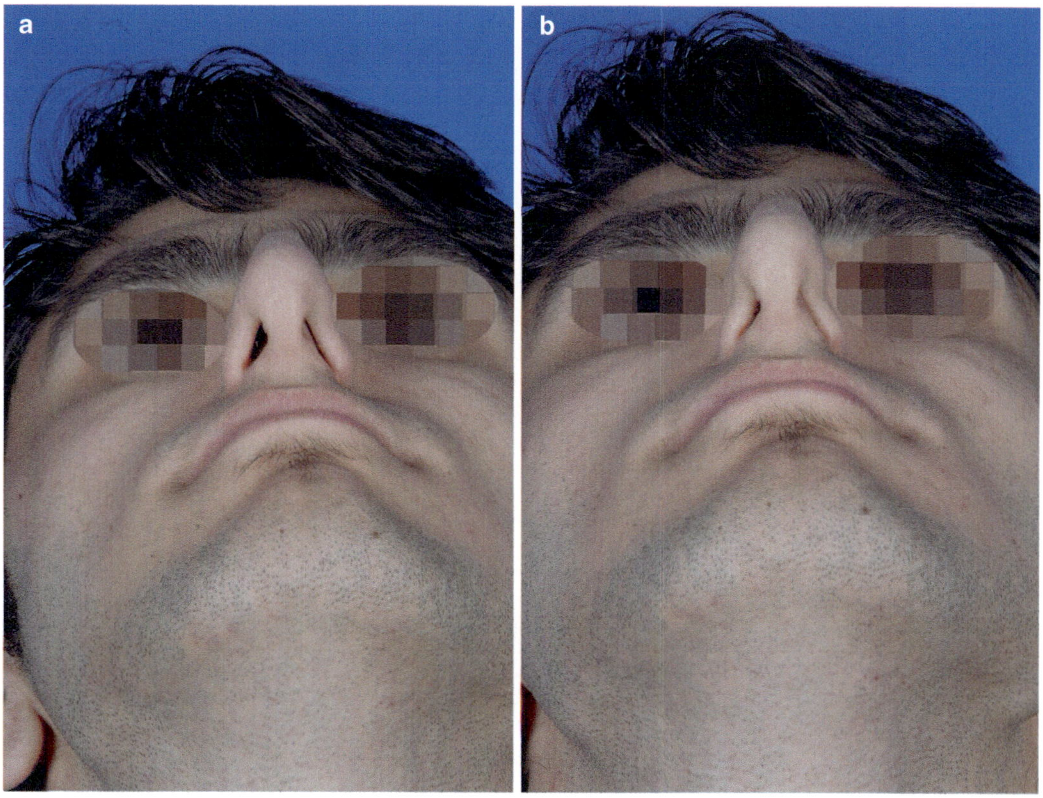

Fig. 4.3 The external collapse can be seen when the patient is breathing peacefully (**a**) or with mild force (**b**)

4.3 Palpation

Palpation of the nose is a crucial step in rhinoplasty and septoplasty. Palpation begins with the bony vault to detect its anatomical situation and variations. If the patient has had previous trauma, it is not difficult to palpate the fracture lines and irregularities. Palpation of the middle vault can be very helpful in determining the shape and position of the dorsal septum. A recoil test is performed to feel the support of the caudal septum on the tip. If it is weak, the support of the caudal septum is weak or lacking (Fig. 4.4).

After wearing a glove, the caudal septum and anterior nasal spine should be palpated (Fig. 4.5). The position of the caudal septum and anterior nasal spine is noted to determine whether they are in or off the midline. The relationship between the caudal septum and the anterior nasal spine is also critical for palpation. If these structures are in a favorable position, the surgeon may choose not to disturb this relationship.

The alae are palpated to feel their strength. A Cottle test can be added to this examination to determine if pulling the cheek next to the ala makes any difference during breathing (Fig. 4.6). In fact, it can be a deceptive maneuver in most patients, and that is why I do not like to use it. The use of an ear curette to lateralize the ala from the inside is a more helpful test for evaluating the internal nasal valve (Fig. 4.7).

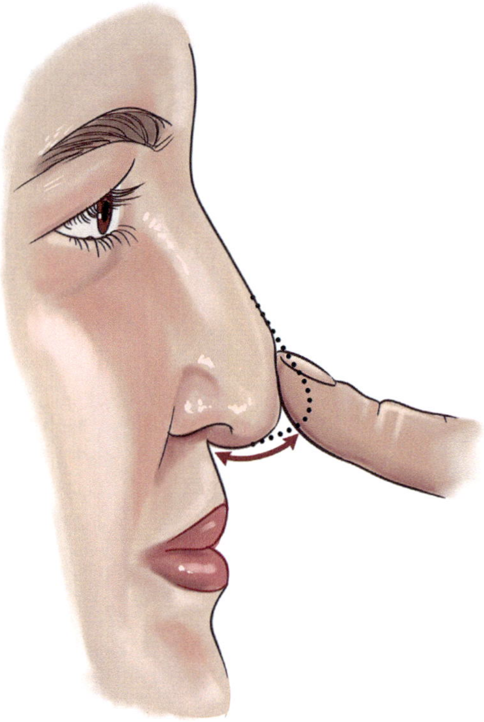

Fig. 4.4 In a recoil test, the surgeon presses on the tip of the nose to see its resistance

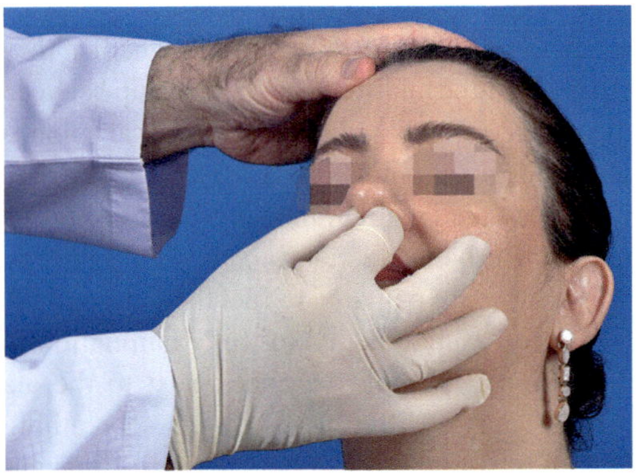

Fig. 4.5 After wearing a glove, the caudal septum and anterior nasal spine are palpated

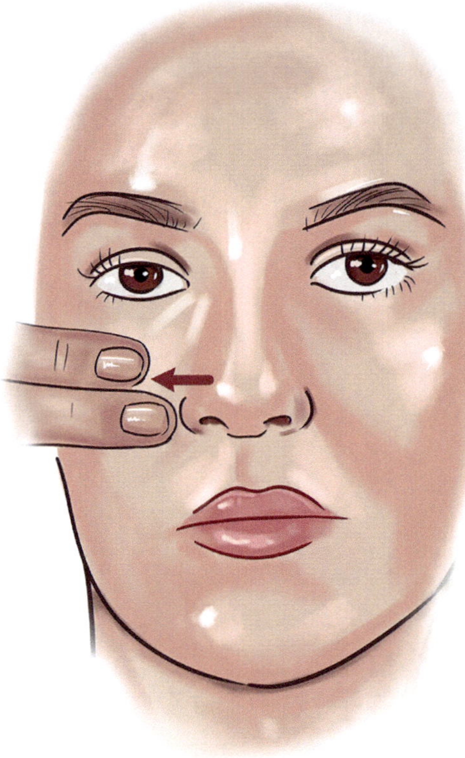

Fig. 4.6 Cottle test can be added to this examination to determine if pulling the cheek next to the ala makes any difference during breathing

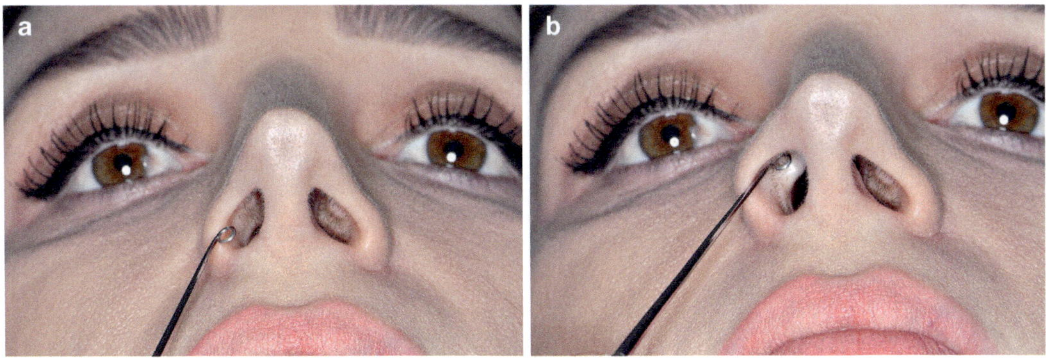

Fig. 4.7 Ear curette to lateralize the ala from the inside is a more helpful test to evaluate the internal nasal valve

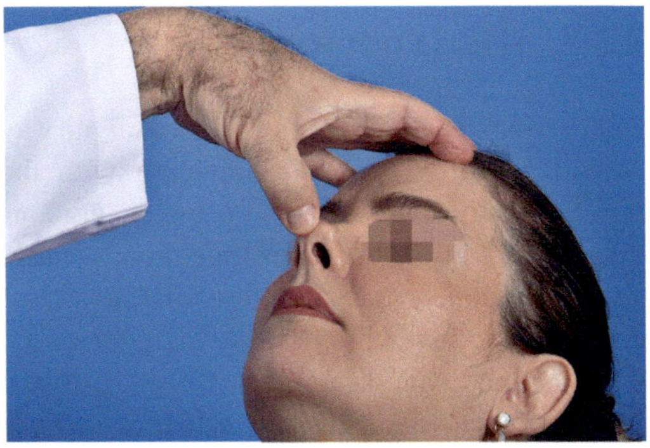

Fig. 4.8 The best way to examine the nostrils and internal nasal valve is to use the left hand, placing the four fingers on the forehead, while the thumb gently elevates the tip of the nose

4.4 Anterior Rhinoscopy

Examination starts while the patient is sitting on an ENT examination chair. After detailed inspection and palpation, the patient's head is tilted backward. The surgeon should use a headlight at this stage. He should use his left hand, placing the four fingers on the forehead, while the thumb is used to gently elevate the tip of the nose. It is possible to see and examine the nostrils, external valve, internal valve, and position of the caudal septum (Fig. 4.8). At the internal valve, there can be mucocutaneous changes, such as adhesions or strictures, and septal or upper lateral cartilage changes, such as thickening, deflection, or twisting [8].

The patient's head is brought to the neutral position, and a nasal speculum is used to further examine the inside of the nose at different positions and angles (Fig. 4.9). If deviation, inferior turbinate, or mucosal congestion blocks visualization of the nasal passages, a decongestant, such as oxymetazoline, can be used to see deeper structures. At 0°, it is possible to see the inferior meatus, inferior turbinates, and the lower part of the nasal septum. If there is no septal deviation, inferior turbinate hypertrophy, or mucosal congestion, the nasal passage can be seen up to the nasopharynx. At 30°, the middle meatus and middle turbinate can be seen. Septal deviation, concha bullosa, and purulent discharge from the sinuses can be identified in this position. At 60°, the upper portion of the nasal passages, nasal septum, and middle turbinate is visible.

The nasal septum is examined, and the type, site, and severity of any deviation are noted. The type of septal deviation can be simple, spur, subluxation, or fractured. I have been using an SL classification to describe the septal deviation site for more than 20 years [9]. In this classification, the site of deviation is described according to Cottle zones, namely, (1) vestibulum nasi, (2) nasal valve, (3) attic, (4) anterior turbinate area, (5) posterior turbinate area [10] (Fig. 4.10). The severity of deviation should be noted as mild, moderate, or severe. The type of crooked nose, such as linear, cartilaginous linear, C-shaped, or S-shaped, should also be noted.

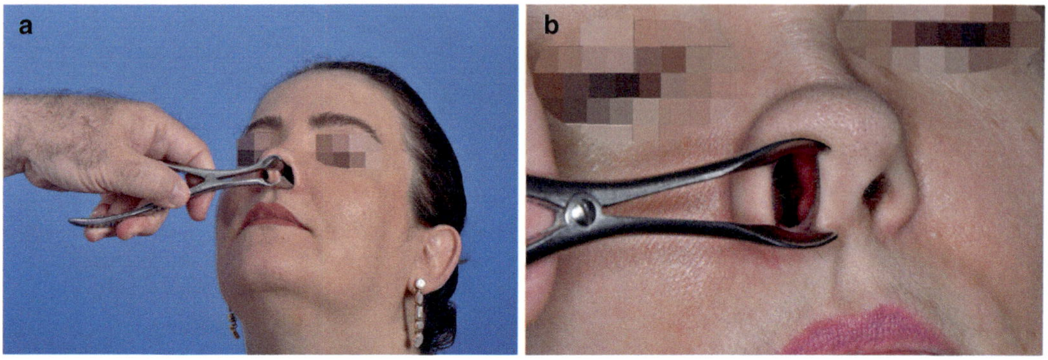

Fig. 4.9 Anterior rhinoscopy is performed by using a nasal speculum to examine the inside of the nose at different positions and angles

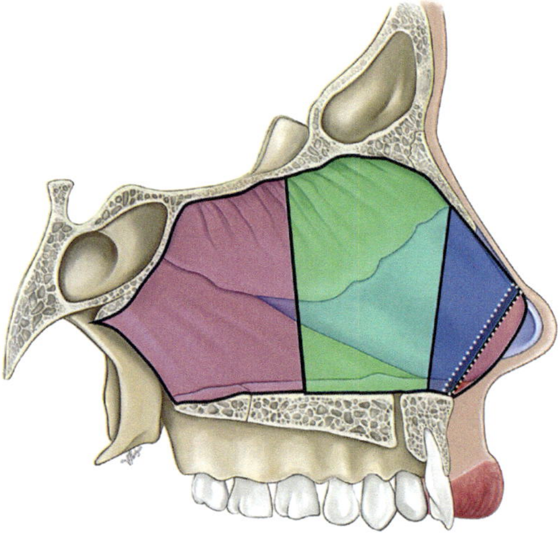

Fig. 4.10 Cottle zones are depicted in this illustration: (1) vestibulum nasi, (2) nasal valve, (3) attic, (4) anterior turbinate area, (5) posterior turbinate area

The existence of polyp(s), septal perforation, synechia, bleeding sites, mucopus, scarring, dryness, inferior turbinate hypertrophy, concha bullosa, adenoid hypertrophy, color of the mucosa, ulceration, crusting, and any other pathological conditions must be noted. At the end of this examination, the estimated degree of nasal airway obstruction for both passages should be recorded as a percentage.

4.5 Nasal Endoscopy

Endoscopic examination of the nasal airway should be followed by examination with the nasal speculum. In fact, some younger surgeons may find traditional nasal examination by nasal speculum unnecessary because of the use of endoscopes. I use both because the endoscopic examination can sometimes give distorted images due to the wide angle. I like using a 6-cm long 0° 4 mm Hopkins straight otoscopic telescope for routine examination instead of the standard 14-cm long telescope for two reasons: it is much easier to manipulate, and the patient shows less anxiety when they see the shorter telescope (Fig. 4.11a). When an endoscopic camera is attached to the telescope, the examination can be recorded on a computer along with other examination findings (Fig. 4.11b). The mucosa can be anesthetized and decongested to observe the nasopharynx and posterior portion of the nasal airway. If a flexible endoscope of 3 mm in diameter is used, the patient can tolerate the endoscopic examination without topical anesthesia (Fig. 4.11c). Therefore, any lesion of the nasopharynx, such as hypertrophy of the tail of the inferior turbinate, adenoid hypertrophy, choanal atresia, nasopharyngeal tumor, and nasopharyngeal

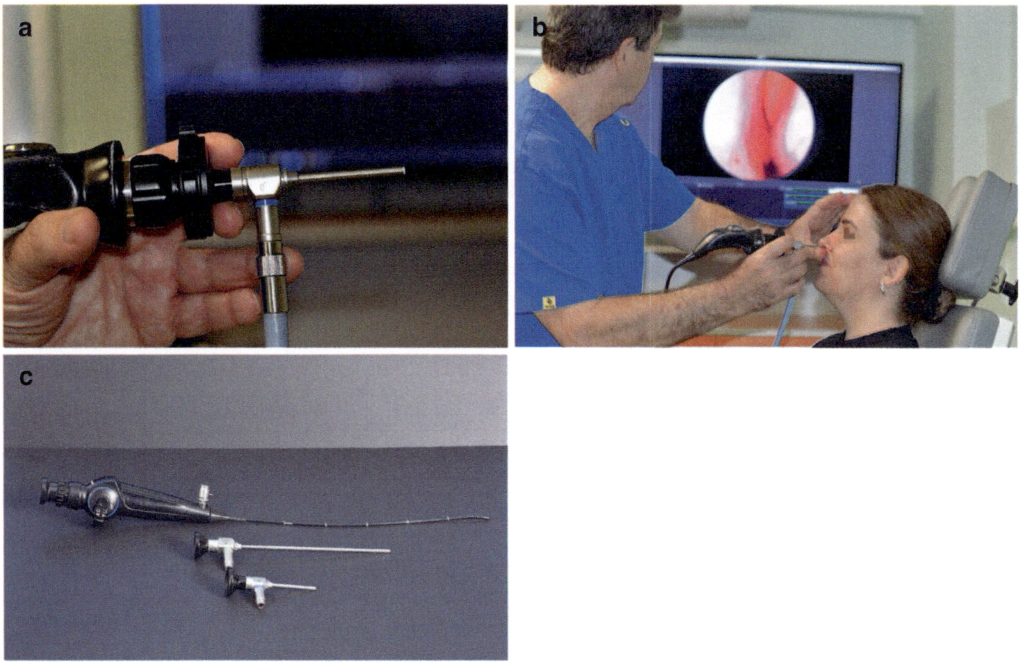

Fig. 4.11 (**a**) Nasal endoscopy using a 6-cm long 0° 4 mm Hopkins straight otoscopic telescope. (**b**) Endoscopic camera attached to the telescope helps the surgeon show the findings to the patient and record them. (**c**) A flexible endoscope of 3 mm is well tolerated during the endoscopic examination without topical anesthesia

angiofibroma, can be identified. I would like to emphasize that I have seen all these lesions in patients who were candidates for rhinoplasty. Therefore, the surgeon should attempt to explore the entire nasal cavity during endoscopic examination.

4.6 Functional Diagnostic Tests

4.6.1 Peak Nasal Inspiratory Flow

This is a measurement of nasal permeability that provides nasal flow data expressed in liters per minute. It can be obtained by an inspiratory maneuver. It is a simple and rapid technique that can be performed using a portable device [11]. We used it in some clinical studies.

4.6.2 Rhinomanometry

In this technique, simultaneous measurement of pressure debit and variations of airflow in the nasal passages during the breathing cycle is performed. In anterior rhinomanometry, the measurement systems are placed at the level of the nasal nostril. An intraoral device is used to register choanal pressure in posterior rhinomanometry [12]. In four-phase rhinomanometry, acceleration and deceleration in the inspiratory and expiratory phases can be measured. In addition to obtaining quantitative values, this study aims to introduce the measurement of parameters that correlate better with the subjective sensation of nasal breathing [13]. We have been using four-phase rhinomanometry in my department for clinical research (Fig. 4.12a, b).

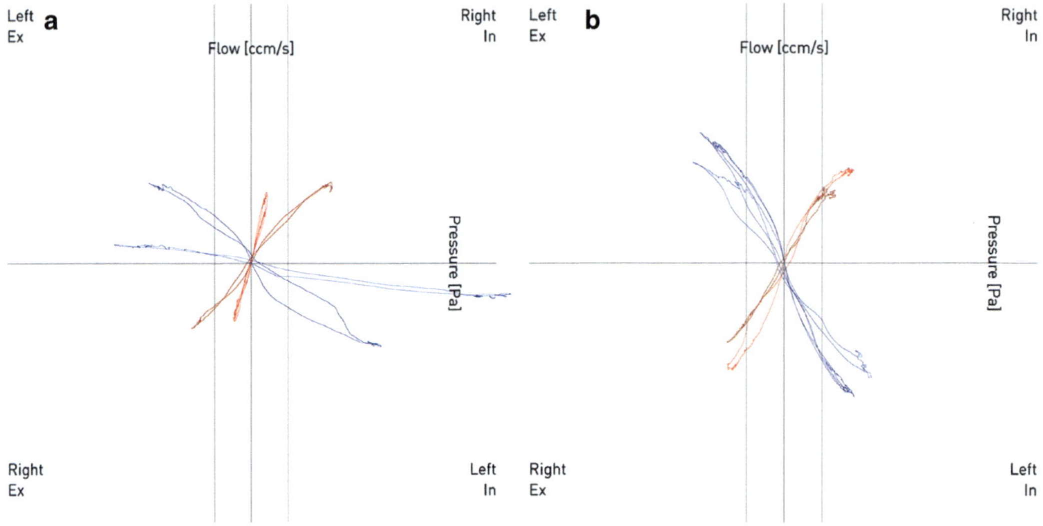

Fig. 4.12 (**a**) This is the rhinomanometric of a patient with severe septal deviation to the left. In curve a, it is seen that all phases occur with a very strong flow against low pressure. In curve b, which represents the deviated left nasal cavity, it is seen that the flow slows down considerably due to the increase in pressure. In particular, Phase 2 in curve b, which expresses the subjective feeling of congestion, is quite prolonged in the direction of pressure. The logarithmic pressure value in the left nasal cavity was rated very high at 1.84. (**b**) This is the rhinomanometric diagram of the same patient 6 months after surgery. It is observed that the flow of the patient increased due to the decrease in intranasal pressure in all measurement phases, and especially in Phase 2, which creates the subjective feeling of obstruction, accelerated considerably. The logarithmic pressure value in both nasal cavities approached each other and was rated at a low-pressure level

4.6.3 Acoustic Rhinometry

This objective method for exploring the geometry of the nasal cavity enables the analysis of the acoustic reflection of a sound wave that travels along the nasal cavity and the measurement of areas and volumes at different points in the nasal fossa [14]. We used it for some time in our department for clinical research, but we do not use it anymore.

4.7 Radiological Studies

4.7.1 Computerized Tomography

This is the traditional and most rewarding imaging modality for the nose and paranasal sinuses during the last two decades. It is possible to obtain information regarding the anatomy and variants of the nasal septum, airway, lateral nasal wall, and paranasal sinuses using this modality (Fig. 4.13a–d). It is possible to make measurements of the septal cartilage, ethmoid, and vomer, which can be very helpful before surgery [15]. In addition, inferior turbinate hypertrophy, concha bullosa, septal deviation, nasal polyps, sinus infections, and nasopharyngeal tumors can be more easily diagnosed in detail. Therefore, the surgeon can perform some measurements and preoperative planning based on CT images [16]. In recent years, cone beam CT has become so popular that some surgeons use it as a standard preoperative analysis tool. The target area can be chosen, which is why there is less radiation exposure than traditional CT, and the cost is less [17]. Recently, McIntosh et al. presented the "Rhinoplasty Cephalometric Evaluation for Radiologic pre-operative systematization" protocol to present guidelines for radiologists to report relevant nasal anatomy in the context of preoperative rhinoplasty evaluation [18].

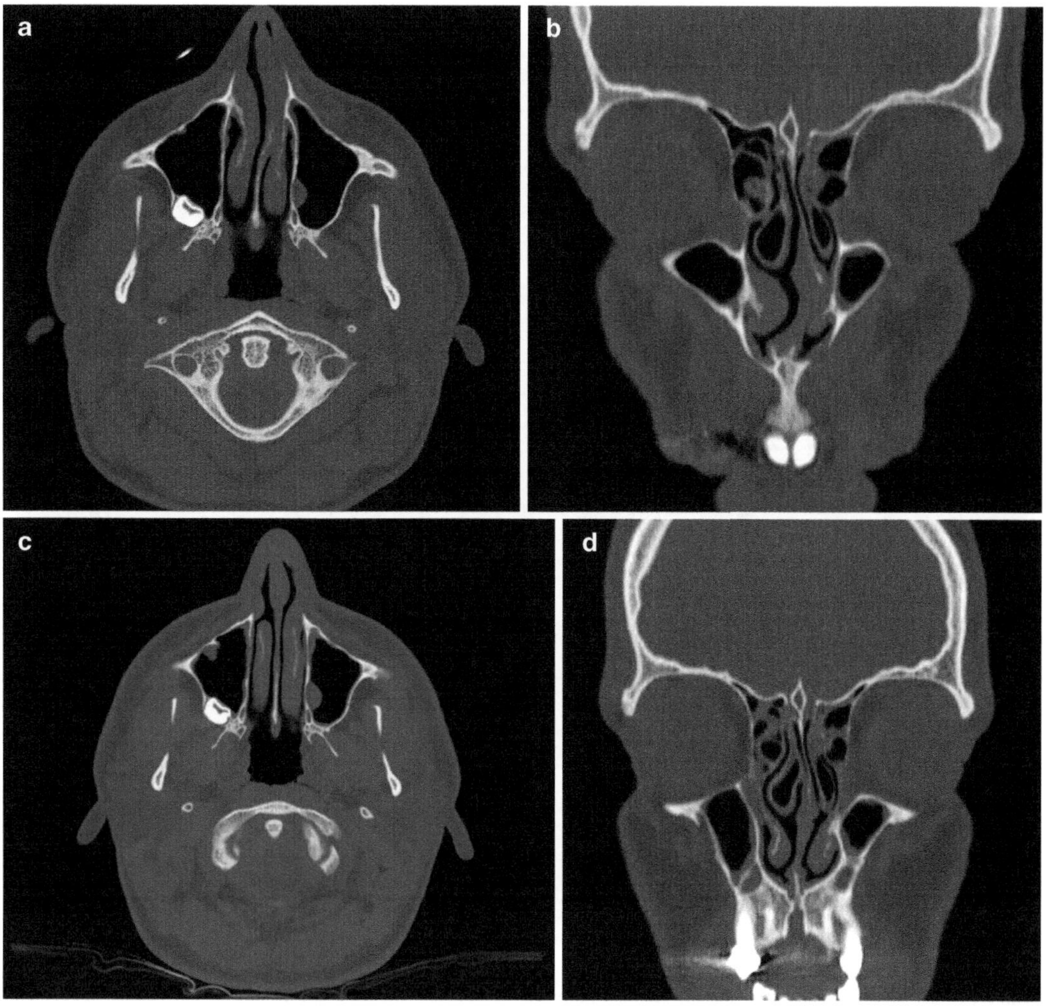

Fig. 4.13 The preoperative (**a**, **b**) and postoperative (**c**, **d**) computerized tomography images of the patient

4.7.2 Computational Fluid Dynamics

This involves creating three-dimensional computational models of nasal airways using imaging data from CT or MRI. These models are processed using special computer programs by mechanical engineers to calculate the velocity of nasal airflow, nasal resistance, heat transfer, and humidification. It can help to determine the location of the nasal obstruction and its effect on the patient [19–21]. It can even be used to simulate airway surgery and/or rhinoplasty and see the results before surgery [22]. We have been working with a team of mechanical engineers using this modality in recent years. It takes days to create the models and perform the calculations (Fig. 4.14a–d). In addition, powerful computers and expensive software are required.

In summary, examination of the nose is a critical step before any rhinoplasty or septoplasty. The surgeon should follow all the steps mentioned in this chapter and record all the data thoroughly.

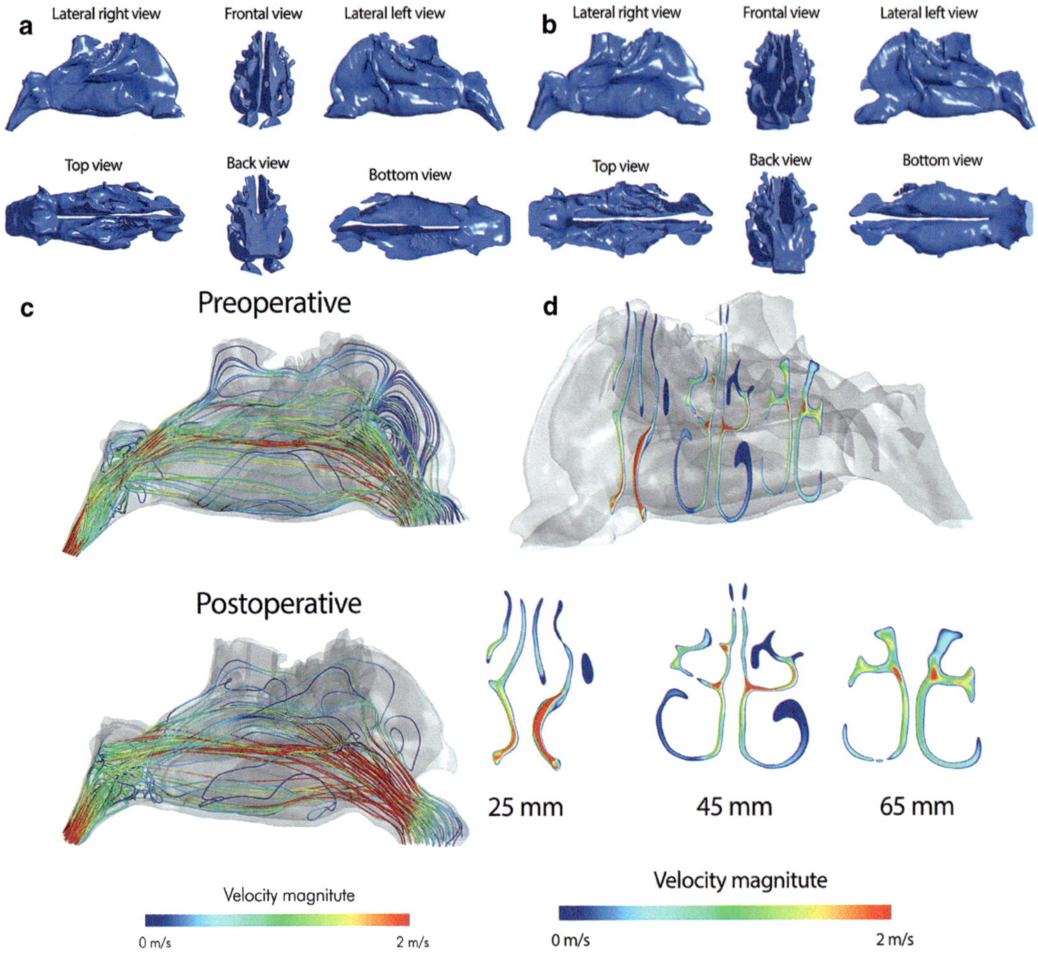

Fig. 4.14 (**a**) The 3D reconstruction model of a patient from different views by using the preoperative computerized tomography data. (**b**) The 3D reconstruction model of the same patient from different views by using the postoperative computerized tomography data. (**c**) This image shows the velocity contour in the nasal airways of the same patient by using computational fluid dynamics. It is set to display speeds between 0 and 2 m/s. 0 m/s is expressed in dark blue, while 2 m/s and higher speeds are expressed in red. (**d**) The streamline is visible in these images. Velocities between 0 and 2 m/s are shown in color. Dark blue indicates 0 m/s, while red indicates speeds of 2 m/s and higher. A certain amount of flow is sent through the nostrils, and the trajectory of the airflow in the nose can be examined

References

1. Stewart MG, Witsell DL, Smith TL, Weaver EM, Yueh B, Hannley MT. Development and validation of the Nasal Obstruction Symptom Evaluation (NOSE) scale. Otolaryngol Head Neck Surg. 2004;130:157–63.
2. Alsarraf R, Larrabee WF Jr, Anderson S, Murakami CS, Johnson CM Jr. Measuring cosmetic facial plastic surgery outcomes: a pilot study. Arch Facial Plast Surg. 2001;3:198–201.
3. Lohuis PJFM, Hakim S, Duivesteijn W, Knobbe A, Tasman AJ. Benefits of a short, practical questionnaire to measure subjective perception of nasal appearance after aesthetic rhinoplasty. Plast Reconstr Surg. 2013;132:913e–23e.
4. Klassen AF, Cano SJ, East CA, Baker SB, Badia L, Schwitzer JA, Pusic AL. Development and psychometric evaluation of the FACE-Q scales for patients undergoing rhinoplasty. JAMA Facial Plast Surg. 2016;18:27–35.
5. Moubayed SP, Ioannidis JPA, Saltychev M, Most SP. The 10-item standardized cosmesis and health

nasal outcomes survey (SCHNOS) for functional and cosmetic rhinoplasty. JAMA Facial Plast Surg. 2018;20:37–42.
6. Lekakis G, Picavet VA, Gabriëls L, Grietens J, Hellings PW. Body dysmorphic disorder in aesthetic rhinoplasty: validating a new screening tool. Laryngoscope. 2016;126:1739–45.
7. Gode S, Ozturk A, Sahin M, Berber V, Apaydin F. Turkish validation of the standardized cosmesis and health nasal outcomes survey. Facial Plast Surg. 2019;35:397–9.
8. Kasperbauer JL, Kern EB. Nasal valve physiology. Implications in nasal surgery. Otolaryngol Clin North Am. 1987;20:699–719.
9. Apaydın F. A new documentation standard in the nose examination: SL classification. Facial Plast Surg. 2013;29:449–54.
10. Cottle MH. Rhino-sphygmo-manometry and aid in physical diagnosis. Intern Rhinol. 1968;6:7–26.
11. Ottaviano G, Fokkens WJ. Measurements of nasal airflow and patency: a critical review with emphasis on the use of peak nasal inspiratory flow in daily practice. Allergy. 2016;71:162–74.
12. Eccles R. A guide to practical aspects of measurement of human nasal airflow by rhinomanometry. Rhinology. 2011;49:2–10.
13. Vogt K, Jalowayski AA, Althaus W, Cao C, Han D, Hasse W, Hoffrichter H, Mösges R, Pallanch J, Shah-Hosseini K, Peksis K, Wernecke KD, Zhang L, Zaporoshenko P. 4-Phase-Rhinomanometry (4PR)—basics and practice 2010. Rhinol Suppl. 2010;21:1–50.
14. Grymer LF, Hilberg O, Pedersen OF, Rasmussen TR. Acoustic rhinometry: values from adults with subjective normal nasal patency. Rhinology. 1991;29:35–47.
15. Moon KM, Cho G, Sung HM, Jung MS, Tak KS, Jung SW, Lee HB, Suh IS. Nasal anthropometry on facial computed tomography scans for rhinoplasty in Koreans. Arch Plast Surg. 2013;40:610–5.
16. Eravci FC, Özer H, Arbağ H, Eryilmaz MA, Aricigil M, Dündar MA. Computed tomography analysis of nasal anatomy in dorsal preservation rhinoplasty. Aesthet Surg J. 2022;42:249–56.
17. Robotti E, Daniel RK, Leone F. Cone-beam computed tomography: a user-friendly, practical roadmap to the planning and execution of every rhinoplasty—A 5-year review. Plast Reconstr Surg. 2021;147:749e–62e.
18. McIntosh C, Stutterheim J, Prinsloo H, Randall M, Toman J, Pisapia F. The RhinoCEROS guidelines: a practical tool for reporting nasal anatomy on computed tomography pertaining to rhinoplasty. Facial Plast Surg. 2023;39:362–71.
19. Rhee JS, Pawar SS, Garcia GJ, et al. Toward personalized nasal surgery using computational fluid dynamics. Arch Facial Plast Surg. 2011;13(5):305–10.
20. Pawar SS, Gacia GJ, Kimbell JS, et al. Objective measures in aesthetic and functional nasal surgery: perspectives on nasal form and function. Facial Plast Surg. 2010;26:320–7.
21. Garcia GJ, Rhee JS, Senior BA. Septal deviation and nasal resistance: an investigation using virtual surgery and computational fluid dynamics. Am J Rhinol Allergy. 2010;24:e46–53.
22. Radulesco T, Meister L, Bouchet G, Varoquaux A, Giordano J, Dessi P, Perrier P, Michel J. Computational fluid dynamics and septal deviations—Virtual surgery can predict post-surgery results: a preliminary study including two patients. Clin Otolaryngol. 2020;45:286–91.

Preoperative Planning for Septorhinoplasty

5

5.1 Introduction

Rhinoplasty is an operation of details, and the surgeon should plan all steps like a chess player before surgery. Therefore, preoperative planning is quite important in rhinoplasty and septoplasty. It is ideal that this plan is performed after thorough history taking and detailed examination. The patient should be informed about the reasons for nasal obstruction. It must always be mentioned that this is not an obligatory surgery, and it can be performed to make breathing more comfortable through the nose. The patient should be informed about the physiology and anatomy of the nose. I always try to teach the patients about the four valves, namely the external valve, internal valve, septal valve, and conchal valve, and their importance for breathing [1] (Table 5.1).

Patients sometimes have the wrong impression that the appearance of the nose will change after septal surgery. Because 95% of my patients seeking a remedy for nasal obstruction also demand rhinoplasty, the equilibrium between function and esthetics is explained in detail. The patients are usually not aware that if the nose becomes smaller, the airway also gets smaller. Therefore, patients should understand the trade-off between the function and aesthetics of the nose. The surgeon should try his/her best to describe functional rhinoplasty.

Table 5.1 Four valves in the nose that are very important for functional rhinoplasty

1.	External valve
2.	Internal valve
3.	Septal valve (nasal septum)
4.	Conchal valve (turbinates)

I do my best to explain the importance of projection and rotation in rhinoplasty. Imaging performed on patients' pictures can ease decision-making by the patient and surgeon. Projection can be preserved, increased, or decreased. Rotation can be preserved and can be changed upward or downward. The patient should be informed if she/he will undergo rhinoplasty, septoplasty, or septorhinoplasty.

Another important issue to note is whether it will be a primary or revision surgery for the patient. It can look like a very easy step, but I have seen cases in which the patients were simply not aware of any previous nasal surgeries and did not inform the surgeon. Therefore, I would always like to obtain consent from the patient about conchal and/or rib harvest if an unexpected situation is confronted.

The first decision is the approach to be used to reach the nasal septum. During rhinoplasty, there can be an endonasal approach such as hemitransfixion, Killian, transfixion incision, or an external approach. If there is no septal deviation, the nasal septum can be left undisturbed. Hemitransfixion incision is my favorite incision when I want to perform any kind of basic septal

© The Author(s), under exclusive license to Springer Nature Switzerland AG 2025
F. Apaydın, *Septal Surgery Challenges in Rhinoplasty*,
https://doi.org/10.1007/978-3-031-74734-2_5

surgery in the beginning or harvest cartilage. The Killian incision was the only incision that I have learned during my residency years. I have almost abandoned its use during the last two decades. I have been using transfixion incision very rarely during the endonasal approach. If the problem is a badly deviated spur at the rear part of the nose where the anterior half is straight, direct incision on the spur and resection of the spur is performed with the help of loupes or endoscopic surgery. Transcartilaginous or intercartilaginous incisions can also be planned if the nasal tip is fine and should be bypassed or slightly bulbous.

External incision is routinely used by many surgeons in all cases. In my daily routine rhinoplasty, I use the external approach in 90% and the endonasal approach in 10% of my cases. I strongly believe that rhinoplasty surgeons should learn to use both approaches. When the external approach is used, the nasal septum can be reached in three ways: (1) Hemitransfixion incision; (2) Dissecting the soft tissues between the medial crura; (3) Opening the middle vault by either resecting the hump or dissecting the upper lateral cartilages from the nasal septum. There are times when a combination of these three is used as well. I also abandoned the use of the traditional delivery approach within the last decade because I found that only marginal incision is good enough to perform any procedure on the tip and nasal dorsum.

It should also be noted what type of septal procedure is possible in each individual case. In some selected cases where there is a nasal hump and the tip has a mild deformity, it is possible to keep the nasal septum intact and use the resected hump as a graft. In case of an isolated spur at the posterior part of the nasal septum, endoscopic resection of a limited area can be performed. However, in most cases, septoplasty or submucous resection is performed.

One of the main decisions to make during preoperative planning is which kind of septal correction is needed and if cartilage harvest is required to obtain grafts. Structural rhinoplasty techniques have been the most popular techniques during the last two decades, and that is why cartilage harvest usually means submucous resection. The Cottle type of septoplasty is very seldom used. However, in recent years, preservation rhinoplasty techniques have started gaining popularity. I have also started using these techniques in selected cases. One of the main advantages of dorsal preservation techniques is that the use of spreader grafts or flaps is not needed, so more septal cartilage can be preserved, or the grafts can be used for different purposes.

The position, strength, length, and condition of the caudal septum should be evaluated immediately before surgery. It is a tradition originating from Joseph techniques to resect the caudal portion of the caudal septum. Depending on the situation, different portions of the caudal septum can be resected. The only time I resect the caudal septum is in the case of a very long caudal septum in tension noses. Otherwise, I prefer using the caudal septum as an anchor platform for septocolumellar sutures.

The surgeon should also plan what to do with the nasal dorsum and profile: to keep the dorsum as it is, reduce, or augment. This plan should also be discussed with the patient and informed accordingly.

The surgeon should look at the frontal view and evaluate the width of the nasal dorsum. It can be undisturbed, widened, or narrowed.

On the tip, the surgeon should plan the approach to the lateral crura, domes, and medial crura. The lateral crura can be kept intact or more traditionally trimmed cephalically. In addition, a lateral crural turn-in flap or a similar flap technique can be planned. In rare cases, the lateral crura can be divided and overlapped or repositioned in cases of cephalically positioning. Various suture techniques, such as domal suture, hemitransdomal suture, dome equalization suture, and transdomal suture, can be planned for use on domes. Although I am not fond of dome division techniques, they are listed here because there are still some surgeons using this technique. The medial crura are evaluated before surgery. They are usually kept intact. However, they can be sutured to the caudal septum to change rotation and/or projection, a columellar strut can be placed between them, or partial resections or overlap can be performed.

The nasal dorsum is an important part of the profile and requires special planning before surgery. If there is a need for dorsal reduction, which is one of the main problems in many parts of the world, will it be a bony and/or cartilaginous reduction? Will there be a need for augmentation, and with which material? What about the radix? Should we keep it as it is, or is there a need for reduction or augmentation?

After hump removal or in the case of a crooked nose, osteotomies are usually necessary. The side, type, route, and types of osteotomies should be planned and noted. In crooked noses, correction of septal deviation is very important, but the bony pyramid must be mobilized to bring the nose into the midline.

In structural rhinoplasty, and especially in revision cases, there is a need to use grafts. Depending on each individual case, the type of grafts, such as spreader, shield, columellar strut, and lateral crural strut grafts, should be planned. Only after careful planning can the surgeon decide about the source of the grafts and explain the situation to the patient accordingly.

At the end of surgery, if the nasal tip is deprojected or if there is a flaring before, alar base surgery may be needed. This need should be seen before surgery, and the technique and possible scar should be explained to the patient. If the surgeon misses this small detail, the patient may suffer from an unexpected surgical maneuver.

If there is a septal deviation limited to the cartilaginous septum, a quilting suture is sufficient, and no splints or packing are necessary. This small detail must be shared with the patient because some patients may be worried about packing after surgery.

If there is hypertrophy of the inferior turbinate, the surgeon should choose the modality of treatment that he/she feels is best for the patient. Although radiofrequency cauterization is the most popular and my preferred technique, lateralization, submucous resection, or turbinoplasty can also be preferred by the surgeon. If there is a concha bullosa, paradoxically bent middle turbinate, polyps, or another pathology, the operative plan should be performed after a detailed endoscopic examination and CT examination of the nose and paranasal sinuses.

It is not unusual for patients to demand additional surgery during rhinoplasty. If the patient asks for injectables, blepharoplasty, facelift, or any other procedure, the time for surgery will be longer, and this should also be planned.

A preoperative planning sheet is listed in Table 5.2, which is also part of Rhinobase [2]. This is a quick checklist that can help the surgeon complete a detailed plan in a short time. It is recommended that each surgeon customize such a checklist for himself. Besides, a preoperative planning diagram is also very useful to visualize the operative plan (Figs. 5.1 and 5.2).

A serious surgeon should accept each rhinoplasty as a project and spend time listening to the patient's demands, for examination, and for careful planning.

Table 5.2 Preoperative planning sheet

Operative planning			
Projection	[ ] Do not disturb	[ ] Increase	[ ] Decrease
Rotation	[ ] Do not disturb	[ ] Upward rotation	[ ] Downward rotation
Type of procedure	[ ] Rhinoplasty	[ ] Septoplasty	[ ] Septorhinoplasty
	[ ] Cleft lip nose	[ ] Closed fracture reduction	[ ] Other
Procedure	[ ] Primary	[ ] Secondary	[ ] Revision
Inferior turbinate surgery	[ ] Partial resection	[ ] Total resection	[ ] Submucous resection
	[ ] Turbinoplasty	[ ] Bipolar cauterization	[ ] Monopolar cauterization
	[ ] Radiofrequency cauterization	[ ] Lateralization	[ ] Other
Inferior turbinate surgery_2	[ ] Partial resection	[ ] Total resection	[ ] Submucous resection
	[ ] Turbinoplasty	[ ] Bipolar cauterization	[ ] Monopolar cauterization
	[ ] Radiofrequency cauterization	[ ] Lateralization	[ ] Other
Incisions			
[ ] Killian	[ ] Hemitransfixion	[ ] Transfixion	[ ] Midcolumellar
[ ] Marginal	[ ] Intercartilagenous	[ ] Transcartilagenous	[ ] Rim
[ ] High transfixion			
Approach	[ ] Delivery	[ ] Nondelivery	[ ] External
Septum	[ ] Undisturbed	[ ] SMR	[ ] Septoplasty
[ ] Cartilage harvest	[ ] Spur excision	[ ] Caudal edge resection	[ ] Total septal reconstruction
Caudal edge resection	[ ] Anterior	[ ] Middle	[ ] Posterior
	[ ] Complete		
Dorsum lateral view	[ ] Undisturbed	[ ] Augmentation	[ ] Reduction
Dorsum frontal view	[ ] Do not disturb	[ ] Widening	[ ] Narrowing
	[ ] Medialize		
Lateral profile changes (mm)	[ ] Radix	[ ] Rhinion	[ ] Middle vault
	[ ] Supratip	[ ] Tip	[ ] Subnasale
Lateral crura	[ ] Undisturbed	[ ] Interrupted strip	[ ] Complete strip
	[ ] Overlap shortening		
Domal sutures	[ ] Left + Right	[ ] Left	[ ] Right
	[ ] None		
Reorientation sutures	[ ] Tongue-in-groove	[ ] Transdomal suture	[ ] Septocolumellar suture
	[ ] Interalar suture	[ ] Intermediate crura sutured together	Footplate narrowing suture
Medial crura	[ ] Caudal margin resection	[ ] Vertical segment resection	[ ] Footplate resection right
	[ ] Footplate resection left	[ ] Footplate resection bilateral	[ ] Overlap shortening
Alar reduction	[ ] Nostril	[ ] Nostril floor	[ ] Alar lobule
Medial osteotomies	[ ] Bilateral	[ ] Right	[ ] Left
Lateral osteotomies	[ ] Bilateral	[ ] Right	[ ] Left
Intermediate osteotomies	[ ] Bilateral	[ ] Right	[ ] Left
Transverse osteotomies	[ ] Bilateral	[ ] Right	[ ] Left
Nasolabial angle	[ ] Do not disturb	[ ] Augmentation	[ ] Reduction
Splint	[ ] Bilateral	[ ] Right	[ ] Left
Merocel	[ ] Bilateral	[ ] Right	[ ] Left
Vaseline gauze	[ ] Bilateral	[ ] Right	[ ] Left

(continued)

Table 5.2 (continued)

Operative planning			
Other procedures	[ ] Mentoplasty	[ ] Blepharoplasty	[ ] Closure of septal perforation
Miscellaneous	[ ] Quilting suture	[ ] Division of depressor septi muscle	[ ] Vestibular skin resection
Grafts			
[ ] Shield	[ ] Columellar strut	[ ] Spreader graft	[ ] Lateral crural graft
[ ] Lateral crural strut graft	[ ] Tip graft (Peck)	[ ] Spreader flap	[ ] Caudal septal extension
[ ] Rim graft	[ ] Alar batten graft	[ ] Radix graft	
Camouflage			
Radix	[ ] Soft-tissue fascia	[ ] Soft-tissue perichondrium	[ ] Cartilage dust
[ ] Diced cartilage	[ ] Morselized cartilage	[ ] Thinned cartilage	[ ] Filler
Middle third	[ ] Soft-tissue fascia	[ ] Soft-tissue perichondrium	[ ] Cartilage dust
[ ] Diced cartilage	[ ] Morselized cartilage	[ ] Thinned cartilage	[ ] Filler
Tip	[ ] Soft-tissue fascia	[ ] Soft-tissue perichondrium	[ ] Cartilage dust
[ ] Diced cartilage	[ ] Morselized cartilage	[ ] Thinned cartilage	[ ] Filler

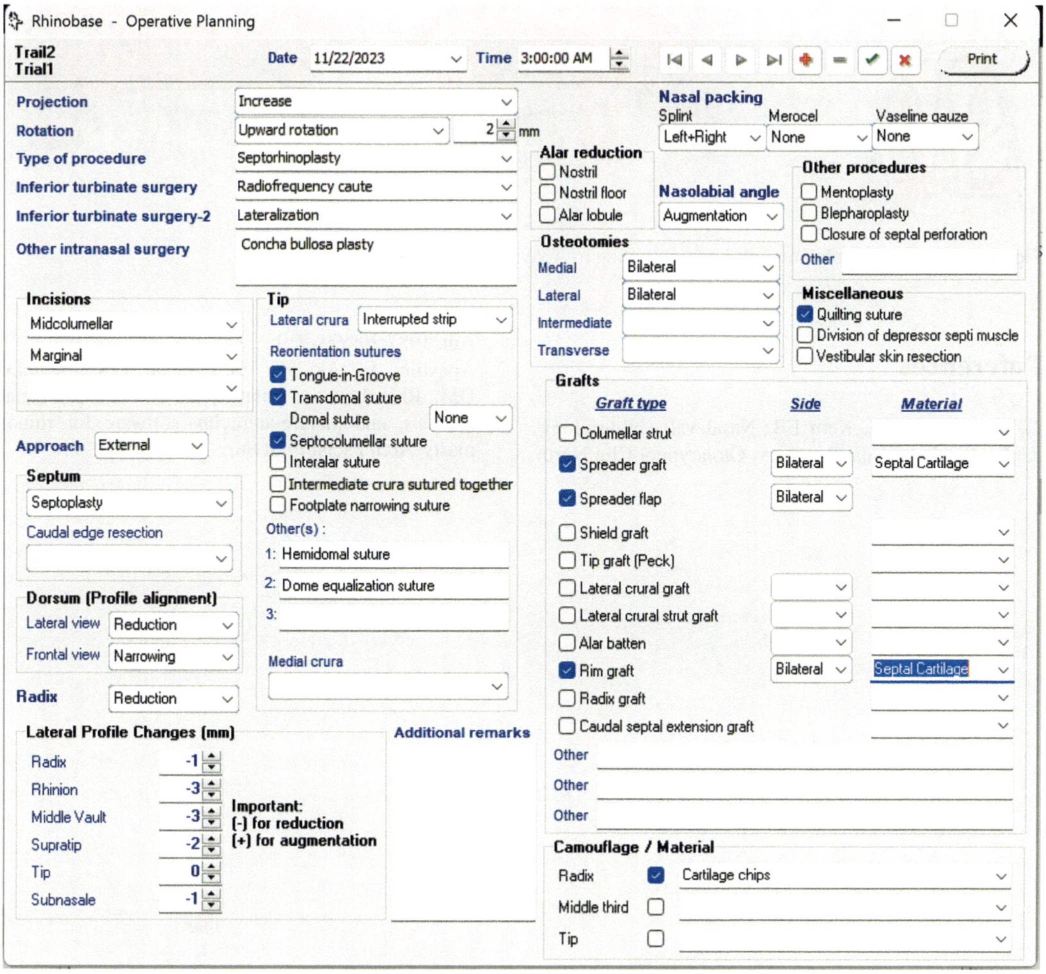

Fig. 5.1 Preoperative planning sheet in Rhinobase 2.2

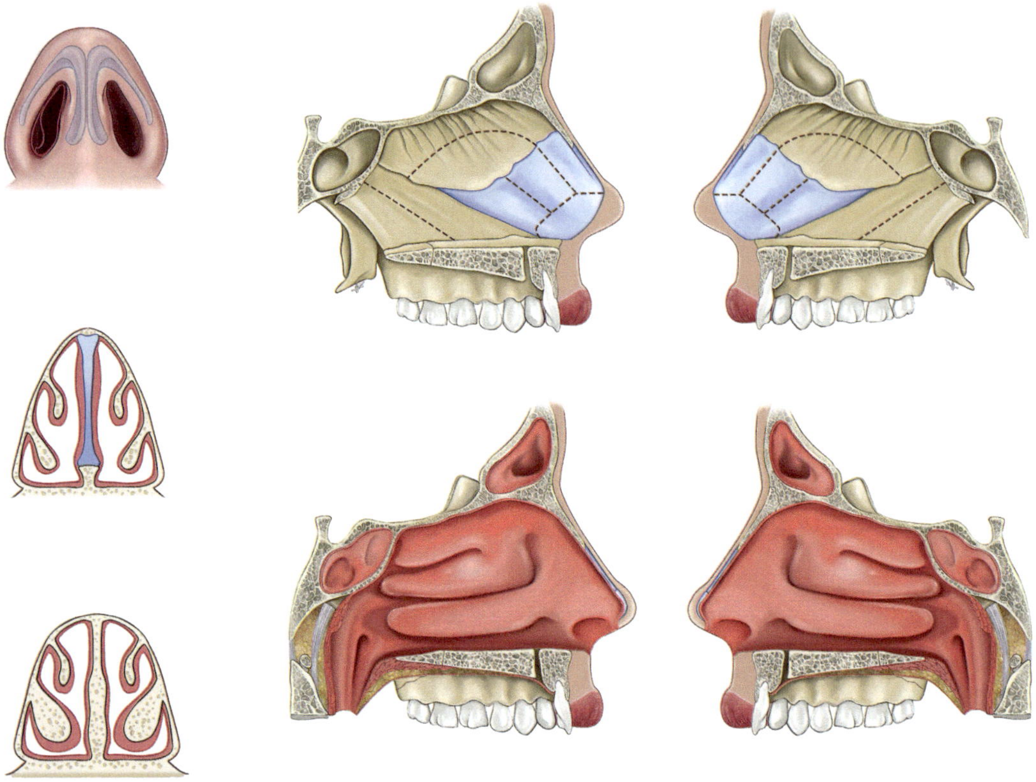

Fig. 5.2 Preoperative planning diagram according to Apaydin

References

1. Kasperbauer JL, Kern EB. Nasal valve physiology. Implications in nasal surgery. Otolaryngol Clin North Am. 1987;20:699–719.
2. Apaydin F, Akyildiz S, Hecht DA, Toriumi DM. Rhinobase: a comprehensive database, facial analysis, and picture-archiving software for rhinoplasty. Arch Facial Plast Surg. 2009;11:209–11.

6 Classification of Septal Deviations

6.1 Introduction

Currently, there is no widely accepted method of classifying septal deviations. An important challenge after a detailed nasal examination is to record the findings in a systematic manner. The data obtained are usually written on a sheet of paper and sometimes recorded in a computer program. In recent years, endoscopic examination instruments have become so sophisticated that it is very easy to examine nasal cavities using rigid or flexible endoscopes. The images can be recorded using full HD or 4 K systems. Imaging systems using computerized tomography or magnetic resonance imaging have made diagnosing the problems of the nasal cavities and paranasal sinuses much easier. However, there is still a need to classify the deviations to make progress in clinical research and maintain more details regarding the examination findings.

If standardization can be attained for recording the examination findings, there will be less need for using handwriting, and documentation will be easier, more efficient, and reliable.

In fact, septal surgery is usually accepted as a minor procedure, and its detailed documentation is not considered as a serious task in daily routine. Some studies have been conducted to classify the condition of the nasal septum and the lateral nasal wall [1–3].

Lawson classified the twisted nose as C-shaped and S-shaped [1] (Fig. 6.1). Guyuron made a classification of six different types of septal deviation. He described septal tilt and S-shaped anteroposterior deviations as the most common ones. The other deformities were C-shaped cephalocaudal, C-shaped anteroposterior, S-shaped cephalocaudal, and localized deviations or large spurs in his classification [2] (Fig. 6.2).

Mladina divided septal pathologies into seven types. The first four types refer to vertical deformities, types 5 and 6 to horizontal deformities, and type 7 to a combination of the previous groups. Type 1 was a mild, unilateral, vertical septal ridge in the valve region. Type 2 was a more severe form of type 1 that compromised breathing. Type 3 was a unilateral vertical ridge at the junction of the quadrangular and perpendicular laminae. Type 4 was an S-shaped deviation. Type 5 was a simple horizontal spur with an almost flat septum. Type 6 was a massive unilateral bone spur. Type 7 combined types 2–6 (Fig. 6.3) [3].

Radulesco et al. conducted a very interesting study recently by using 3D segmentation models extracted from CT scans and geometric morphometrics [4]. After detailed analysis, they classified the septal deviation as C-shaped and S-shaped, as by Lawson in 1978 [1].

Many other classifications have been published in the literature with some modifications of the above-mentioned studies. I designed my own classification system for describing pathologies in the nasal cavity. I have been using SL

© The Author(s), under exclusive license to Springer Nature Switzerland AG 2025

F. Apaydın, *Septal Surgery Challenges in Rhinoplasty*,
https://doi.org/10.1007/978-3-031-74734-2_6

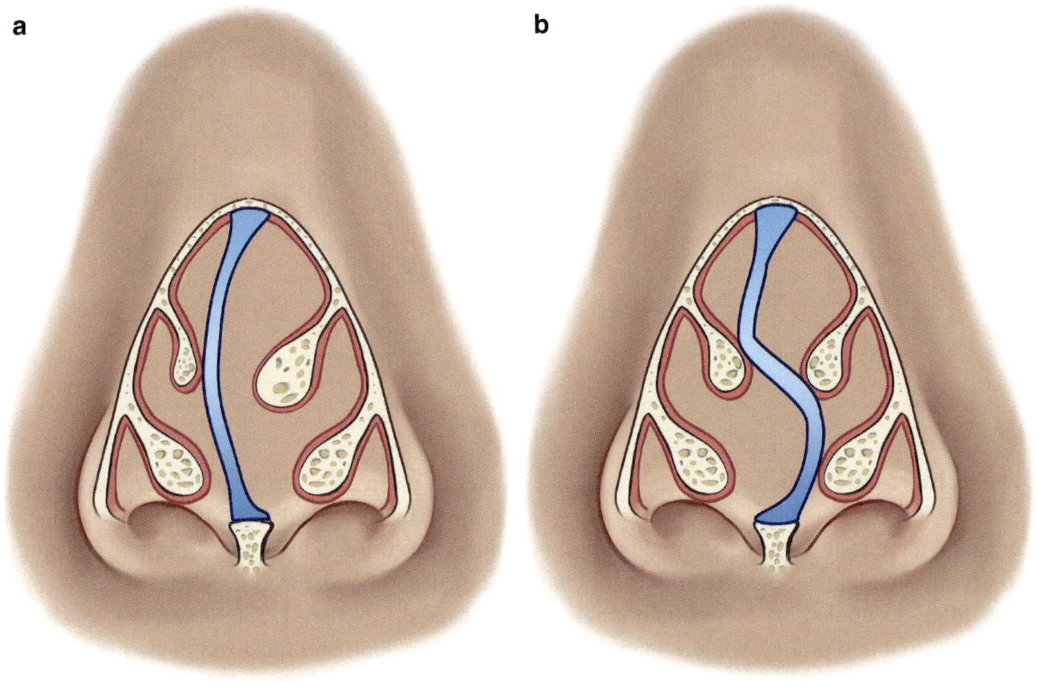

Fig. 6.1 The twisted nose is classified as C-shaped and S-shaped according to Lawson

classification for more than 20 years and published it in 2013 [5, 6]. It was developed by using the Cottle classification of nasal septum [7] (Fig. 6.4), diagnostic endoscopy of the nose [8], TNM cancer staging [9], and the Gunter sheet for rhinoplasty [10].

The SL system has been created with three levels of data recording. The first level was designed for routine usage in outpatient clinics (Table 6.1). In my opinion, it is a very practical way of recording the findings of a nose examination in 10–15 s. In the second level, an advanced form of the Gunter sheet is added (Fig. 6.5). This is for those who would like to show more details of the pathologies on a graphic sheet. The third level is mainly designed for those with an academic interest in their operative records. It is a very detailed questionnaire that covers almost all aspects of the examination of the nose and nasal cavity.

A classification system should be simple to use and serve the important needs of the surgeon. Levels 2 and 3 were not as practical as the first. Therefore, the first level of SL classification has remained my choice throughout the recent two decades. In this classification, the numbers used in the "S" section denote the septal areas described by Cottle. Pathologies on the lateral nasal wall have been abbreviated to facilitate their use in this system (Tables 6.2 and 6.3).

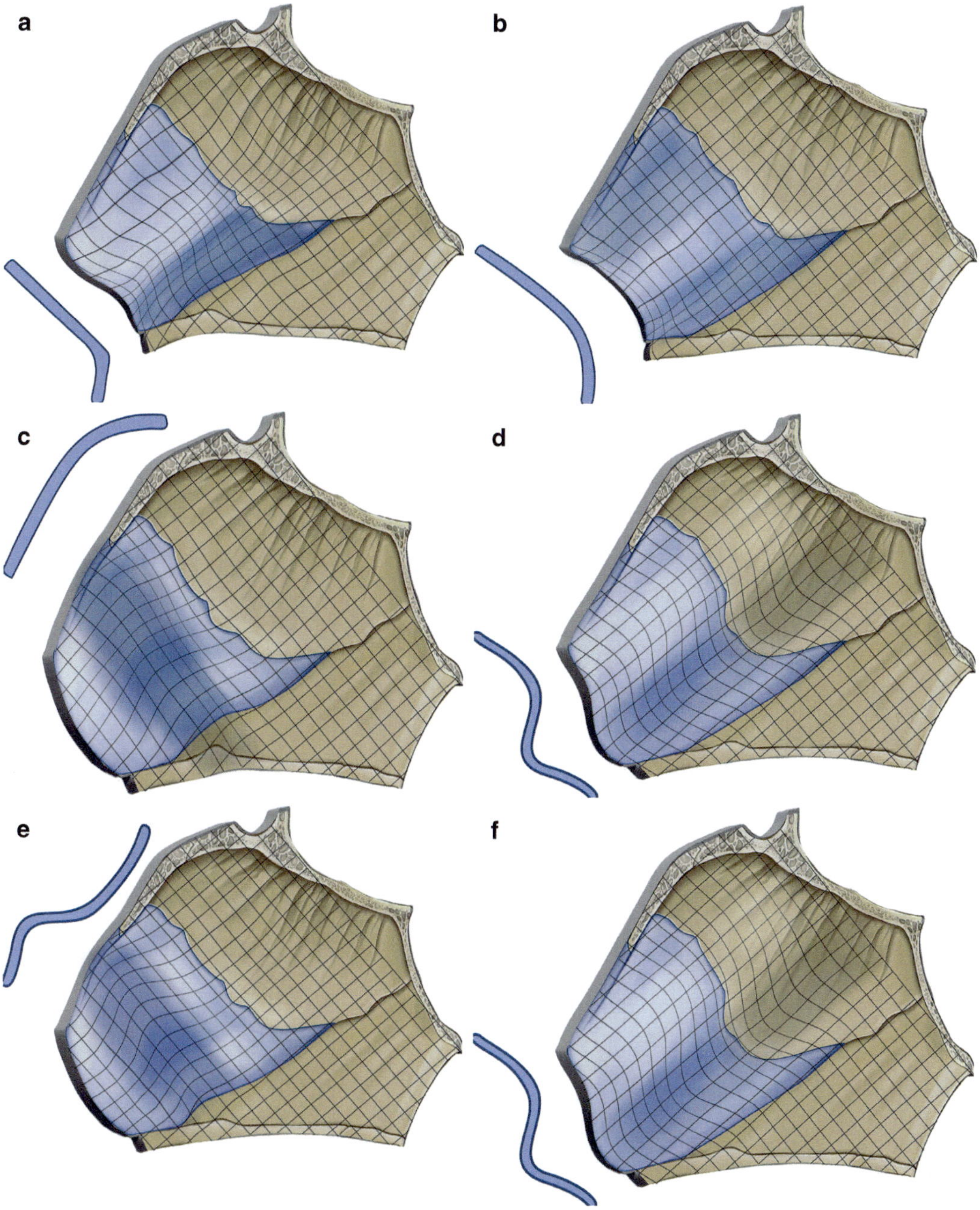

Fig. 6.2 In the Guyuron classification, there are six different types of septal deviation: (**a**) septal tilt, (**b**) C-shaped anteroposterior, (**c**) C-shaped cephalocaudal, (**d**) S-shaped anteroposterior, (**e**) S-shaped cephalocaudal. The sixth type is not shown here

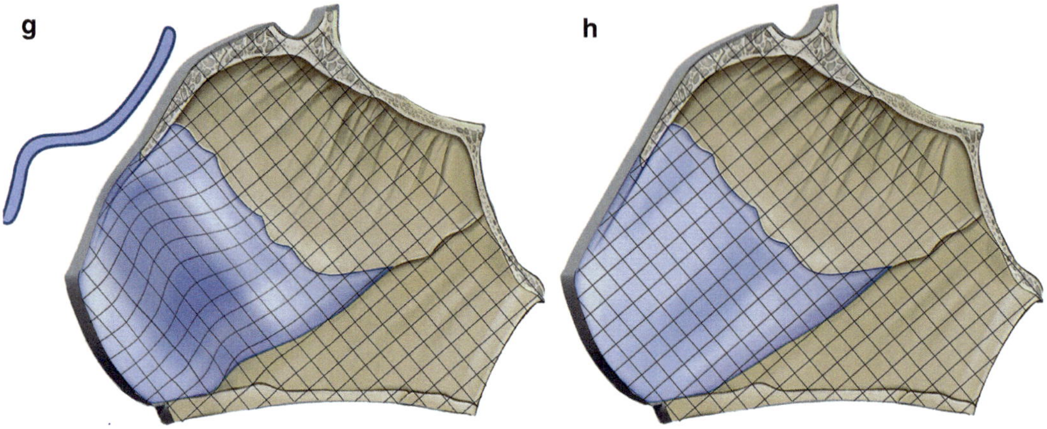

Fig. 6.2 (continued)

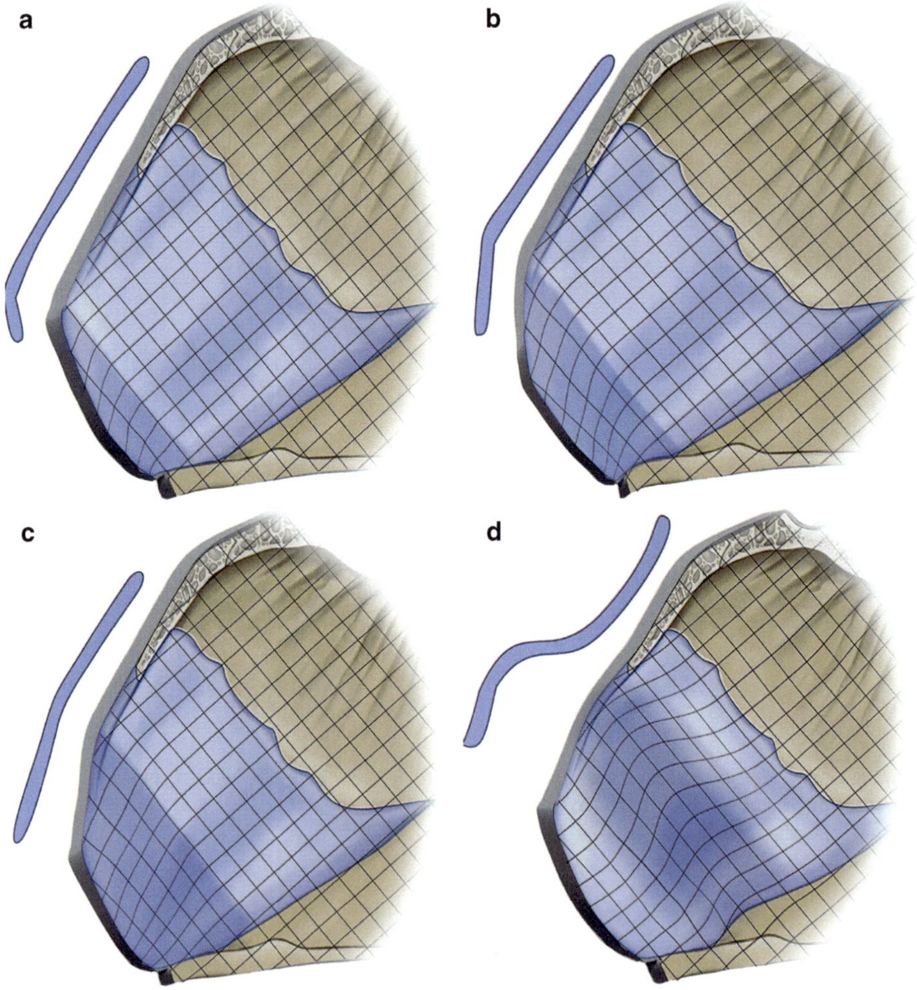

Fig. 6.3 Mladina divided septal pathologies into seven types: (**a**) mild unilateral vertical septal ridge in the valve region, (**b**) more severe form of type 1 that compromises breathing, (**c**) a unilateral vertical ridge at the junction of the quadrangular and perpendicular laminae, (**d**) S-shaped deviation, (**e**) a simple horizontal spur with an almost flat septum, (**f**) massive unilateral bone spur, (**g**) combined types 2 to 6 (which is not shown here)

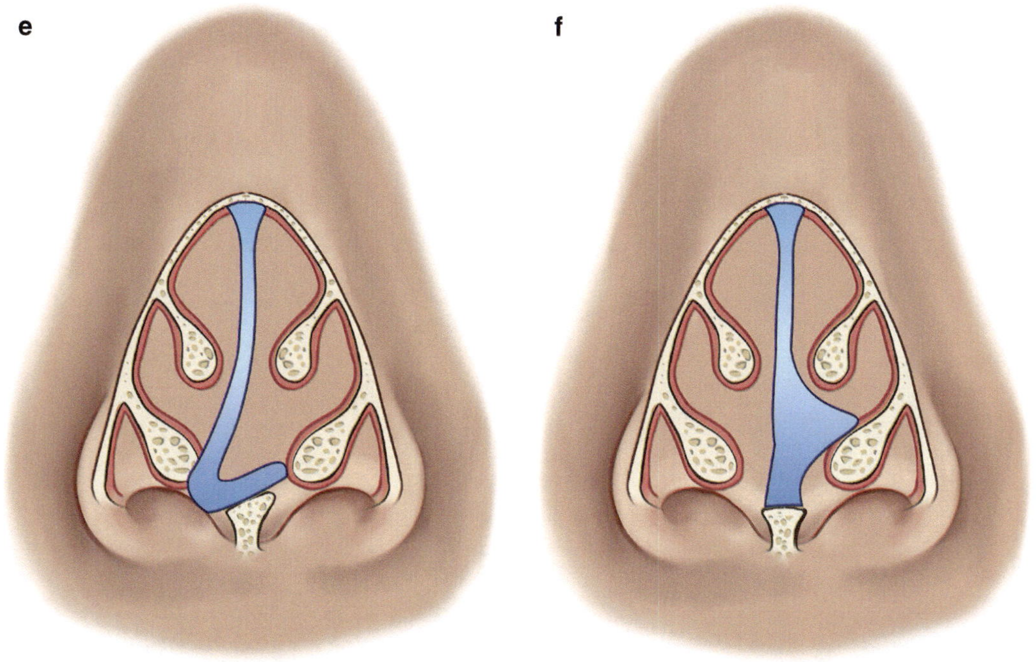

Fig. 6.3 (continued)

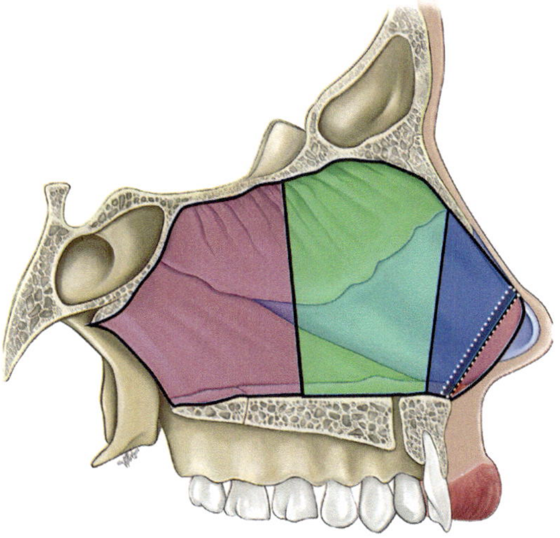

Fig. 6.4 The Cottle areas of the nasal cavity: (1) nostril; (2) nasal valve; (3) attic, the area underneath the bony and cartilaginous vault; (4) anterior aspect of the nasal cavity, including the heads of the turbinates and the infundibulum; (5) the posterior aspect of the nasal cavity, including the tails of the turbinates

Table 6.1 SL classification is used to record the pathologies inside the nose (first level of data recording)

S: Septum nasi
0: No evidence of septal deformity
1: Septal deviation confined to the vestibulum nasi
2: Septal deviation confined to the nasal valve area
3: Septal deviation confined to the attic
4: Septal deviation confined to the anterior turbinate region
5: Septal deviation confined to the posterior turbinate area
X: Minimum requirements to assess septal deviation cannot be met
L: Lateral nasal wall
n: No evidence of pathology confined to the lateral nasal wall
p(s): Polyp (polyposis nasi)
c: Concha bullosa
h: Inferior turbinate hypertrophy
t: Tumor
r: Rhinitis
x: Minimum requirements to assess the septal deviation cannot be met
o: Other_______________

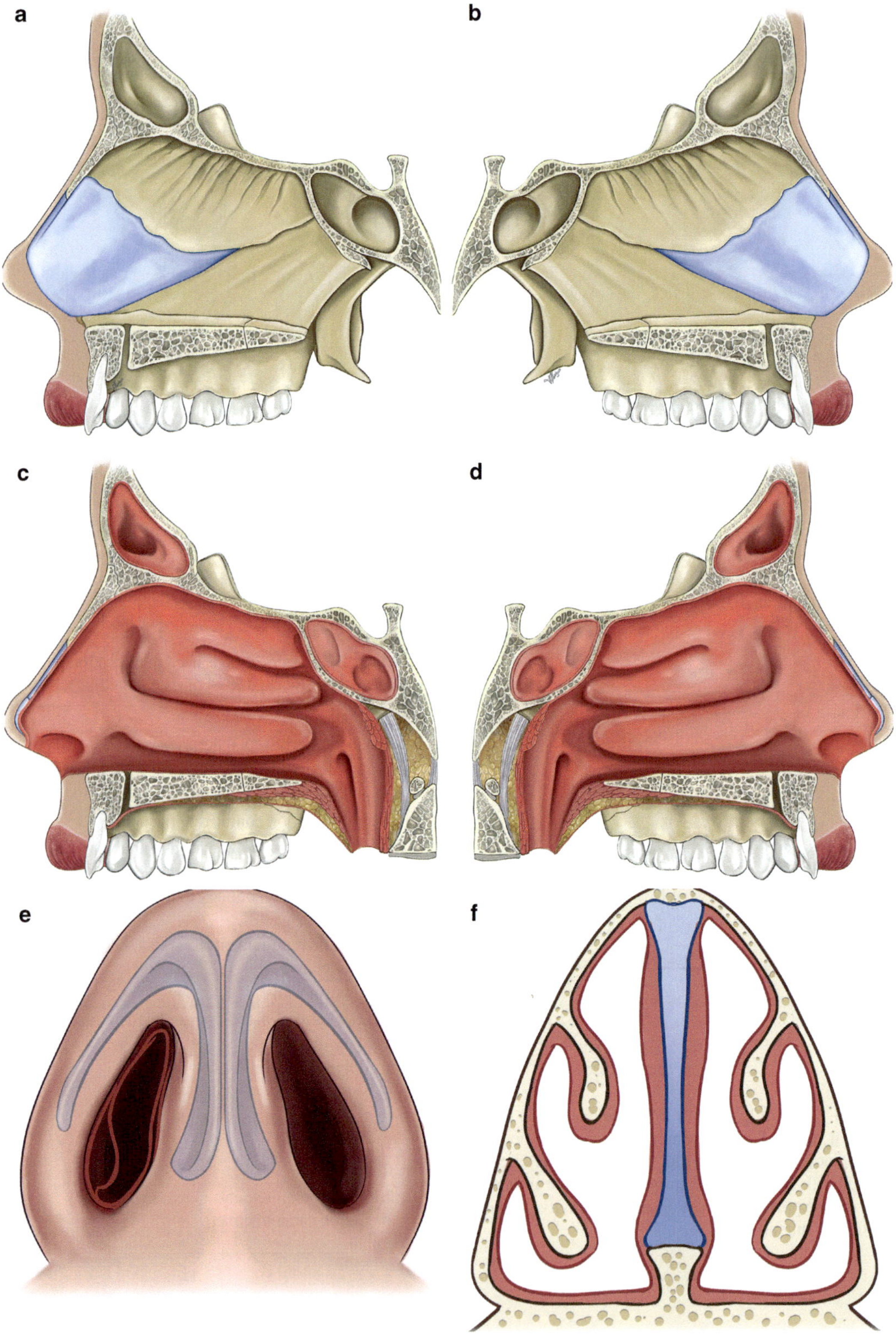

Fig. 6.5 In the second level of SL classification, an advanced form of the Gunter diagram is added to show more details about the pathologies inside the nose on a graphic sheet

g

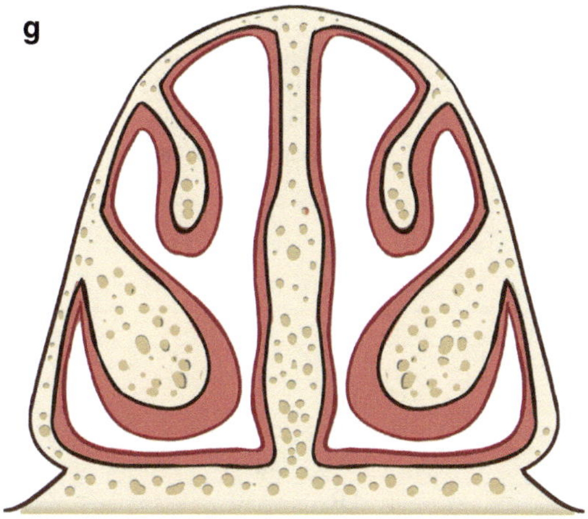

Fig. 6.5 (continued)

Table 6.2 Examples of the use of SL classification (first level of data recording)

SL classification	Explanation
$S_{2,3}L_{n(R)} + S_1L_{h(L)}$	Septal deviation confined to the nasal valve region and attic; no pathology confined to the lateral wall on the right side. Septal deviation confined to the vestibulum nasi and hypertrophy of the inferior turbinate on the left side
$S_{1-3}\ L_{n(R)} + S_0L_{ps(L)}$	Septal deviation confined to the vestibulum nasi, nasal valve area, and anterior turbinate area on the right side. No septal pathology, but polyposis nasi on the left side

Note: When more than one area is involved and if these are consecutive areas, a hyphen is placed between the lowest and the highest number. If different areas are involved, they are separated by commas
L left nasal passage, *R* right nasal passage

Table 6.3 The detailed questionnaire used in the third level of recording in addition to SL-classification and the schematic drawing

1. Dynamic nasal examination	2. Tip ptosis upon animation	3. Tip recoil
[ ] Internal valve collapse	[ ] None	[ ] Normal
[ ] External valve collapse	[ ] Minimal	[ ] Weak
	[ ] Moderate	[ ] Strong
	[ ] Severe	
4. Internal valve changes		
Mucocutaneous	Septal	Upper lateral cartilages
[ ] Normal	[ ] Absent	[ ] Absent
[ ] Swollen	[ ] Thickened	[ ] Thickened
[ ] Adhesion	[ ] Deflected	[ ] Deflected
[ ] Stricture	[ ] Twisted	[ ] Twisted
5. Septal deviation site (Cottle classification)		
1 (Vestibulum nasi)	[ ] R	[ ] L
2 (Nasal valve)	[ ] R	[ ] L
3 (Attic)	[ ] R	[ ] L
4 (Anterior turbinate area)	[ ] R	[ ] L
5 (Posterior turbinate area)	[ ] R	[ ] L
6. Septal deviation type	7. Caudal deflection type	

(continued)

Table 6.3 (continued)

[ ] Simple septal deviation (tilt)	[ ] Isolated caudal deflection (subluxation)	
[ ] Spur formation	[ ] C-shaped deformity	
[ ] Subluxation	[ ] S-shaped deformity	
[ ] Tension septum (overprojected nose)		
[ ] Caudal border fracture		
[ ] Septal crushes		
[ ] Saddling		
[ ] Other		
8. Other intranasal findings		
Nasal polyp	[ ] R	[ ] L
Nasal polyposis	[ ] R	[ ] L
Septal perforation (size)	___ ___ cm	
Epistaxis	[ ] R	[ ] L
Mucopus	[ ] R	[ ] L
Scarring	[ ] R	[ ] L
Dryness	[ ] R	[ ] L
Inferior turbinate hypertrophy	[ ] R	[ ] L
Concha bullosa	[ ] R	[ ] L
Adenoid hypertrophy	[ ]	
Mucosa color	[ ] Normal [ ] Pale [ ] Red [ ] Bluish	
Ulceration	[ ] R	[ ] L
Crusting	[ ] R	[ ] L
Other ______________	[ ] R	[ ] L
9. Estimated degree of nasal airway obstruction	R ____% (VAS)	L ____% (VAS)

References

1. Lawson VG. Management of the twisted nose. J Otolaryngol. 1978;7:56–66.
2. Guyuron B, Uzzo CD, Scull H. A practical classification of septonasal deviation and an effective guide to septal surgery. Plast Reconstr Surg. 1999;104:2202–9.
3. Subarić M, Mladina R. Nasal septum deformities in children and adolescents: a cross sectional study of children from Zagreb, Croatia. Int J Pediatr Otorhinolaryngol. 2002;63:41–8.
4. Radulesco T, Hazbri D, Dessi P, Adalian P, Michel J. Geometric morphometric contribution to septal deviation analysis. Surg Radiol Anat. 2019;41:823–31.
5. Apaydin F, Akyildiz S, Hecht DA, Toriumi DM. Rhinobase: a comprehensive database, facial analysis, and picture-archiving software for rhinoplasty. Arch Facial Plast Surg. 2009;11(3):209–11.
6. Apaydın F. A new documentation standard in the nose examination: SL classification. Facial Plast Surg. 2013;29:449–54.
7. Beeson WH. Septal surgery. In: Daniel RK, editor. Rhinoplasty. Boston: Little-Brown and Company; 1993. p. 595–611.
8. Stammberger H. Nasal and paranasal sinus endoscopy. A diagnostic and surgical approach to recurrent sinusitis. Endoscopy. 1986;18:213–8.
9. Weymuller AE. Head and neck cancer staging. In: Cummings CW, editor. Otolaryngology head & neck surgery. St. Louis: Mosby-Year Book; 1998. p. 136–44.
10. Gunter JP. A graphic record of intraoperative maneuvers in rhinoplasty: the missing link for evaluating rhinoplasty results. Plast Reconstr Surg. 1989;84:204–12.

Incisions and Approaches for Septal Surgery

7

7.1 Introduction

The surgeon can access the nasal septum in many ways during rhinoplasty. There are mainly two surgical approaches in rhinoplasty: endonasal and external. The incisions can be classified as alar cartilage, septal, and transcolumellar.

7.2 Approaches

7.2.1 Endonasal

The traditional classification includes nondelivery and delivery approaches. However, the nasal septum can also be approached endonasally, which will be detailed in the incision section. The focus of this book is on the nasal septum, and these two approaches are mainly for the nasal dorsum and tip.

7.2.2 External

It is the most comfortable way to reach the nasal tip, dorsum, and nasal septum. Transcolumellar and marginal incisions are performed for this approach. In my opinion, this is the best approach for operating on difficult, traumatic, and crooked noses. First, it gives the surgeon the opportunity to identify the underlying problems that can be difficult using endonasal approaches. Second, it gives me the chance to solve problems under direct vision and without any distortion in a wider field of work. In addition, it provides a great opportunity to teach residents, fellows, and colleagues. This is the best approach for recording using photography and/or videography. However, there are some disadvantages to this approach. It creates a scar on the columella. In my own experience, this scar is difficult to see and is well tolerated by patients. Some surgeons find this approach more aggressive and claim that a wider region of dissection can result in a scar. Having analyzed the scar in many cases, I can easily say that if properly closed, the scar is inconspicuous in nearly all the cases.

7.3 Incisions

7.3.1 Alar Cartilage Incisions

7.3.1.1 Intercartilaginous

This is performed between the caudal portion of the upper lateral cartilage and the cephalic margin of the lateral crus [1]. The incision should be placed 2–3 mm lateral to the caudal margin of the upper lateral cartilage in order not to create a scar at the internal valve area. I prefer this incision to

Supplementary Information The online version contains supplementary material available at https://doi.org/10.1007/978-3-031-74734-2_7. The videos can be accessed individually by clicking the DOI link in the accompanying figure caption or by scanning this link with the SN More Media App.

© The Author(s), under exclusive license to Springer Nature Switzerland AG 2025

F. Apaydın, *Septal Surgery Challenges in Rhinoplasty*,
https://doi.org/10.1007/978-3-031-74734-2_7

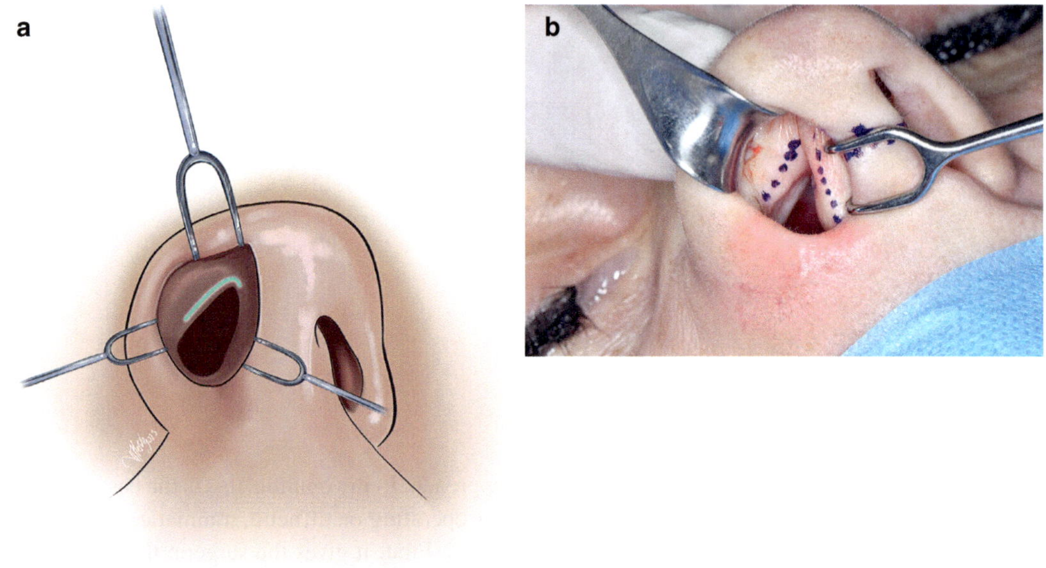

Fig. 7.1 An intercartilaginous incision is made between the caudal portion of the upper lateral cartilage and the cephalic margin of the lateral crus (**a**, **b**)

reach the nasal dorsum directly. I also like to combine it with the hemitransfixion or partial hemitransfixion incision to reach the nasal septum (Fig. 7.1a, b).

7.3.1.2 Transcartilaginous (Intracartilaginous, Cartilage Splitting) [1, 2]

The incision is placed 4–5 mm lateral to the caudal margin of the upper lateral cartilage. Cephalic trimming of the lateral crus can be performed simultaneously with the incision. However, I prefer to make the incision on the mucosa first, skeletonize the lateral crus, and then trim it. I have found that I have more control over the amount of resection with this method (Figs. 7.2a, b, and 7.3).

7.3.1.3 Marginal

This incision follows the caudal border of the lower lateral cartilages [1, 2]. It has become extremely popular in recent years, providing a full approach to the nasal tip and even to the nasal dorsum (Fig. 7.4a, b). However, it is more limited when approaching the nasal septum. Therefore, it is usually combined with a transcolumellar or hemitransfixion incision to reach the nasal septum.

7.3.2 Septal Incisions

7.3.2.1 Killian

It was published by Gustave Killian in 1905 [3]. Originally, it starts about half a centimeter back of the caudal edge of the septum from below and courses obliquely to the caudal septum, where the upper end is 1 cm or more distant from the anterior septal angle. This was the incision I first learned in 1988 as a resident, and it was the only incision for septal surgery that I performed until 1993. In this incision, the caudal septum is preserved and bypassed (Fig. 7.5).

This is a good incision if the caudal septum is straight and its relationship with the columella is good. It has two drawbacks: the deflections of the caudal septum cannot be addressed, and the mucociliary clearance is violated and can stop at this point when the mucosa is violated. I use this incision very rarely.

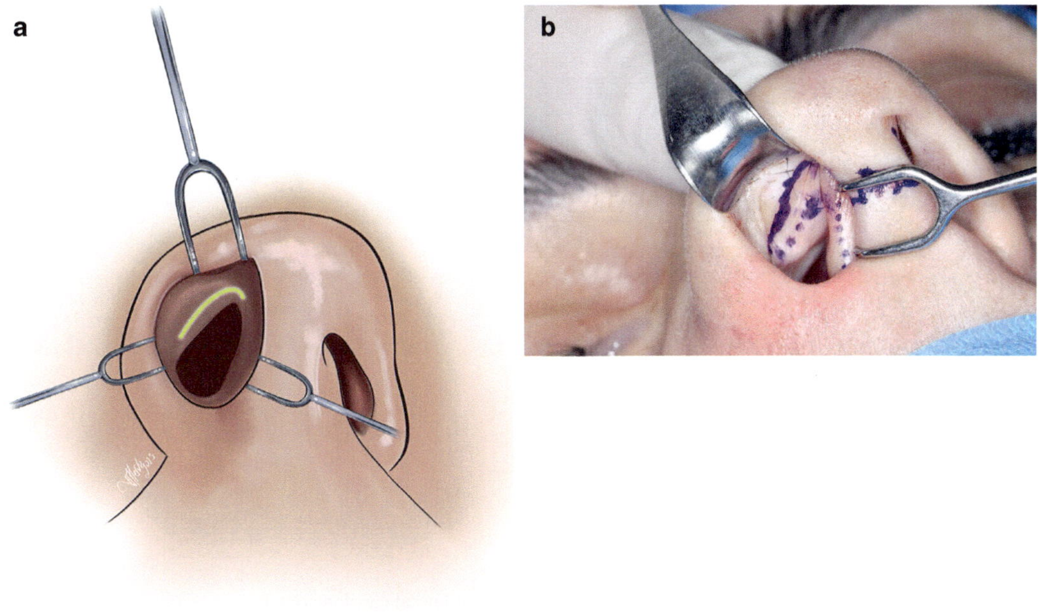

Fig. 7.2 A transcartilaginous incision is placed 4–5 mm lateral to the caudal margin of the upper lateral cartilage (**a**, **b**)

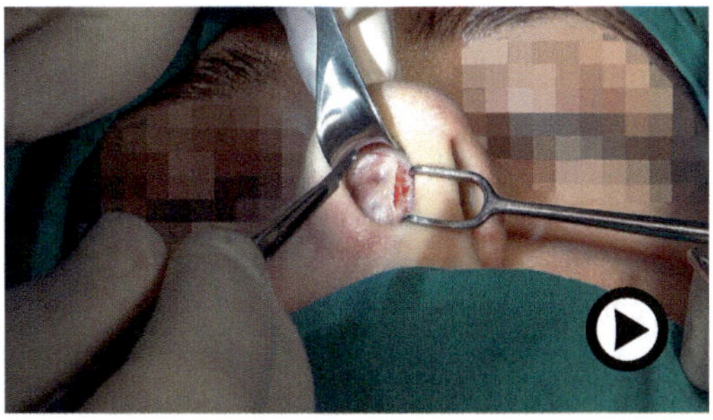

Fig. 7.3 Transcartilaginous incision (▶ https://doi.org/10.1007/000-dya)

7.3.2.2 Hemitransfixion Incision

This is performed on the skin overlying the caudal end of the cartilaginous septum (Fig. 7.6a–c) [4]. It should start 2 mm behind the caudal end below and remain parallel to the caudal septum. This is the best incision for accessing the entire septum starting from the caudal portion. I use a wide double-prong hook with sharp ends to expose the caudal septum and pull the skin to the caudal edge, along with an alar retractor to widen the exposure (Fig. 7.7). In my experience, it has two drawbacks: (1) the straight caudal septum can accidentally be violated during surgery; (2) the strong junction of the caudal septum with the anterior nasal spine can also be accidentally destroyed.

7.3.2.3 Complete Transfixion

It is used to separate the caudal end of the septum from the membranous columella and medial crura [1, 2]. It is mainly used to decrease tip projection and shorten the nose (Fig. 7.8). It is not specifically designed for septal surgery.

7.3.2.4 Partial Transfixion

It courses around the anterior septal angle but not beyond the medial crural attachments to the caudal septum (Fig. 7.9). The tip support mechanisms are preserved. I like using this incision when I want to reach the nasal dorsum, either subperichondrially or supraperichondrially. It is relatively easy to rasp a bony hump, resect dorsal humps, and insert spreader grafts. However, its use is limited for correcting septal deviations, except for deviations of the dorsal segment. Spreader grafts can be easily inserted through this incision.

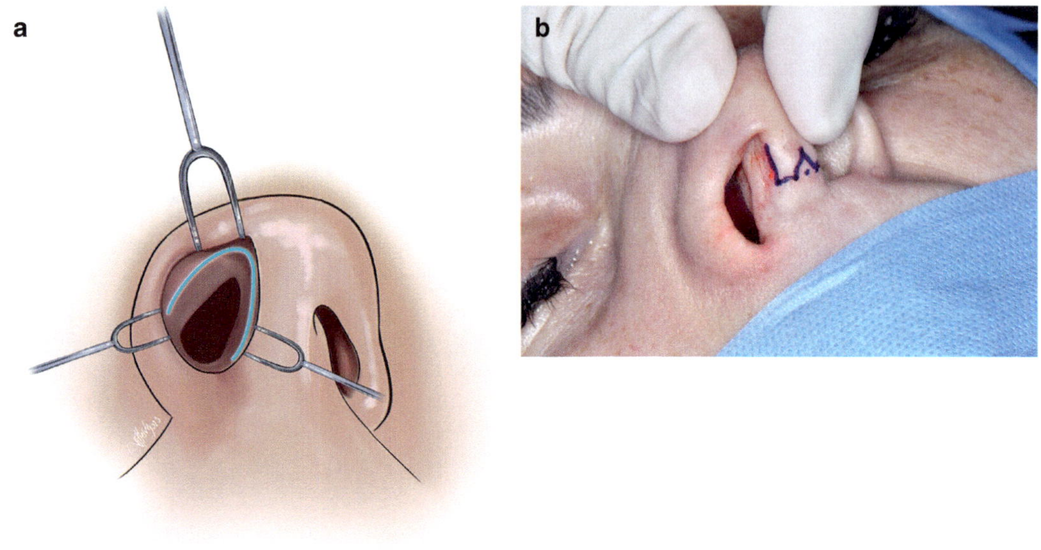

Fig. 7.4 Marginal incision follows the caudal border of the lower lateral cartilages (**a**, **b**)

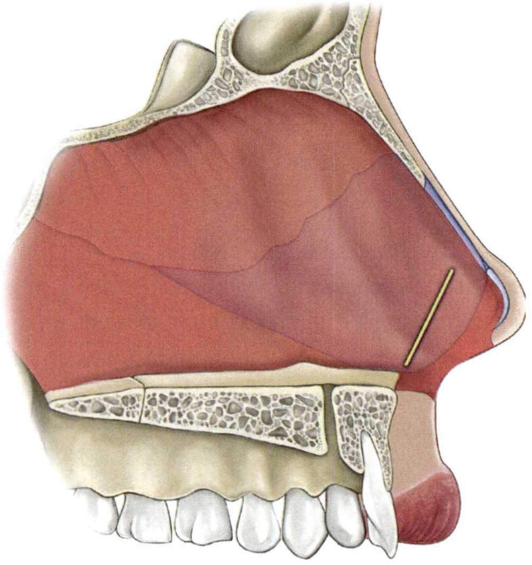

Fig. 7.5 Killian incision starts 5 mm back from the caudal edge of the septum from below and courses obliquely to the caudal septum, where the upper end is 1 cm from the anterior septal angle

7.3.2.5 Over the Spur

When there is a very severe spur, especially at the bony septum, an incision directly on the mucosa overlying the spine can be helpful to get direct access to the deviated portion without touching the anterior part of the nasal septum (Fig. 7.10) [5]. It can be criticized for making an incision on the mucosa, which can hinder mucociliary clearance. However, in most cases, the mucoperichondrium is lacerated during exposure of this area because the mucosa overlying the sharpest part of the spur is very thin and tightly adheres to the septum. Therefore, although it does not look like a physiological incision, its use can be justified and can be used in selected cases where there is only a deviation at the posterior part of the nasal septum without disturbing the anterior part. An endoscope can be used to enhance the visualization of the surgeon and work with greater precision.

7.3.3 Transcolumellar Incisions

These incisions can be classified as midcolumellar and lower columellar incisions.

7.3.3.1 Midcolumellar Inverted-V Incision

This is the most popular incision among all transcolumellar incisions. It is also my preferred incision for external rhinoplasty. It is suggested to use it at the narrowest part of the columella to keep the incision and scar as small as possible

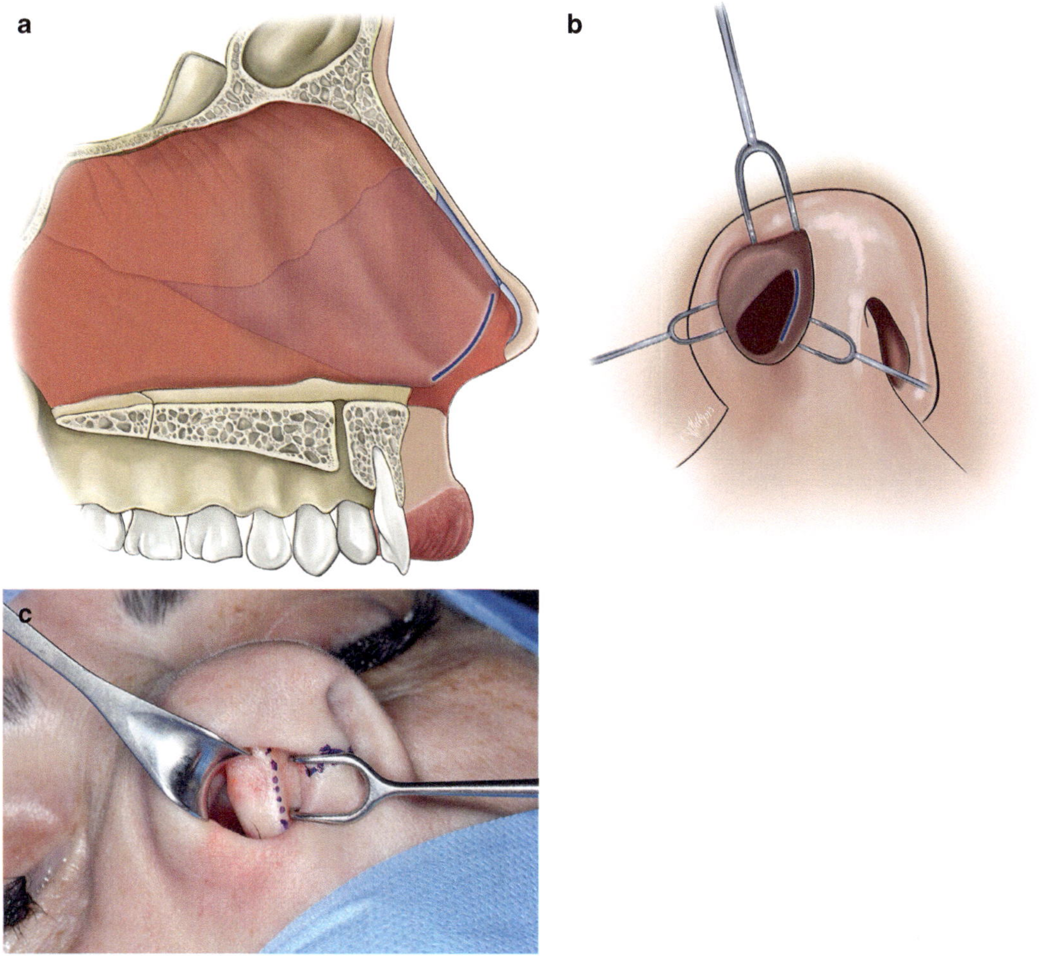

Fig. 7.6 Hemitransfixion incision starts 2 mm behind and parallel to the caudal margin of the caudal septum (**a**–**c**)

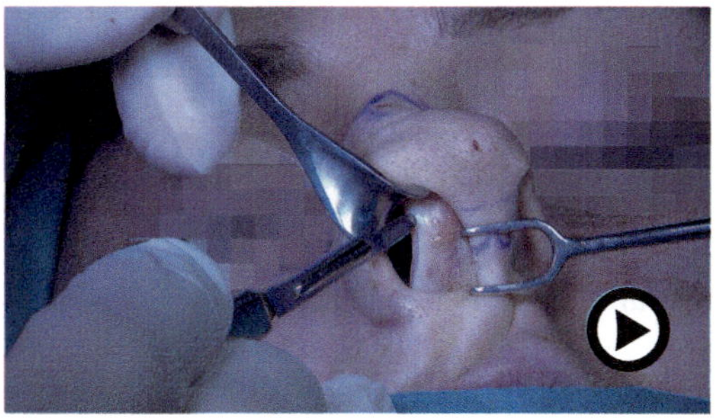

Fig. 7.7 Hemitransfixion incision (▶ https://doi.org/10.1007/000-dy8)

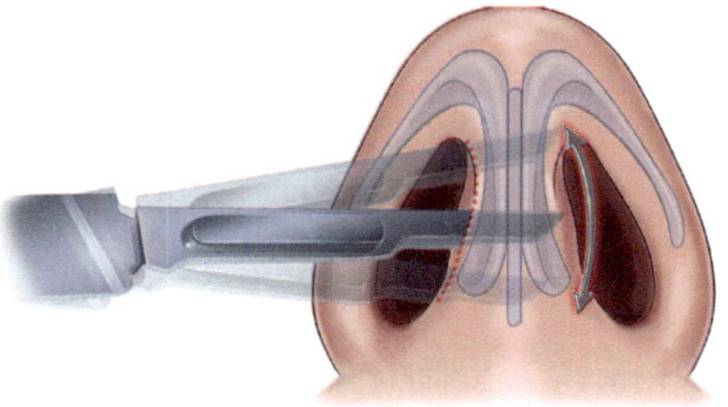

Fig. 7.8 Complete transfixion incision separates the caudal end of the septum from the membranous columella and medial crura. It can be used to deproject the tip

[6]. Although this is the usual trend, I prefer placing the incision at a lower position, at the level where the footplates start flaring (Figs. 7.11 and 7.12). By doing so, I aim to reduce the chance of visibility, especially from the frontal view. One of the major complaints of rhinoplasty patients I

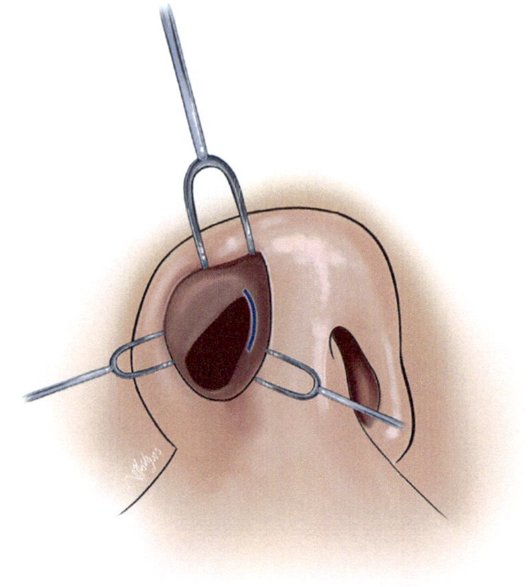

Fig. 7.9 Partial transfixion courses around the anterior septal angle but not beyond the medial crural attachments to the caudal septum

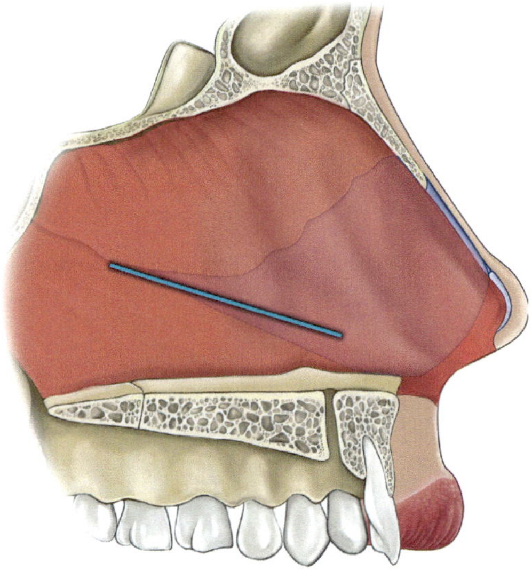

Fig. 7.10 Over-the-spur incision is used when there is a severe spur located at the rear part of the nasal septum. The incision goes through the peak of the spur

operate on is a droopy tip. When the tip is rotated and if the incision is closer to the infratip lobule, it becomes visible from the frontal view. The idea of placing the incision at a lower level is to eliminate this problem. This incision is usually combined with a marginal incision.

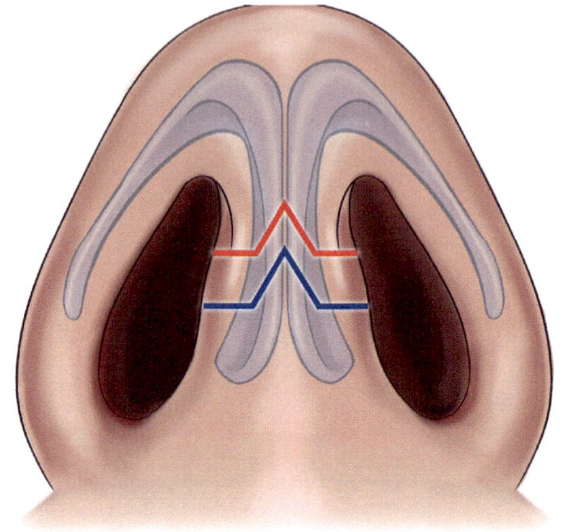

Fig. 7.11 A midcolumellar inverted-V incision is traditionally placed at the narrowest part of the columella (red line). In my opinion, it should be at the point where the footplates start flaring (blue line). The main reason is to prevent visibility of the incision if the tip is rotated upward

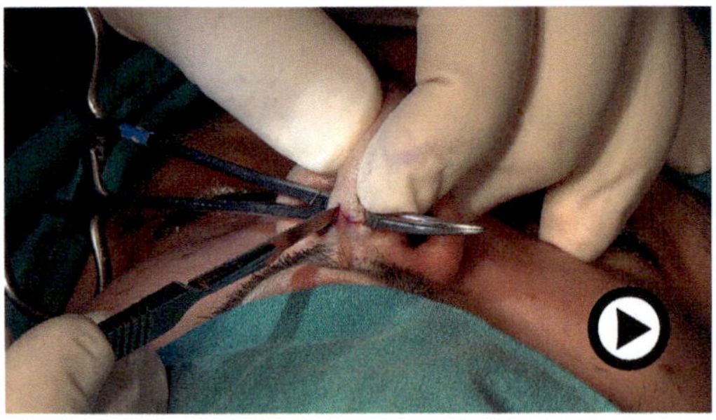

Fig. 7.12 Midcolumellar inverted-V incision (▶ https://doi.org/10.1007/000-dy9)

I have been using the six-dot technique for a long time to mark the incision lines (Figs. 7.13 and 7.14). The first two dots are marked at the lateral points of the columella where the footplates start flaring. The third dot is placed in the midline between these dots. The fourth dot is placed 2–3 mm above the midline dot. The fifth and sixth dots are marked between the middle dot and the lateral dots. Then, an inverted-V is drawn between these dots using a pen with a thin tip. The marginal incision line is drawn 2 mm away from the columellar margin (Fig. 7.15a–n). When

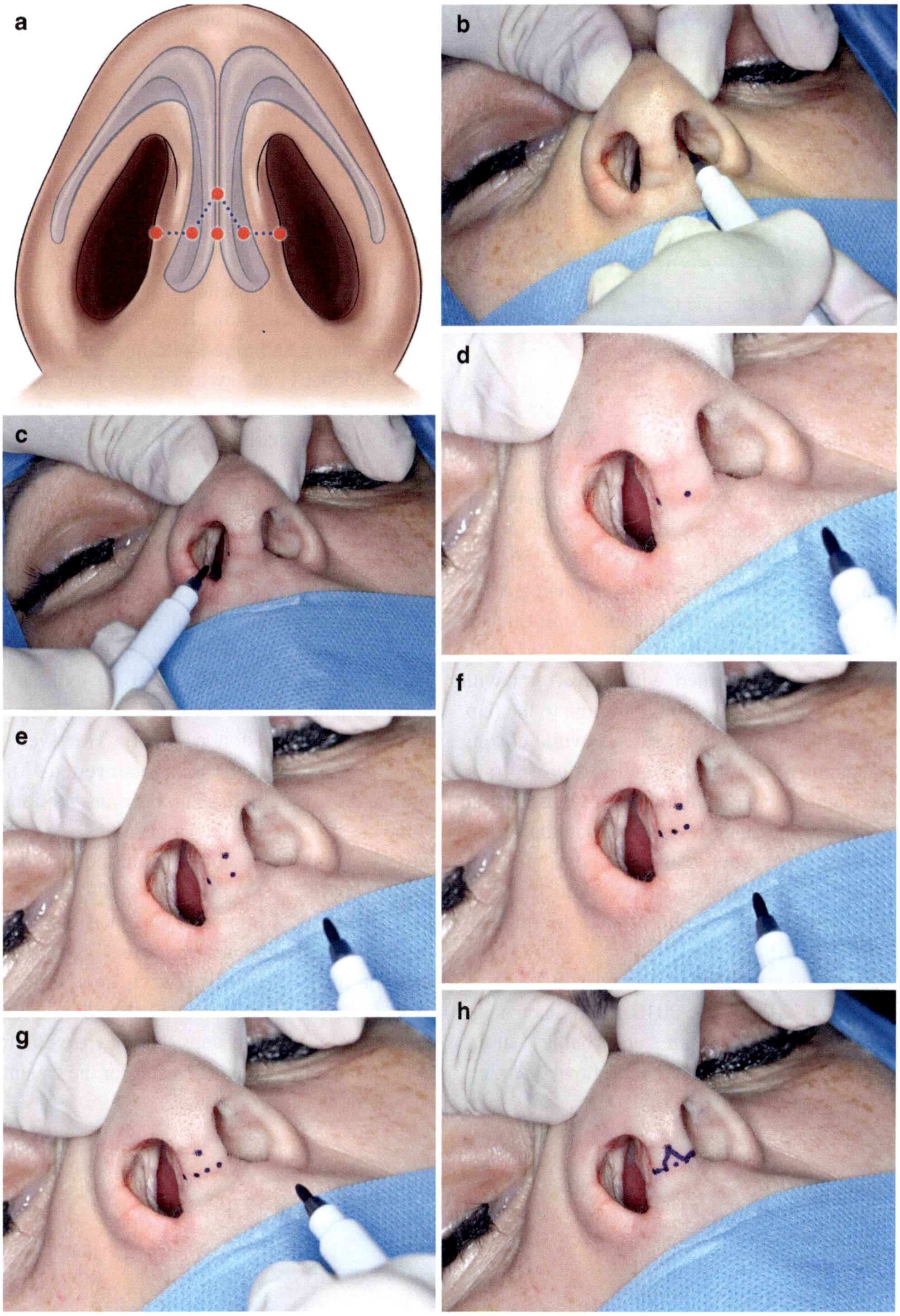

Fig. 7.13 Six-dot technique for midcolumellar inverted-V incision. The first two dots are marked on the lateral points of the columella where the footplates start flaring. The third dot is placed in the midline between these dots. The fourth dot is placed 2–3 mm above the midline dot. The fifth and sixth dots are marked between the middle dot and the lateral dots. Then, an inverted-V is drawn between these dots using a pen with a thin tip. The marginal incision line is drawn 2 mm away from the columellar margin (**a**–**h**)

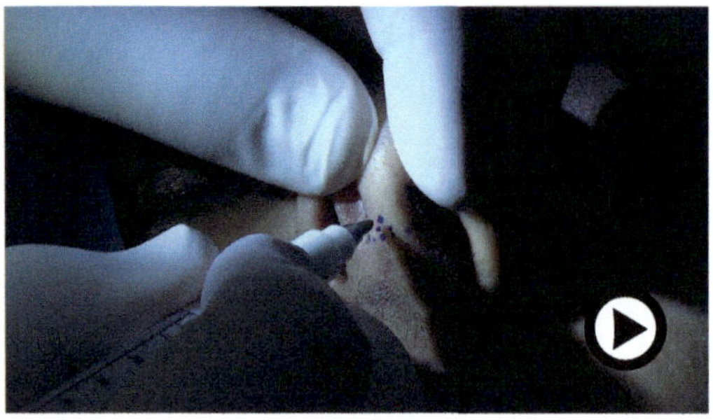

Fig. 7.14 Six dot technique for marking the inverted-V midcolumellar incision (▶ https://doi.org/10.1007/000-dy7)

the columella is short, the dots are designed for a W-incision (Fig. 7.16).

What are the prerequisites for an inconspicuous scar? First, I use curved sharp scissors to cut perpendicularly and elevate the flap above the medial crura. Second, I try to avoid raising a thin flap, i.e., the columellar flap should be as thick as possible. Third, the handling and elevation of the flap should be performed with hooks, not with forceps, which can cause more trauma to the flap. Fourth, I like to have a flat surface while closing the incision; therefore, I usually suture a long, curved, and strong columellar strut whose caudal margin is at the same level as the medial crura. Fifth, I use five corner mattress stitches to obtain eversion of the wound edges and add six more simple sutures between and around the mattress sutures (Fig. 7.17).

As the suture material, I used 6-0 Prolene® from 1999 to 2010. Since 2010, I have been using 6-0 Vicryl Rapid®, an absorbable suture (Fig. 7.18). Some of my patients showed anxiety about suture removal, and one of them ran away because of her fear.

7.3.3.2 Stairstep Incision

The stairstep incision is in the shape of a stair that starts at the narrowest part of the columella and ends at the upper part of the crural footplate [7]. This was the most popular incision among plastic surgeons 20 years ago. I used this incision only in three revision cases where the first surgeon had performed the incision. It would not be fair to comment on a technique with my limited experience. At least I can say that it was more difficult to reach the anterior nasal spine and footplates of the medial crura compared to the inverted-V incision (Fig. 7.19a, b).

7.3.3.3 "V" Incision

This incision is placed at the lower end of the columella where the columella joins the lip [1]. The main rationale behind this incision is the chance to bury the incision scar in the lower margin of the columella (Fig. 7.20). It looks like a good idea, and I know a few prominent surgeons who use this incision routinely. However, the incision is much longer than the inverted-V incision, and the columellar flap becomes too long in some cases. I use the "V" incision as a V-to-Y in cases of short columella if I want to lengthen the columella (Fig. 7.17) [8].

The choice of approach and incisions mainly depends on the surgeon's choice and expertise. The days of heavy debates between approaches are over. In my opinion, surgeons should choose the best approach and incisions that they are comfortable with to obtain the best result for the patient.

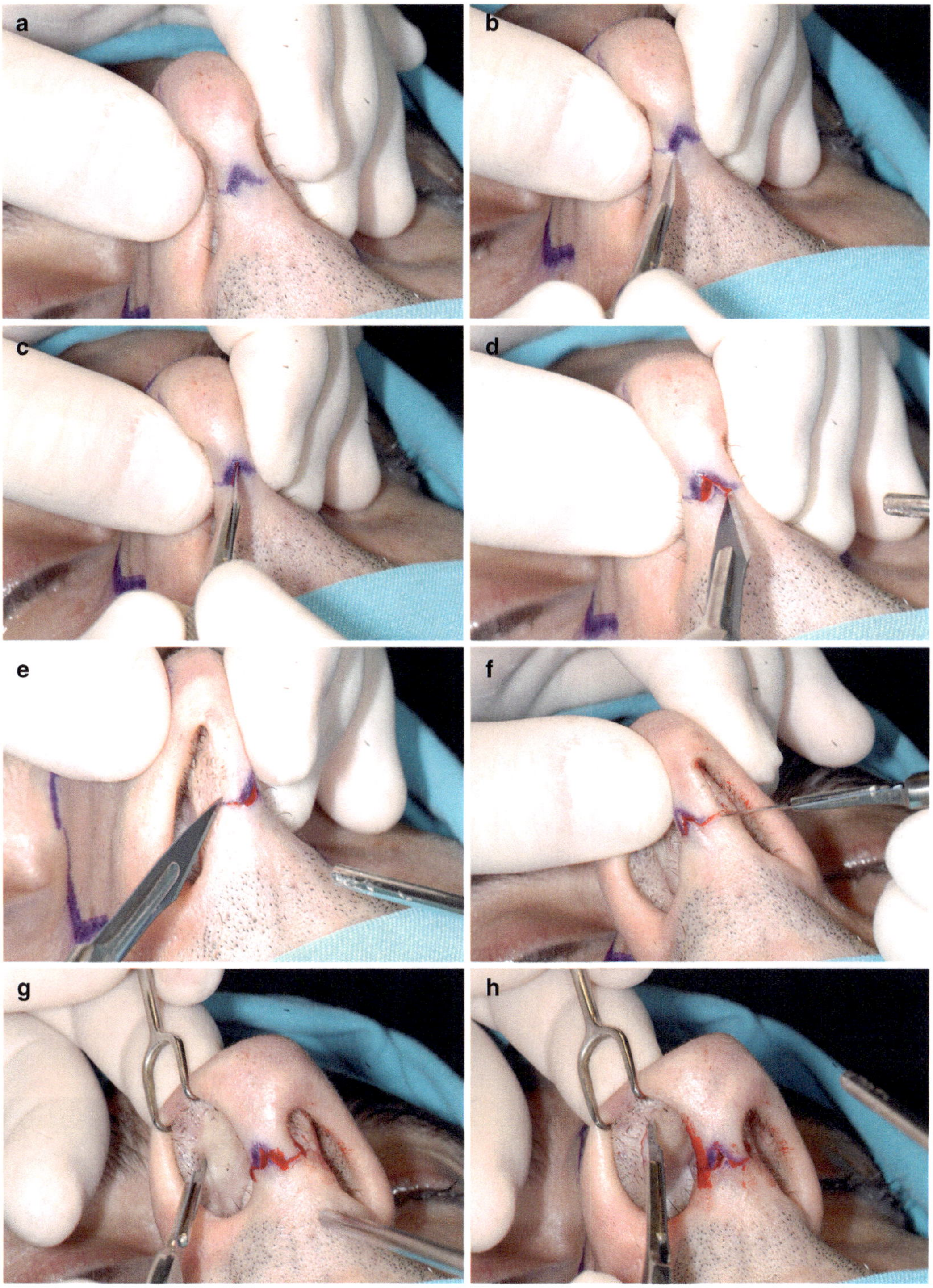

Fig. 7.15 The tip of the nose and the columella should be fixed with the thumb, index finger, and third finger. A #11 blade is used perpendicular to the skin for the midcolumellar incision. The incision starts deep in the midline and continues superficially laterally. The lateral cut of the marginal incision is performed to combine with the medial cut. The columellar flap is elevated, exposing the medial crura. The smooth surface under the columellar flap is obtained by using a long, curved, and strong columellar strut whose caudal margin is at the same level as the medial crura (**a**–**n**)

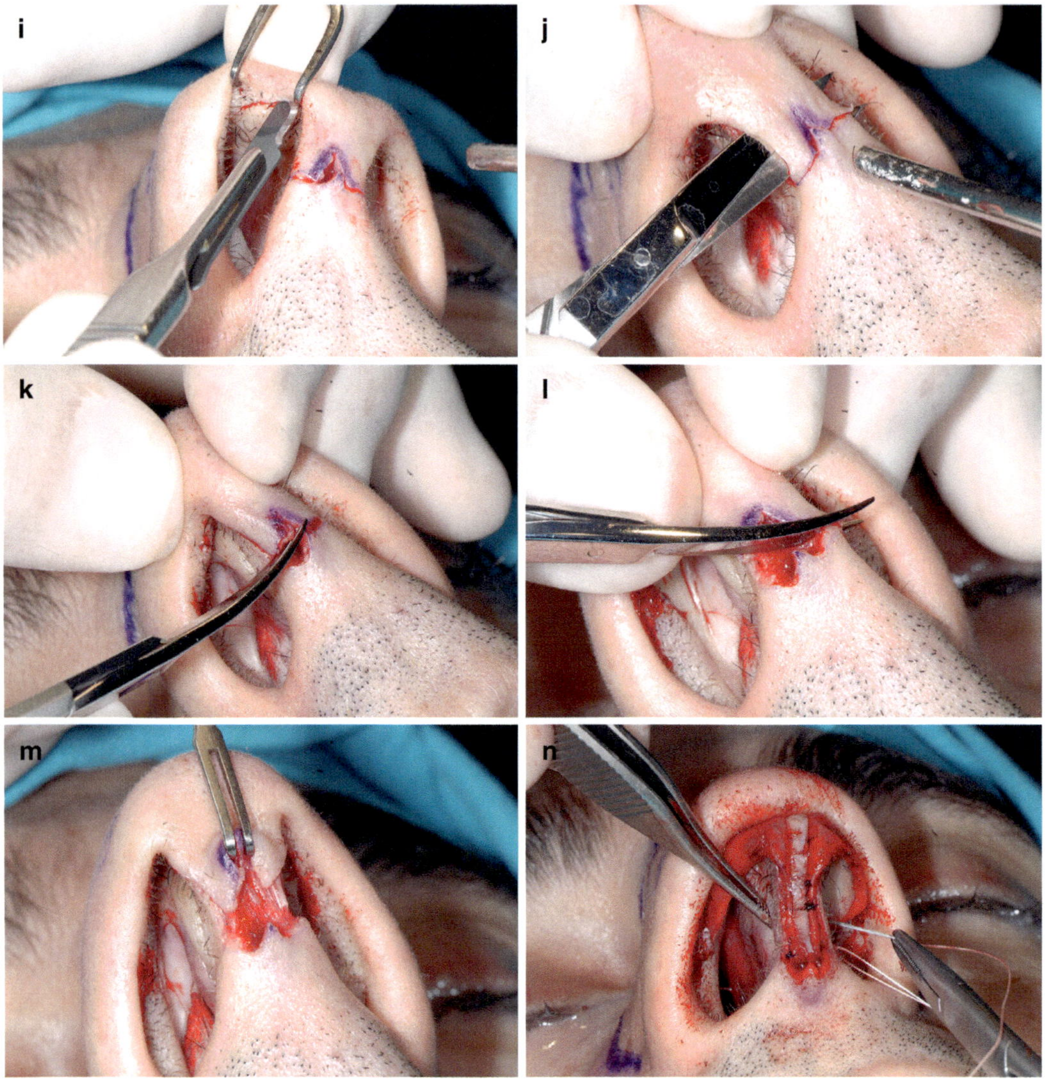

Fig. 7.15 (continued)

Fig. 7.16 W-incision as a columellar incision
(▶ https://doi.org/10.1007/000-dyb)

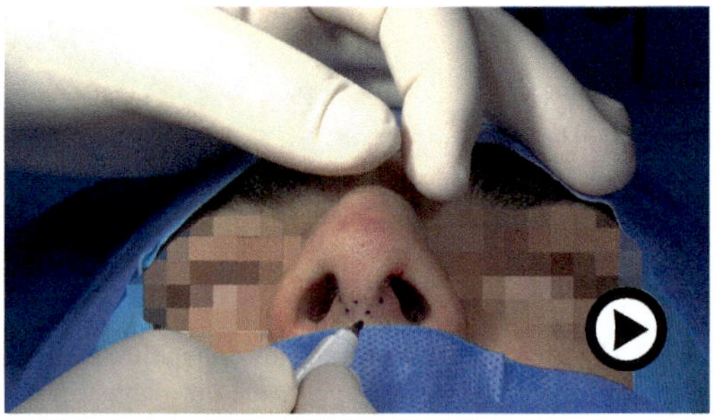

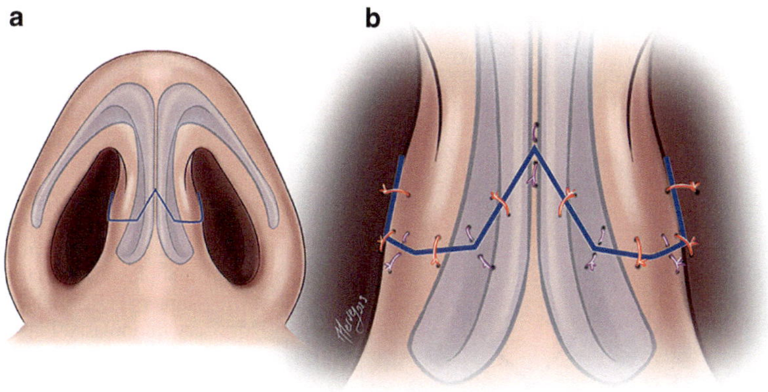

Fig. 7.17 Suturing the columellar flap should be a meticulous job to obtain an inconspicuous scar. I like using five corner mattress stitches to obtain eversion of the wound edges and adding six more simple sutures between and around the mattress sutures (**a**, **b**)

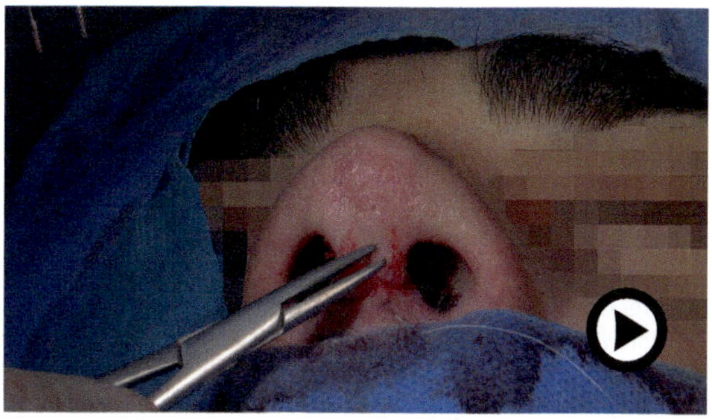

Fig. 7.18 Closure of midcolumellar incision (▶ https://doi.org/10.1007/000-dyc)

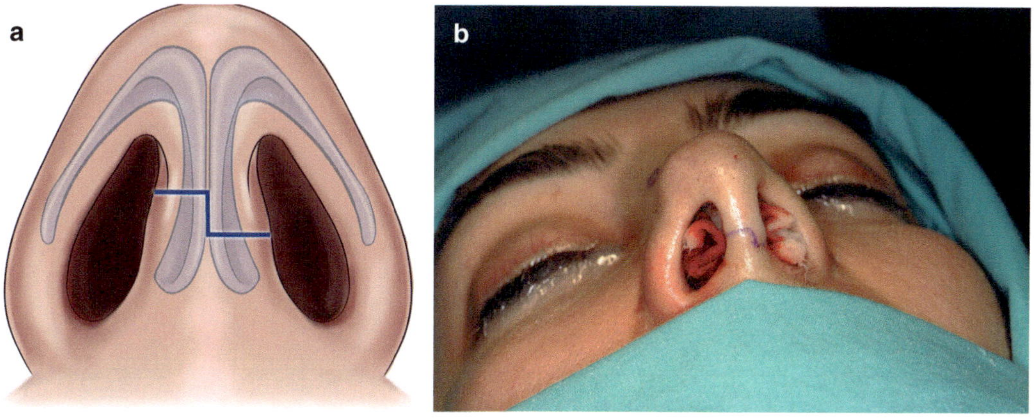

Fig. 7.19 Stairstep incision is in the shape of a stair that starts at the narrowest part of the columella and ends at the upper part of the crural footplate

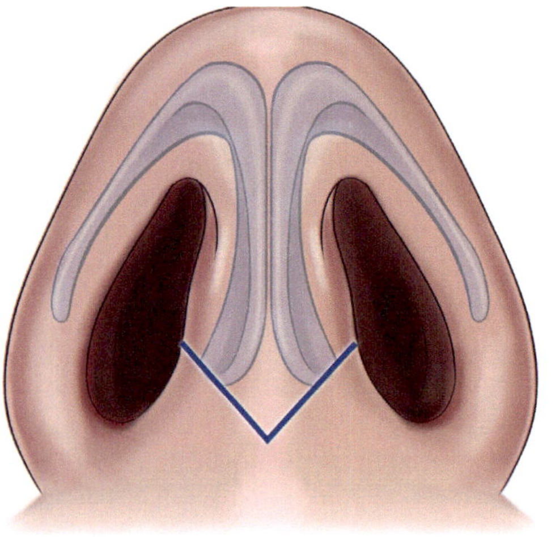

Fig. 7.20 "V" incision is placed at the lower end of the columella where the columella joins the lip

References

1. Denecke HJ, Meyer R. Plastic surgery of head and neck. Berlin Heidelberg: Springer; 1967. https://doi.org/10.1007/978-3-642-87875-6.
2. Tardy ME. Rhinoplasty: the art & the science. Philadelphia: Saunders; 1997.
3. Killian G. The submucous window resection of the nasal septum. Ann Otol Rhinol Laryngol. 1905;14:384.
4. Cottle MH, Loring RM, Fischer GG, Gaynon IE. The "maxilla-premaxilla" approach to extensive nasal septum surgery. AMA Arch Otolaryngol. 1958;68:301–13.
5. Lanza DC, Kennedy DW, Zinreich SJ. Nasal endoscopy and its surgical applications. In: Lee KJ, editor. Essential otolaryngology: head and neck surgery. 5th ed. New York: Medical Examination; 1991. p. 373–87.
6. Goodman WS, Charbonneau PA. External approach to rhinoplasty. Laryngoscope. 1974;84:2195–201.
7. Gunter JP, Rohrich RJ. External approach for secondary rhinoplasty. Plast Reconstr Surg. 1987;80:161–74.
8. Cronin TD, Upton J. Lengthening of the short columella associated with bilateral cleft lip. Ann Plast Surg. 1978;1:75–95.

8 Traditional Surgical Methods for Septal Surgery

8.1 Introduction

Surgery of the deviated nasal septum is one of the main and most frequently performed operations in departments of otorhinolaryngology. In my opinion, the traditional surgical methods for septal deviation are submucous resection and septoplasty. Submucous resection of the nasal septum was the only operation performed for septal deviations during my residency years [1]. I assisted with these surgeries during the first year and then started performing them in the following years. I was taught that the Cottle-type septoplasty technique was not effective and could end with recurrences. I only performed submucous resection of the nasal septum from 1988 to 1993. In 1993, I had a chance to follow and learn about the Cottle-type septoplasty and started using it [2].

8.2 Submucous Resection

I operated on many patients under local anesthesia sitting on an examination chair during my residency years. Although it may look awkward by today's standards, in those years, it was the way we were asked to do it. I have performed almost all nasal septal surgeries under general anesthesia since 1993. In rare situations where the patient is so scared of general anesthesia, I also use monitor-controlled anesthesia. In these cases, after pulverizing the nasal mucosa with Xylocain spray and waiting for a few minutes, cotton pledgets soaked in lidocaine hydrochloride (20 mg/mL) and epinephrine (0.0125 mg/mL) are inserted into the nose on both sides. After 10–15 min, the nose is injected with lidocaine hydrochloride (20 mg/mL) and epinephrine (0.0125 mg/mL) for additional anesthesia and to obtain decongestion. The surgeon can start the operation 15 min after the local injection.

The surgical steps in submucous resection are as follows [1]:

1. Incision
2. Elevation of the mucous membrane
3. Incision of the cartilage
4. Elevation of the mucous membrane on the opposite side
5. Resection
6. Reinsertion of the cartilaginous and bony septum
7. Closure and packing

8.2.1 Incision

The incision can be made from either side. Killian suggested entering from the convex side because it is easier to cut and reach the cartilage [1]. An

Supplementary Information The online version contains supplementary material available at https://doi.org/10.1007/978-3-031-74734-2_8. The videos can be accessed individually by clicking the DOI link in the accompanying figure caption or by scanning this link with the SN More Media App.

© The Author(s), under exclusive license to Springer Nature Switzerland AG 2025

F. Apaydın, *Septal Surgery Challenges in Rhinoplasty*,
https://doi.org/10.1007/978-3-031-74734-2_8

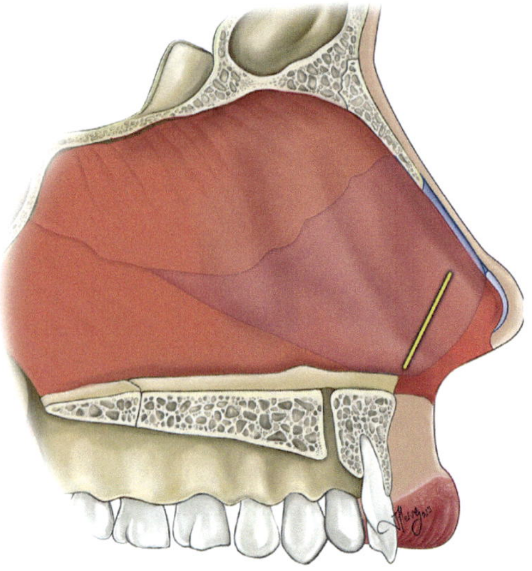

Fig. 8.1 Killian incision starts about half a centimeter behind the posterior septal angle and continues obliquely, ending 1 cm behind the anterior septal angle

alar retractor is applied to pull the ala, and a wide double-prong sharp hook is used to pull the columella. Therefore, a better exposure can be obtained, and it is easier to make the cut on a stretched mucosa. The incision should always be made from the floor of the nose toward the tip, so that the incision line is not obscured by blood. The classical incision described by Killian is about half a centimeter back from the caudal edge of the septum, moving obliquely to the end, 1 cm further back than the edge of the cartilage (Fig. 8.1) [1]. It is fascinating to see that we are still following the suggestions of a pioneer surgeon like Killian, who operated more than a century ago.

8.2.2 Elevation of the Mucous Membrane

Killian has pointed out that the incision should pass completely through the mucous membrane and a little way into the cartilage, so that the mucoperichondrium can be elevated much easier by a sharp Freer elevator [1]. The dissection is later performed using the blunt edge of the Freer elevator further backward, upward, and downward as far back as possible until the bony septum is exposed (Fig. 8.2). Unless there is a spur or marked deviation, it is relatively easy to expose the bony septum, and the surgeon can try to move the elevator from back to front to detach it from the maxillary crest. If there is a spur or marked deviation, it is better to wait for elevation of the contralateral side.

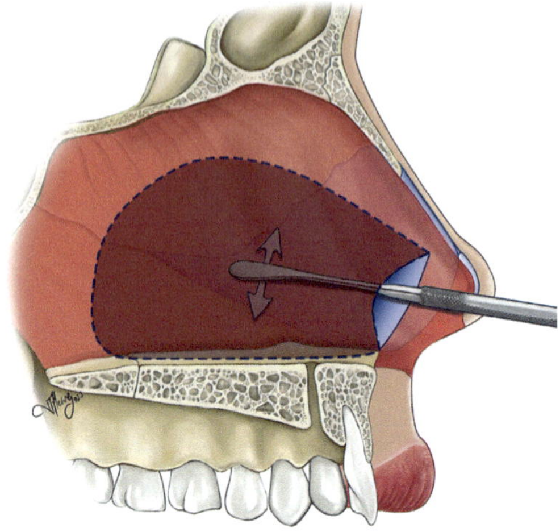

Fig. 8.2 Elevation of the mucous membrane along the cartilaginous and bony septum is performed by using a Freer elevator or suction elevator

8.2.3 Incision of the Cartilage

To elevate the mucoperichondrium on the contralateral side, a partial cut on the cartilage a few millimeters away and parallel to the incision line is performed by keeping a 1-cm intact cartilage under the cartilaginous dorsum (Fig. 8.3).

8.2.4 Elevation of the Mucous Membrane on the Opposite Side

The sharp end of the Freer elevator can be used to complete the cartilaginous incision and dissect the mucoperichondrium on the contralateral side. When the proper cleavage plane is reached, it is easier to elevate the mucoperichondrium using the blunt end of the Freer elevator with upward,

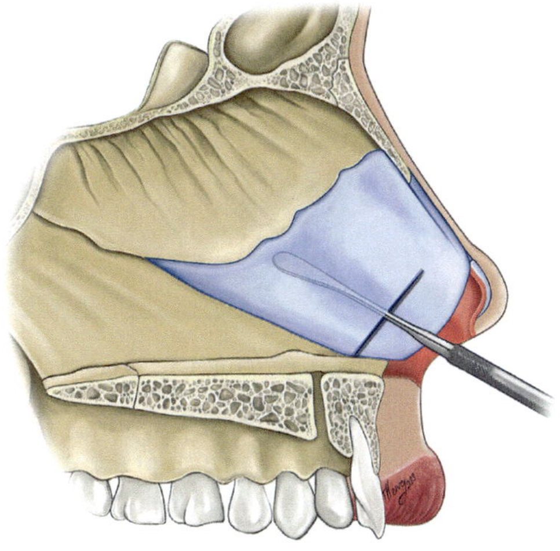

Fig. 8.3 Incision of the cartilage and elevation of the mucous membrane on the opposite side by using a Freer elevator

downward, and forward movements (Fig. 8.3). The bony septum should not be exposed until the cartilage is resected, as suggested by Killian [1]. However, I find it much easier to expose the bone by continuing dissection before resecting the cartilage.

8.2.5 Resection

I used to use a Bellanger knife to resect the cartilage by leaving a 1-cm cartilage under the nasal dorsum until I learned the Cottle type of septoplasty. I know that some surgeons still use the Bellanger knife because it is relatively easy and fast to use. However, the cartilage adjacent to the maxillary crest remains in place after this maneuver. This is one of the main reasons why I abandoned using the Bellanger knife because I want to remove the cartilage under direct vision by including the thicker portion adjacent to the maxillary crest. If I can harvest one big piece of cartilage, then multiple grafts can be sculpted from this big piece.

After this step, the elevation of the mucous membrane on both sides can be performed under direct vision. It is highly recommended to use a Killian speculum with thin blades of 50 mm in length, so that the surgeon's vision is not obstructed with the thicker blades of the Killian speculum. When there is a spur formation or a severe deviation on one side, it is suggested to dissect the mucous membrane on the opposite side first because it is much easier, and it is important to have an intact mucous membrane on at least one side. The surgeon then focuses on the deviated side. The best approach is to dissect the upper and lower parts of the ridge and then make parallel cuts on the bone using Heymann scissors, Kaplan-Meyer bone-cutting scissors or longer Piezo tips. After these cuts, the ridge is mobilized and brought to the midline, which can facilitate its dissection from the mucous membrane and then its resection using Takahashi forceps. If the maxillary crest is also deviated, both sides can be denuded of the mucous membrane. The surgeon can start the elevation from behind, which can be easy with a curved sharp elevator such as a Cottle elevator. Sometimes, a cut with a #15 blade can be done on the lateral wings of the maxillary crest to find a cleavage and go on dissecting downward and posteriorly. The deviated parts of the maxillary crest can be fractured and brought to the midline or resected using bone scissors or a Killian septum gouge. I do not like this method much because it is very easy to mobilize the premaxilla, which is a more delicate tissue than the maxillary crest at the posterior part. I find using Piezotome very useful in this step because it helps me to cut only the deviated portion while preserving the rest of the maxillary crest (Fig. 8.4).

8.2.6 Reinsertion of the Cartilaginous and Bony Septum

This step was not described in the original SMR technique by Killian [1]. This was suggested by Cottle in 1948 [3]. The resected cartilage and bony portions of the nasal septum were checked, reshaped into straight, smaller pieces, and inserted back between the mucoperichondrial flaps. Before insertion, nasal pledgets are inserted into both nasal passages to apply slight pressure

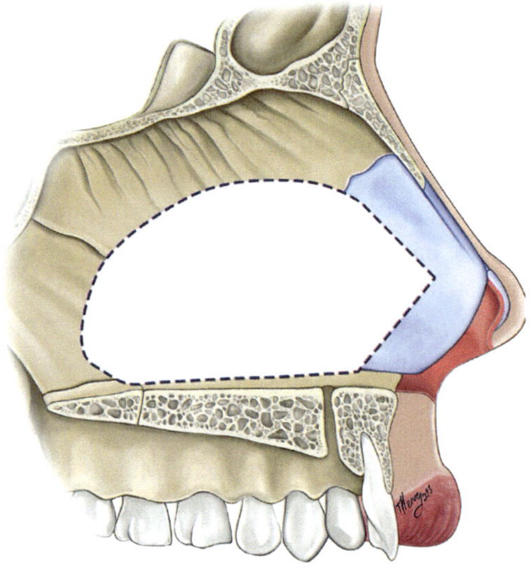

Fig. 8.4 Resection of the deviated cartilaginous and bony septum by leaving 1 cm of dorsal and caudal septal cartilage

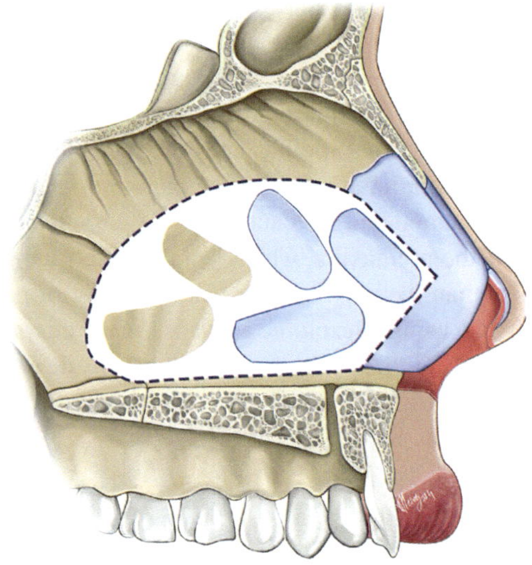

Fig. 8.5 Reinsertion of the fragments of cartilage and bone between the mucoperichondrial flaps

on the mucoperichondrial flaps. Therefore, when the implants of cartilage and bone are inserted, these pledgets are helpful in keeping the implants in place. A second help comes from the oozing blood to keep the implants in place (Fig. 8.5).

The cartilaginous implants can be sutured to each other before insertion. The thicker cartilage portions can be divided into two pieces to increase the surface area and thin the cartilage before insertion.

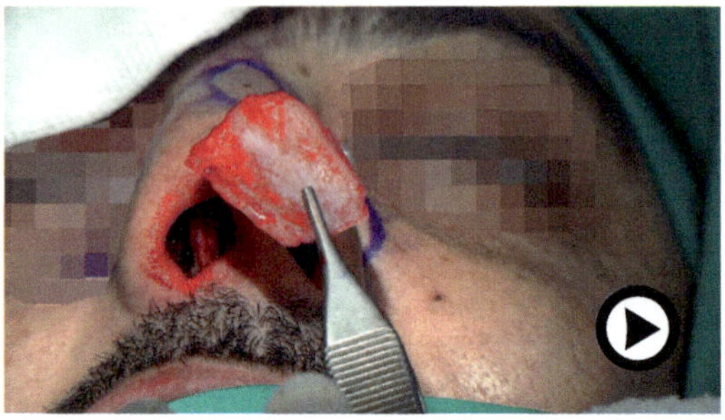

Fig. 8.6 Septoplasty is performed by using spreader grafts (▶ https://doi.org/10.1007/000-dye)

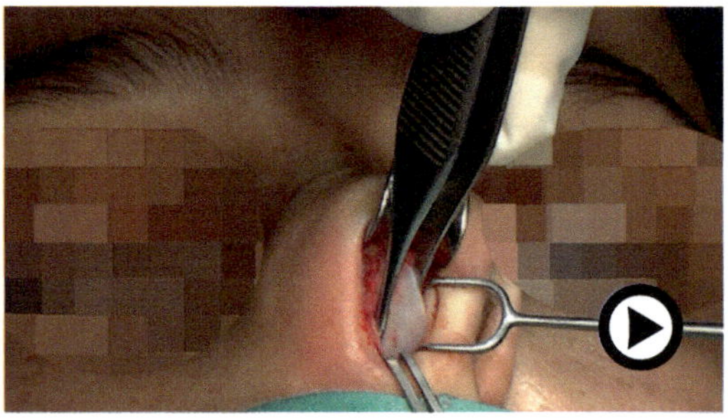

Fig. 8.7 Septoplasty is performed by using L-strut graft and spreader graft (▶ https://doi.org/10.1007/000-dyd)

I used to throw the thick vomer, creating spurs, thinking that I was solving the problem of obstruction. The vomer is a bilaminar bone, and the portion that creates the thicker spur can be resected by rongeurs or powered instrumentation. I call this process "bone recycling." [4] This piece of bone can be reinserted into the nose. These fragments of cartilage and bone can prevent mucosal atrophy and a flagging septum.

At this stage, splinting spreader grafts and/or L-strut grafts can be used to straighten the deviations of the L-strut framework (Figs. 8.6 and 8.7).

8.2.7 Closure and Packing

After the operation site is irrigated and cleaned of any debris, it is checked one more time, and the incision edges are approximated using 5-0 Vicryl Rapide sutures. The quilting sutures by 4-0 Vicryl

Rapide connected to a 13-mm Keith needle help to close the dead space between the mucoperichondrial flaps. If packing is needed, different options are available, which will be discussed in Chap. 17.

Submucous resection has been in use for more than a century. When first described, it was a revolutionary method and remained so for almost half a century until Cottle published his work on septoplasty in 1958 [2]. In fact, having extensive experience with this method, I can easily say that it works well in most cases. The Killian incision bypasses the caudal septum. Therefore, the deflections of the caudal septum cannot be addressed with SMR. In addition, the deviations of the dorsal segment of the nasal septum cannot be addressed either.

It was blamed by many surgeons because of sequelae, and Cottle et al. listed some of them as follows [2]:

1. Sagging of the cartilaginous part of the nose
2. Saddling of the middle vault
3. Broadening of the alar base
4. Columellar retraction and collapse
5. Widening and flattening of the nostrils
6. Ballooning of the internal valve area
7. Septal perforation
8. Mucosal atrophy
9. Absence of the anterior nasal spine

I had the chance to witness all these sequelae during all these years.

8.3 Septoplasty

The Cottle type of septoplasty is conceptualized into six steps after his article on the maxilla–premaxilla approach and coined as functional reconstructive septal surgery [2]:

1. Approach
2. Mobilization
3. Resection
4. Repositioning
5. Reconstruction
6. Fixation

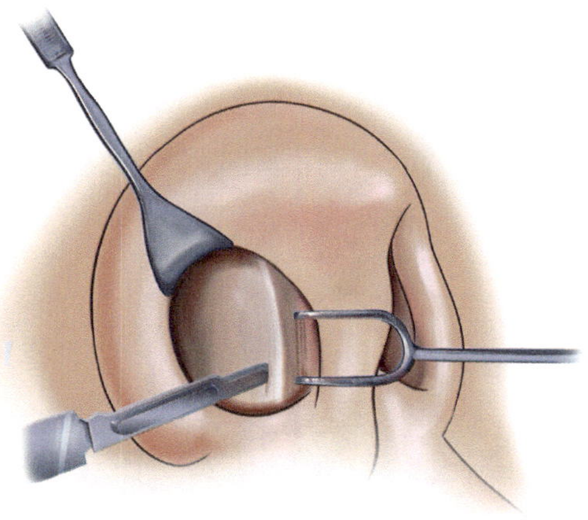

Fig. 8.8 The surgeon should elevate the ala with an alar retractor, and the assistant should pull the columella with a wide two-prong hook to expose the caudal septum and perform the hemitransfixion incision

8.3.1 Approach

Hemitransfixion incision is the preferred approach in this type of septoplasty, and its details are given in Chap. 7 (Fig. 8.8).

8.3.2 Mobilization

After the hemitransfixion incision, the caudal septum is exposed (Fig. 8.9). A #15 blade is used to scratch the caudal septum to expose the cartilage and cut the perichondrium layer. I prefer elevating the first 4–5 mm of the caudal portion with sharp scissors because the mucoperichondrium is very adherent to the caudal septum. A bent, dull-ended Freer elevator is then used to raise the mucosa overlying the cartilaginous septum by up, down, and forward movements of the elevator under direct vision. As soon as the bony septum is reached, the surgeon can feel the characteristic scratchy sound and the transition to the bony surface. When the ethmoid is reached, the elevator can be moved down to elevate the mucosa over the vomer and maxillary crest at the posterior two-thirds of the septum.

In the Cottle approach, the nasal septum is divided into imaginary zones: anterosuperior, anteroinferior, posterosuperior, and posteroinferior.

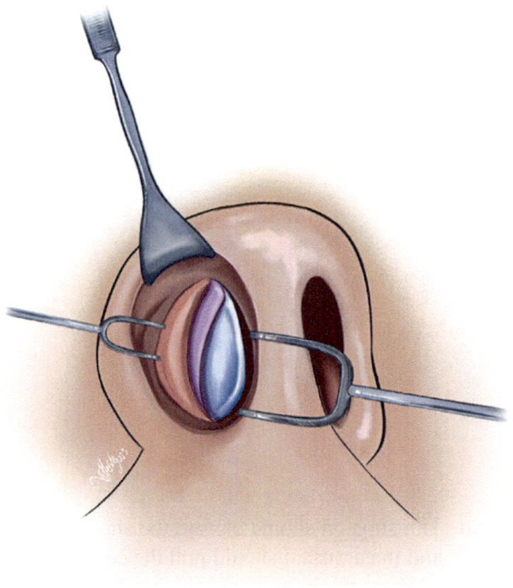

Fig. 8.9 The caudal septum is exposed on the right side after the hemitransfixion incision

A vertical imaginary line passing from the junction of the septal cartilage with the ethmoid divides the nose into anterior and posterior parts, whereas a horizontal line passing from the junction of the septal cartilage with the vomer and maxillary crest divides the nasal septum into inferior and superior parts. The tunnels created during surgery are also named according to these zones [5].

In Cottle septoplasty, there are two-, three-, and four-tunnel approaches. In mild septal deviations limited to the nasal septal cartilage, a two-tunnel approach is enough. In more complex cases, three- or four-tunnel approaches are used [5]. In fact, this kind of terminology is rarely used today. Most structural rhinoplasty surgeons prefer to widely dissect the entire nasal septum to identify the pathological situations better and also harvest cartilage under direct exposure with more precision. I am also in favor of this approach in very difficult septal deviations. However, having used wider dissections for years, I have rarely observed some potential problems, such as detachment of the septal cartilage from the ethmoid after hump removal. Therefore, I decided to use the power of the mucoperichondrium attached to the nasal septum, as our forefathers used, as mentioned in Chap. 1. So, my current preferred approach is a customized approach by using one, two, three, or four tunnels depending on the severity of the septal deviation. I usually start septal surgery by exposing the anterior lower half of the nasal septal cartilage (one tunnel). This approach is more than enough if there is a need for limited cartilage harvest. I cut the septal cartilage with a #15 scalpel or the sharp tip of the Freer elevator and then pass to the opposite side through these incisions to dissect and resect the cartilage. When there is no septal pathology, this is my preferred technique. The cartilage obtained in this way is usually enough for a columellar strut, tip graft, and rim grafts. If the dorsal and/or caudal segments of the nasal septum are deviated, I usually start with opening one- or two-sided inferior tunnels and then bilateral subdorsal tunnels. According to my experience, keeping 3–6 mm of intact mucoperichondrium attached to the septal cartilage has many advantages. The septal cartilage below this intact mucoperichondrium is usually enough to correct most of the septal deviations and also to obtain sufficient cartilage for grafts. The subdorsal tunnels on the other side also have many advantages:

1. It is very easy to insert spreader grafts in these tunnels like a finger in a glove, and one suture is enough to fix the spreader grafts.
2. If spreader grafts are used after hump removal, they do not fall into the nasal cavity because the mucoperichondrium below acts like a barrier and helps to stabilize the spreader graft in place.
3. The septal hump can be more easily resected, and spreader flaps can be turned in much more easily.
4. The original position of the nasal septum is preserved. Suturing of the spreader grafts, flaps, or upper lateral cartilages does not distort the nose, which can be the case when the mucoperichondrial flaps are entirely elevated on both sides.
5. In case the connection of the nasal septum with the ethmoid is damaged during surgery, the mucoperichondrial attachments prevent the total fall of the detached nasal septum. It usually goes down 2–4 mm, and it is much easier to restore the connection.

8.3.3 Resection

Traditionally, a narrow, triangular, vertical strip is resected at the chondroperpendicular junction, keeping the upper 1–1.5 cm of the cartilage intact, which can be called a vertical chondrotomy. A horizontal basal strip of 2–3 mm, which is triangular in shape, is resected to detach the cartilaginous septum from the maxillary crest (horizontal chondrotomy). The cartilage close to the posterior septal angle is spared in order not to lose dorsal support. At this stage, the cartilaginous septum can be detached from the anterior nasal spine to complete the inferior tunnels around the maxillary crest. The deviations and crests can easily be dealt with because all deformities are under good exposure. The crests are usually removed. The cartilaginous deviations are usually addressed by leaving as much as possible in place. However, if rhinoplasty is also part of the procedure, a cartilage harvest may be necessary to use as grafts. Bony deviations are resected at the upper margin using Heymann or Kaplan-Meyer bone-cutting scissors. Floating pieces of bone and/or cartilage can be removed using Takahashi forceps.

8.3.4 Repositioning

If the septal cartilage has been mobilized from the maxillary crest after chondrotomy, it must be sutured back in its place. In fact, when the caudal septum seems to have some tension and concavity, mobilization of it from the anterior nasal spine can solve the problem. Before mobilizing the septal cartilage from the anterior nasal spine, it is suggested to mark the level of the cartilage corresponding to the anterior nasal spine with a drawing pen. Otherwise, the position of the caudal septum can be distorted during its replacement, which can end up with loss of tip projection and rotation. There may be a need for shortening the caudal septum at the attachment to the premaxilla. After this step, the caudal septum should be sutured to the anterior nasal spine. A small trick that makes repositioning much easier is to dissect the mucoperichondrium on one side while keeping the mucoperichondrium attached to the other side of the caudal septum intact. So partial trimming of the lower part of the caudal septum does not mobilize the caudal septum entirely, and suturing and repositioning are much easier.

8.3.5 Reconstruction

Cotton pledgets are inserted into both nasal passages, bringing the mucoperichondrial flaps together in the midline. The resected cartilage and bone fragments are inserted into the defective parts of the nasal septum in a mosaic fashion. The pressure obtained from the cotton pledgets and the oozing blood help these fragments to maintain their position. These fragments are very helpful in preventing unwanted sequelae of SMR, such as perforations, mucosal atrophy, and mucosal fluttering during breathing.

8.3.6 Fixation

To prevent complications such as bleeding, hematoma, ecchymosis, and edema, fixation is needed. Gauze strips, with or without ointment, are the most well-known method, which is rarely used today. Polyvinyl acetate sponges impregnated with oxidized cellulose, silicone splints, and transseptal quilting sutures are popular techniques. The choice depends on the type of surgery performed and the personal preference of the surgeon. These options are discussed in detail in Chap. 17.

The traditional Cottle type of septoplasty has many advantages. The hemitransfixion incision allows us to see and manipulate the whole nasal septum. After horizontal and vertical chondrotomies and strip cartilage resection, more septal cartilage can be preserved. Besides, crosshatching or limited resections of cartilage are possible, which can help solve almost all kinds of deviations. However, sometimes it can be the reason for iatrogenic caudal deflections that were not present before surgery, due to unwanted cuts or trauma to the caudal septum. In this sense, the Killian incision should be kept in mind to employ if the position of the nasal tip and its relation to the caudal septum are good and the surgeon is willing to keep it that way.

Following these two traditional techniques, subtotal reconstruction methods and structural rhinoplasty techniques were described. In particular, structural rhinoplasty techniques require cartilage, which is usually obtained from the septal cartilage. Therefore, during structural rhinoplasty, SMR is the most often used method. However, it is possible to get rid of the disadvantages of SMR by placing cartilaginous and/or bony grafts between the mucoperichondrial flaps (Figs. 8.10, 8.11, 8.12, 8.13, 8.14, 8.15, 8.16, 8.17, 8.18, 8.19, 8.20, 8.21, 8.22, and 8.23).

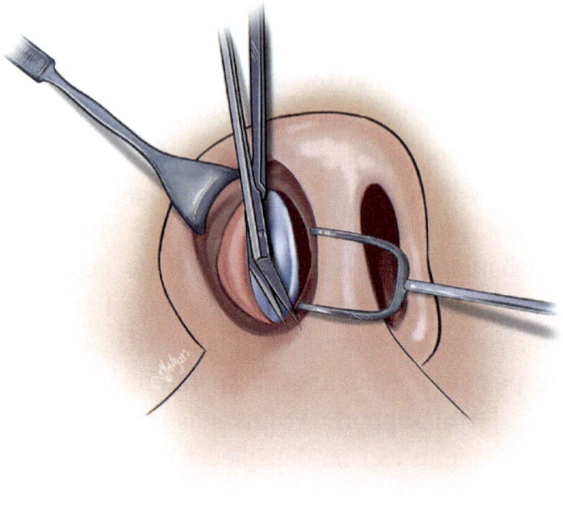

Fig. 8.11 The anterior nasal spine and posterior septal angle are exposed

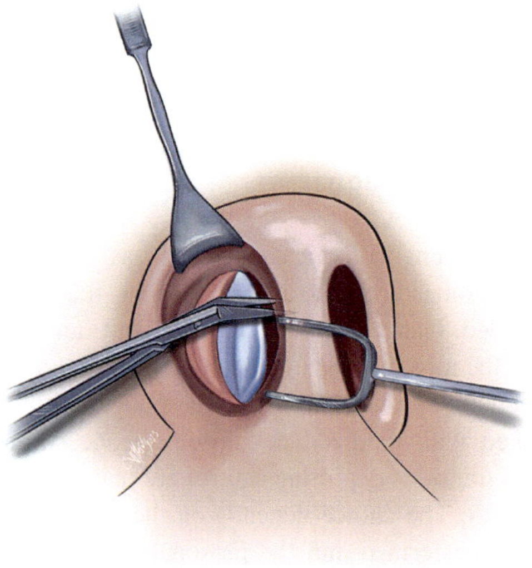

Fig. 8.10 After the caudal margin of the cartilaginous septum is exposed, a small columellar pocket is created

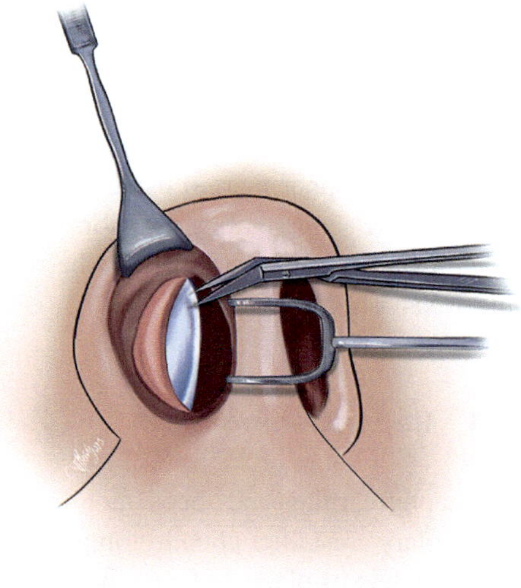

Fig. 8.12 An anterosuperior tunnel is opened on the left side

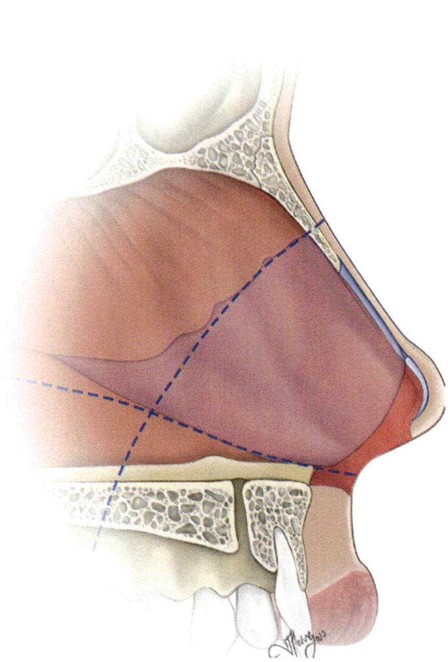

Fig. 8.13 Cottle divided the nasal septum into four imaginary zones by using a vertical and horizontal line: anterosuperior, anteroinferior, posterosuperior, and posteroinferior zones. A vertical imaginary line passes from the junction of the septal cartilage with the ethmoid, and a horizontal line passes from the junction of the septal cartilage with the vomer and maxillary crest. The tunnels created during surgery are named according to these zones

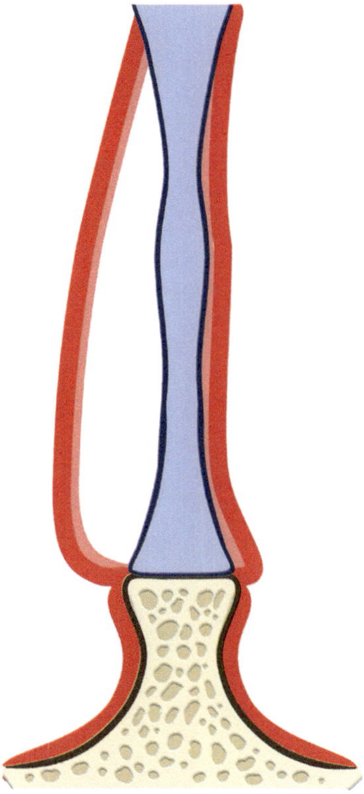

Fig. 8.14 The creation of one tunnel, which is a one-sided anterosuperior tunnel

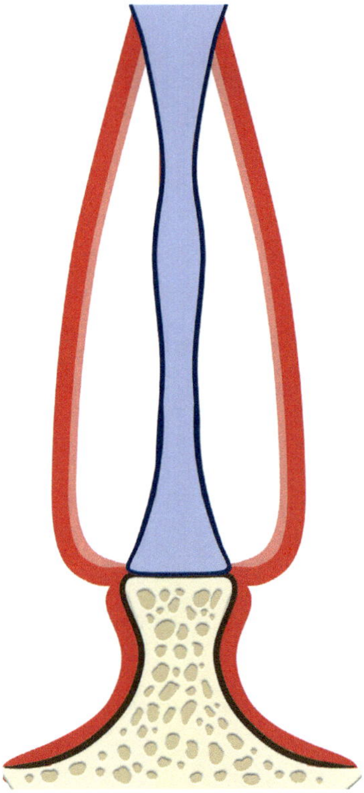

Fig. 8.15 Two anterosuperior tunnels are created

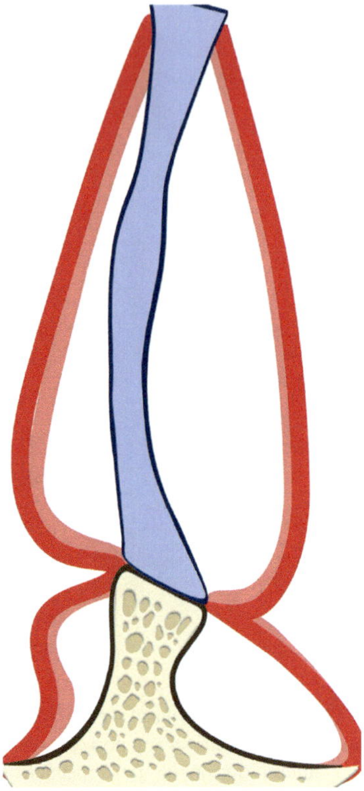

Fig. 8.17 Four-tunnel approach

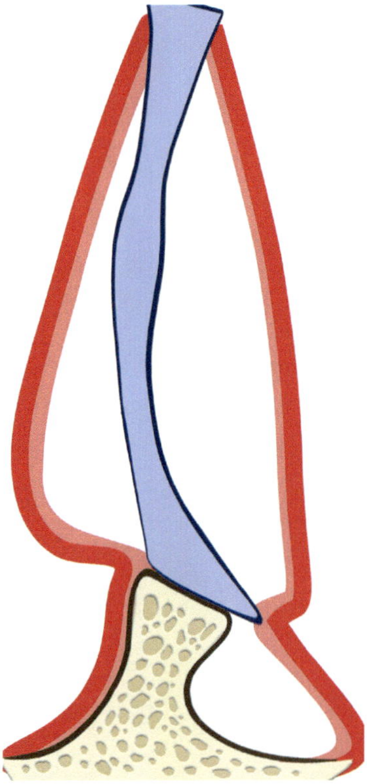

Fig. 8.16 Three tunnels are created when the deviation includes the bony septum

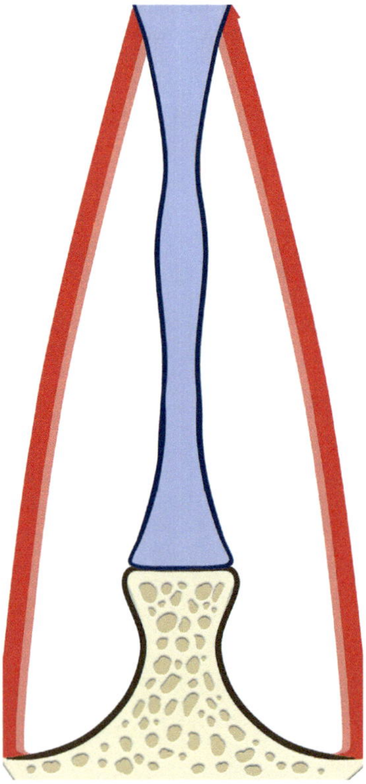

Fig. 8.18 The wide dissection of the entire nasal septum

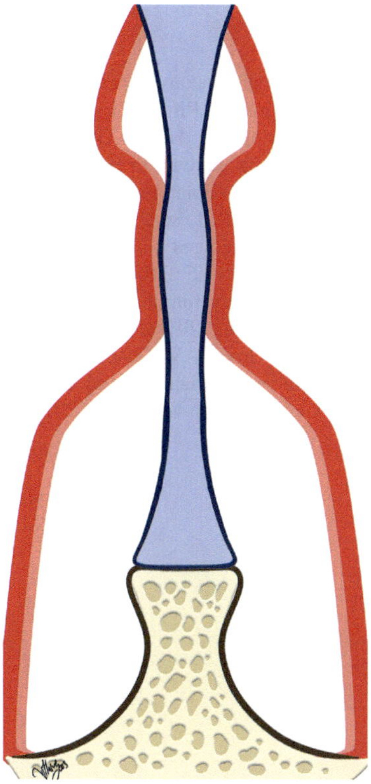

Fig. 8.19 Subdorsal tunnels are created under the middle vault. An intact mucoperichondrium is left between the subdorsal and inferior tunnels

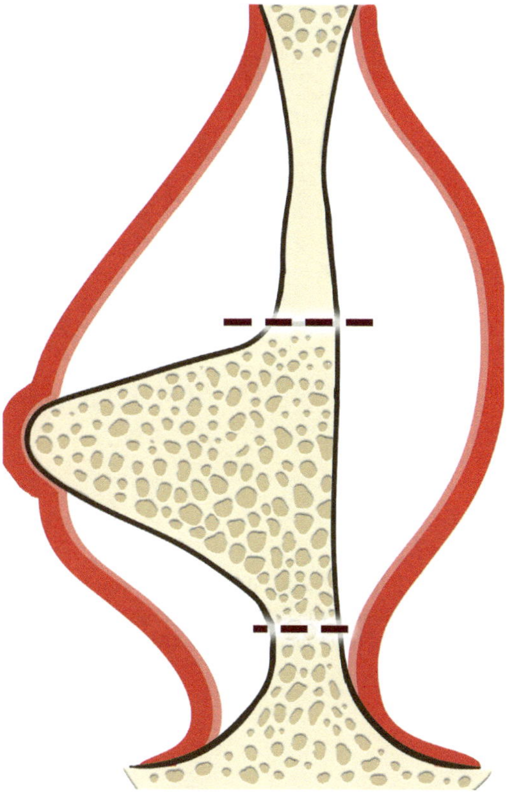

Fig. 8.21 The mucoperichondrium of the upper and lower portions of a bony spur is dissected. Heymann scissors or Kaplan-Meyer bone-cutting scissors can be used to cut the upper and lower parts of the spur

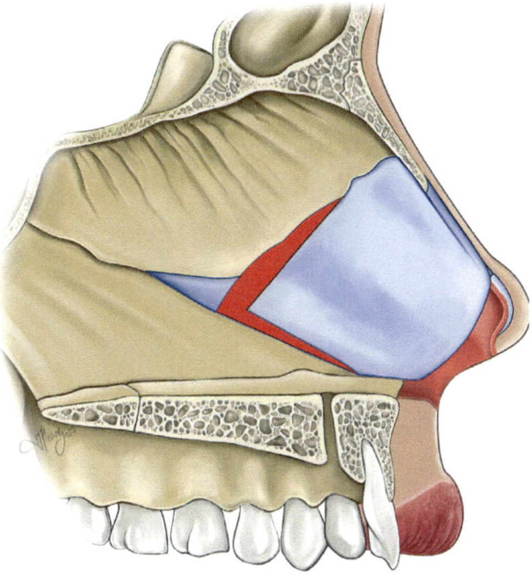

Fig. 8.20 Limited vertical and horizontal chondrotomies can help to get rid of septal deviations while keeping most of the septal cartilage intact

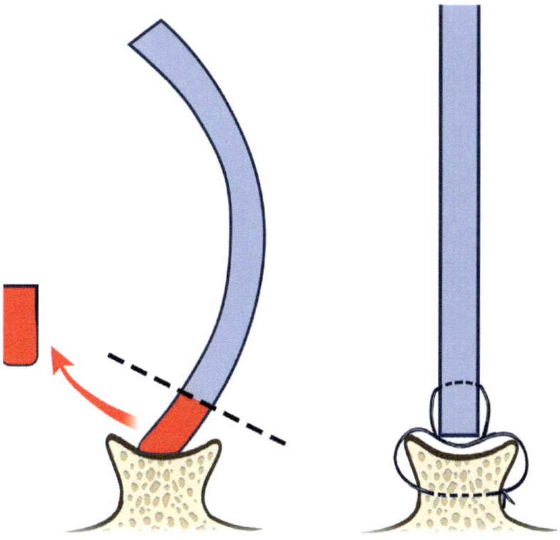

Fig. 8.22 Repositioning and suturing of the caudal septum to the anterior nasal spine with an eight suture after resecting the longer portion of the caudal septum

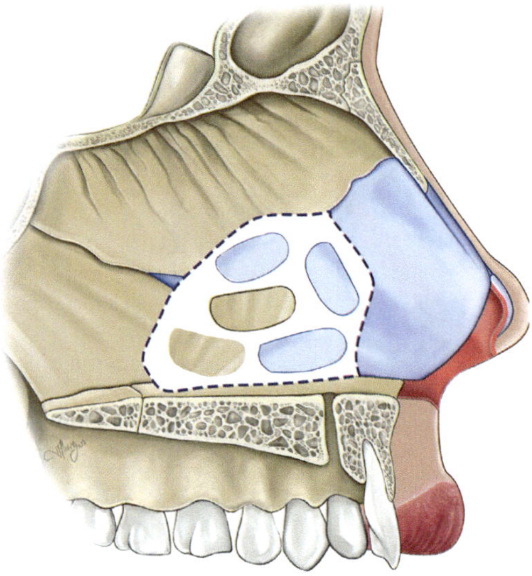

Fig. 8.23 In bigger septal deviations, a wider resection than chondrotomies can be done. However, straight pieces of cartilage and bone should be reinserted

References

1. Killian G. The submucous window resection of the nasal septum. Ann Otol Rhinol Laryngol. 1905;14:384.
2. Cottle MH, Loring RM, Fischer GG, Gaynon IE. The maxilla-premaxilla approach to extensive nasal septum surgery. AMA Arch Otolaryngol. 1958;68:301–13.
3. Cottle MH, Loring RM. Surgery of the nasal septum; new operative procedures and indications. Ann Otol Rhinol Laryngol. 1948;57:705–13.
4. Apaydin F. Bone recycling in nasal septal reconstruction. Facial Plast Surg. 2013;29:473–8.
5. Huizing EH, de Groot JAM. Chapter 5. Septal surgery. In: Functional reconstructive nasal surgery. 2nd ed. Stuttgart: Georg Thieme Verlag KG; 2015.

9 Caudal Septal Deflections

9.1 Introduction

The caudal segment of the nasal septum is the portion of the nose that faces minor and major trauma because the nose is the most prominent part of the face.

In my opinion, the caudal segment is a crucial structure for many reasons:

1. It provides major support for the nasal tip.
2. It is a major cartilaginous structure for the internal and external valves.
3. It has a unique relationship with the anterior nasal spine.
4. It has a loose connection with the membranous septum and the footplates of the medial crura.

Inspection of the tip of the nose on standard rhinoplasty views by the naked eye gives the surgeon many clues about the condition of the caudal septum. It is very easy to diagnose deviation, subluxation, or columellar retraction. The second step is to go for palpation. The surgeon should touch the nasal tip to perform a recoil test to reveal the strength of the tip support. In addition, with gloved fingers, the anterior nasal spine and the caudal septum should be palpated. The position and dimensions of the anterior nasal spine and caudal septum can then be understood.

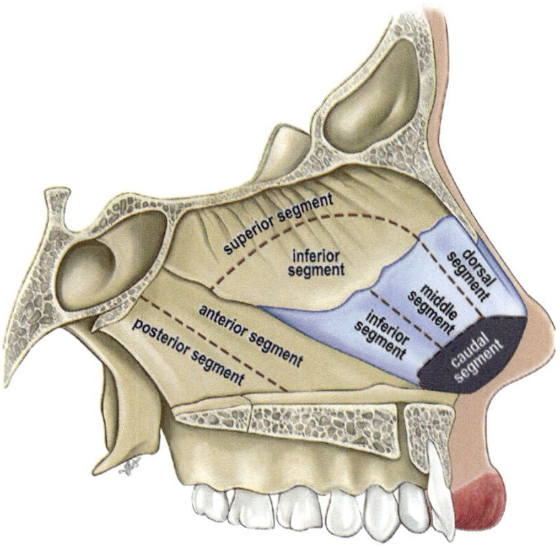

Fig. 9.1 The virtual mapping of the nasal septum according to Apaydin, with the caudal segment of the nasal septum is highlighted in gray

The virtual mapping of the nasal septum is depicted in Fig. 9.1, and in this chapter, the focus will be on the caudal segment (Fig. 9.1). A detailed examination of the nasal septum can reveal the following pathologic conditions.

Supplementary Information The online version contains supplementary material available at https://doi.org/10.1007/978-3-031-74734-2_9. The videos can be accessed individually by clicking the DOI link in the accompanying figure caption or by scanning this link with the SN More Media App.

© The Author(s), under exclusive license to Springer Nature Switzerland AG 2025

F. Apaydın, *Septal Surgery Challenges in Rhinoplasty*,
https://doi.org/10.1007/978-3-031-74734-2_9

9.2 Subluxation

When the caudal segment is off the midline and visible in the basal view, it is called subluxation (Fig. 9.2). This can be due to a linear deviation, C-shaped deviation, or traumatic deviation. Although a lot of preoperative information can be obtained during examination, a real diagnosis can be made after dissecting the mucoperichondrium on both sides of the caudal septum and seeing its relationship with the anterior nasal spine. In addition, the width of the nasal airway on both sides should be evaluated.

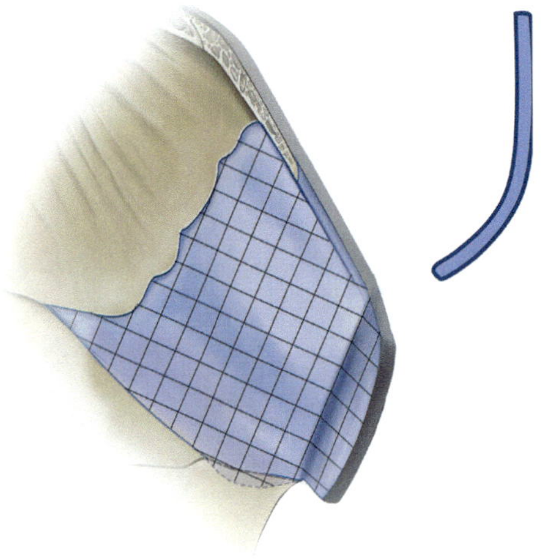

Fig. 9.2 Subluxation of the caudal segment of the septal cartilage

If the anterior nasal spine is in the midline, attention is turned to the caudal septum and the underlying reason causing the subluxation. In my experience, the weakest area causing subluxation is the junction where the caudal septum joins the upper lateral cartilages. It is very easy to observe this situation during surgery when the caudal septum is totally exposed with the rest of the nasal septum during external rhinoplasty. If one draws a vertical line from the junction, it is usually this part that is deviated and subluxated. The caudal septum is usually thinner than the rest of the septal cartilage and is even thinner at this junction point. These clinical observations correlate with the study published by Van Loosen et al., mentioning thicker sphenospinal and sphenodorsal zones and a thinner caudal portion [1]. Metzenbaum used to call it the "angle of deflection of the cartilage," which is still valid today [2]. He summarized the findings in the case of a fractured, dislocated lower end of the septal cartilage as follows (Fig. 9.3):

1. The cartilage is dislocated laterally from the maxillary crest and loses its supporting position in the columella, which could cause a droopy tip and retracted columella.
2. Subluxation can cause slight widening of the ala and nostril.

Fig. 9.3 The subluxation has created a droopy tip, retracted columella, and widening of the ala and nostril

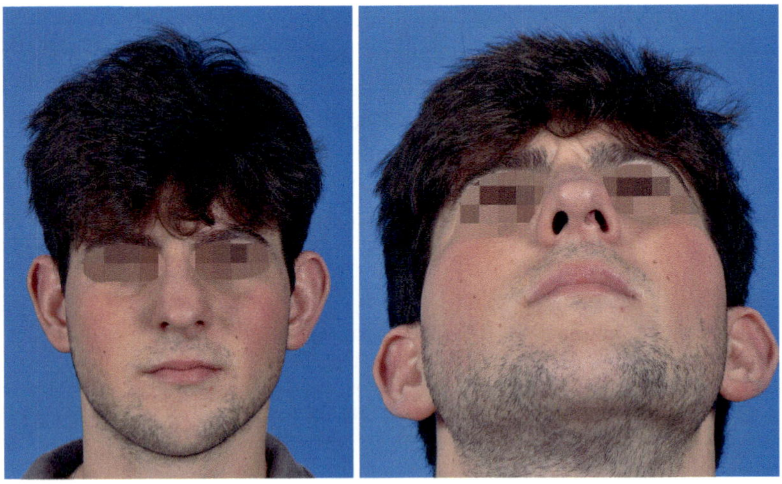

3. Subluxation causes partial or nearly total obstruction of the nostril.
4. A similar obstruction can be seen at the nasal valve on the opposite side due to the sharp angle of deflection.

How can we correct such subluxation? In the method proposed by Metzenbaum [2], after a hemitransfixion incision on the side of the angle of deflection, the caudal septum is exposed. The deflected portion is incised or preferably resected as a thin sliver of cartilage while keeping the mucoperichondrium on the opposite side intact. The Metzenbaum technique was published in 1929 and has been accepted as a revolutionary method since then (Fig. 9.4). With the addition of structural techniques to the surgical armamentarium of the rhinoplasty surgeon, splinting of the dislocated portion using spreader grafts, batten grafts [3], ethmoid bone [4], and/or L-strut grafts [5] has become more popular.

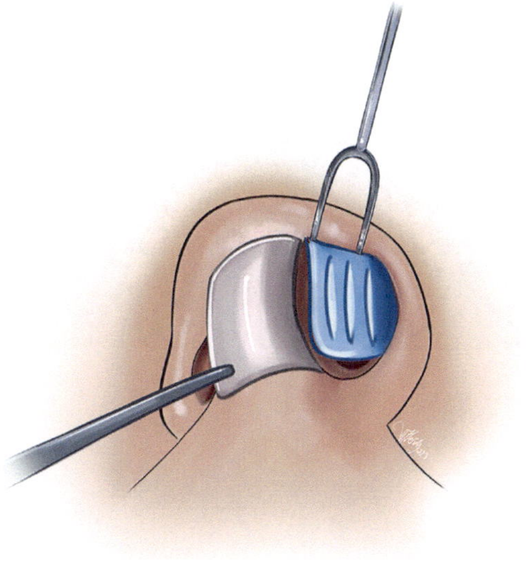

Fig. 9.4 In the Metzenbaum technique, the angle of deflection of the caudal septum is exposed, and the deflected portion is incised or preferably resected as a thin sliver of cartilage while keeping the mucoperichondrium on the opposite side intact

If the caudal septum is also dislocated from the anterior nasal spine, it is sutured to the anterior nasal spine using different suture techniques (Fig. 9.5). Simple suture, suture of eight, mattress suture, and suture through the bone are all options to fix the caudal septum (Fig. 9.6). It can be sutured to the soft tissues around the anterior nasal spine (Fig. 9.7). If the existing groove between the wings of the ANS is not good enough, it is deepened by using scissors, Piezo, or a burr. In addition, a hole can be drilled through the ANS using a thick needle or Piezo, through which a suture can be passed to fix the caudal septum (Figs. 9.8 and 9.9).

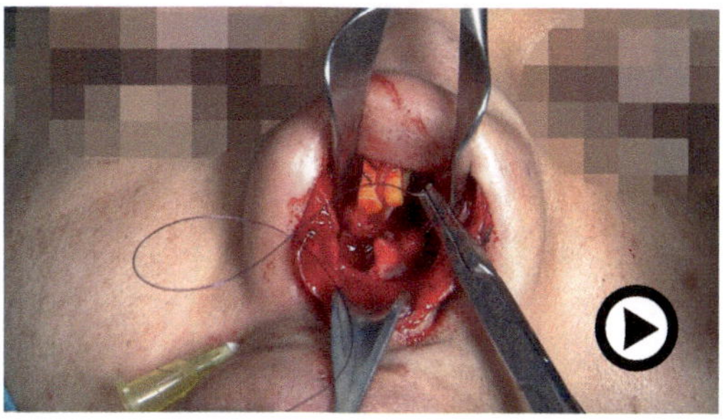

Fig. 9.5 A hole through the Anterior Nasal Spine was performed with an injector needle. Then the needle of the suture was passed through it (▶ https://doi.org/10.1007/000-dyn)

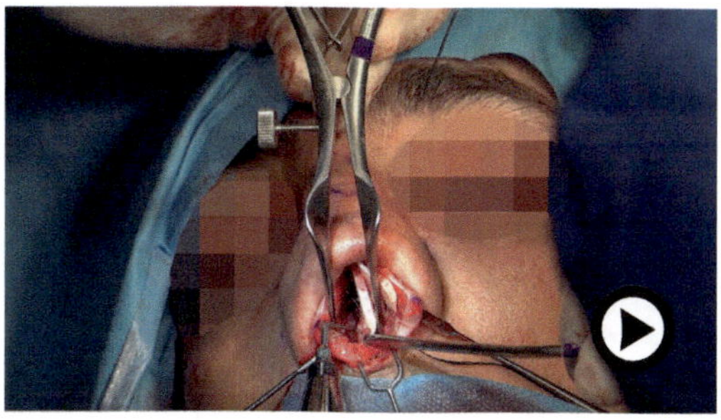

Fig. 9.6 Opening a hole through the anterior nasal Spine by Piezotome (▶ https://doi.org/10.1007/000-dyg)

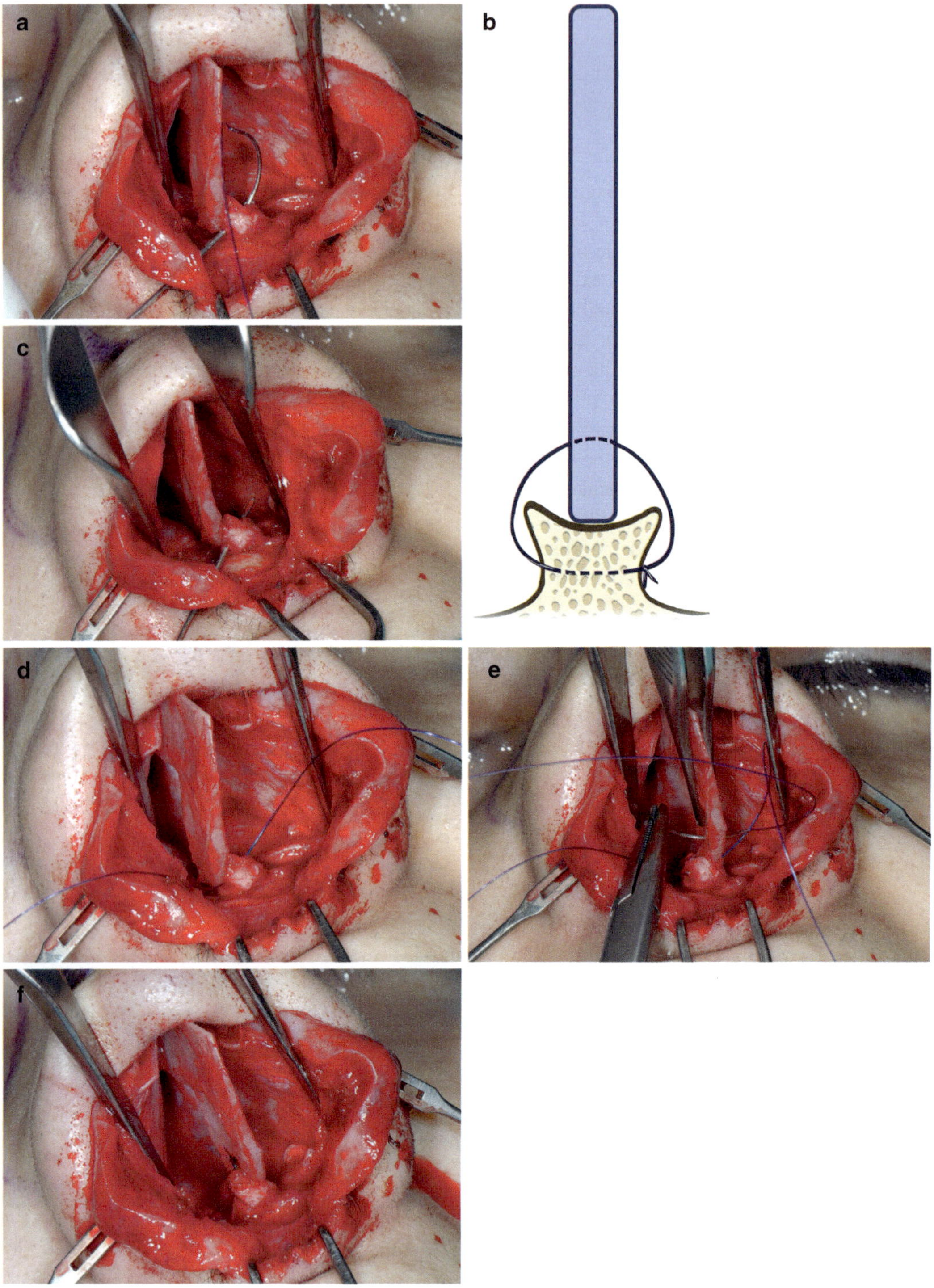

Fig. 9.7 The caudal septum can be sutured to the anterior nasal spine by a suture passing through the bone, and I think this is the most popular method (**a**, **b**). I used to use it routinely in the past by using the needle-in-needle technique (**c**–**f**), but during the last decade, I have preferred suturing the caudal septum to the soft tissues around the anterior nasal spine with a mattress suture (**g**). Simple sutures and figure-of-eight sutures are other options to use (**h**, **i**). As an additional support, I prefer surrounding the caudal septum with a cushion of soft tissues around the anterior nasal spine (**j**)

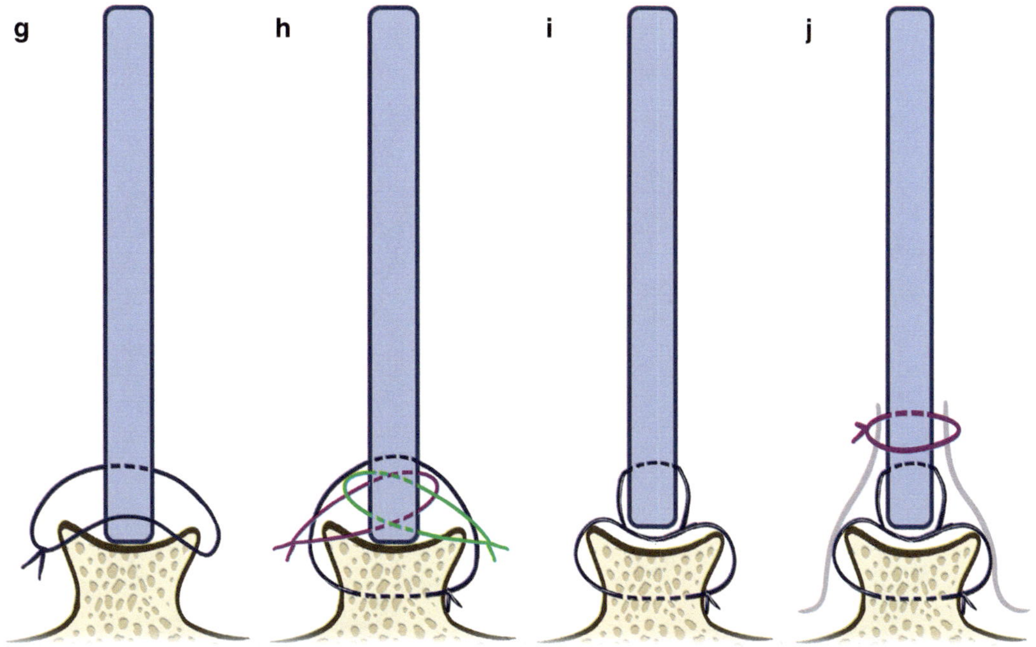

Fig. 9.7 (continued)

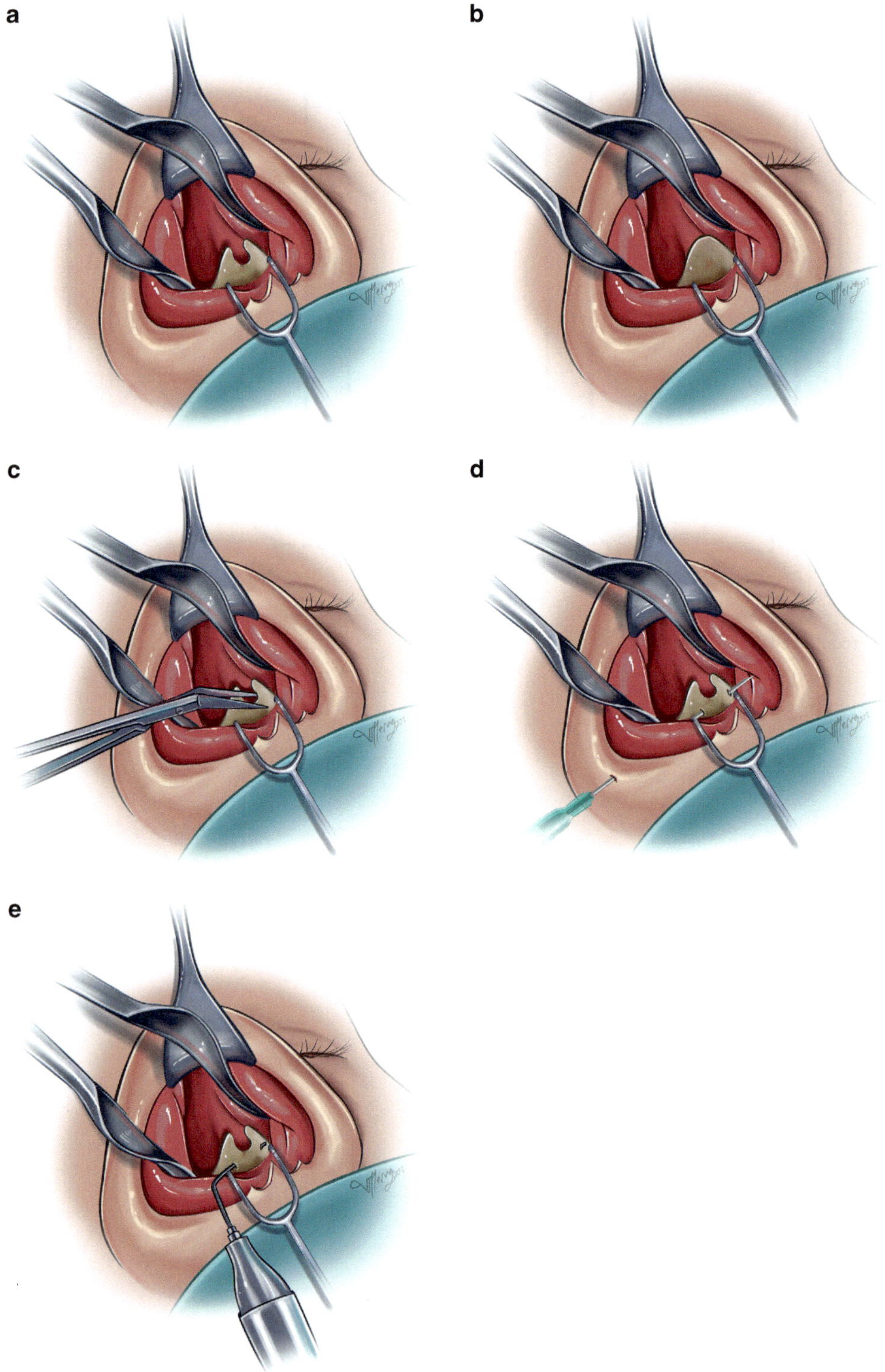

Fig. 9.8 The groove between the wings of the anterior nasal spine is usually in good shape (**a**). If not, it can be deepened by using scissors, Piezo, or a burr (**b**, **c**). Besides, a hole can be drilled through the anterior nasal spine by using a thick needle, Piezotome, or a burr (**d**, **e**)

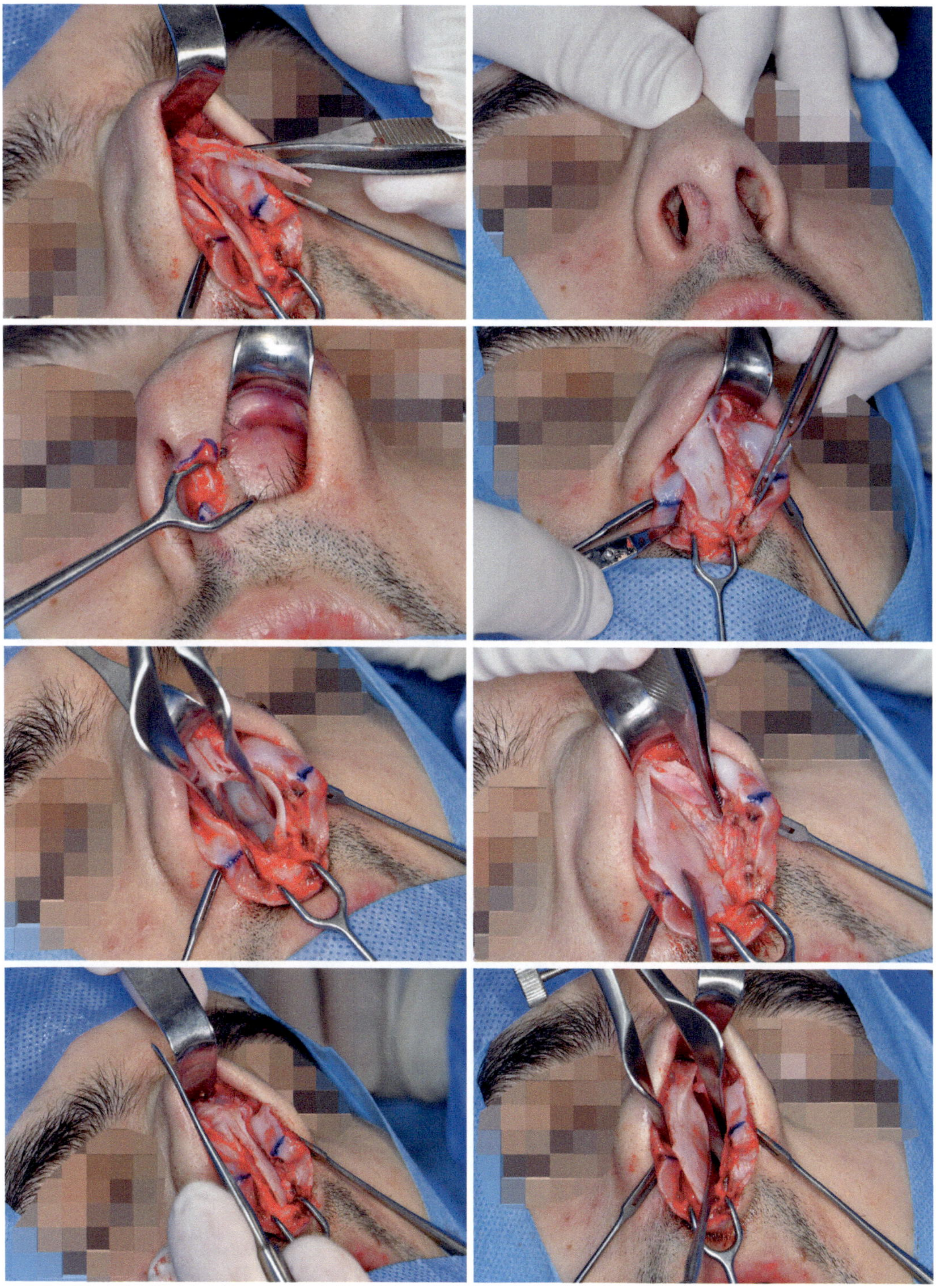

Fig. 9.9 Peroperative and postoperative pictures of a patient with subluxation. An L-strut graft and a spreader graft were used to splint the subluxated caudal septum, which was later sutured to the anterior nasal spine. After 3 months the nose is still swollen. It will get better with time. However, this is a good example to show that the crooked noses do not always heal the way the surgeon likes it. The surgeons should always tell the patients about this fact before surgery. This is a very happy patient, although the nose is still slightly crooked. Because he was informed about this situation before. He can breathe much better, and he likes the esthetic result even though it is still slightly crooked

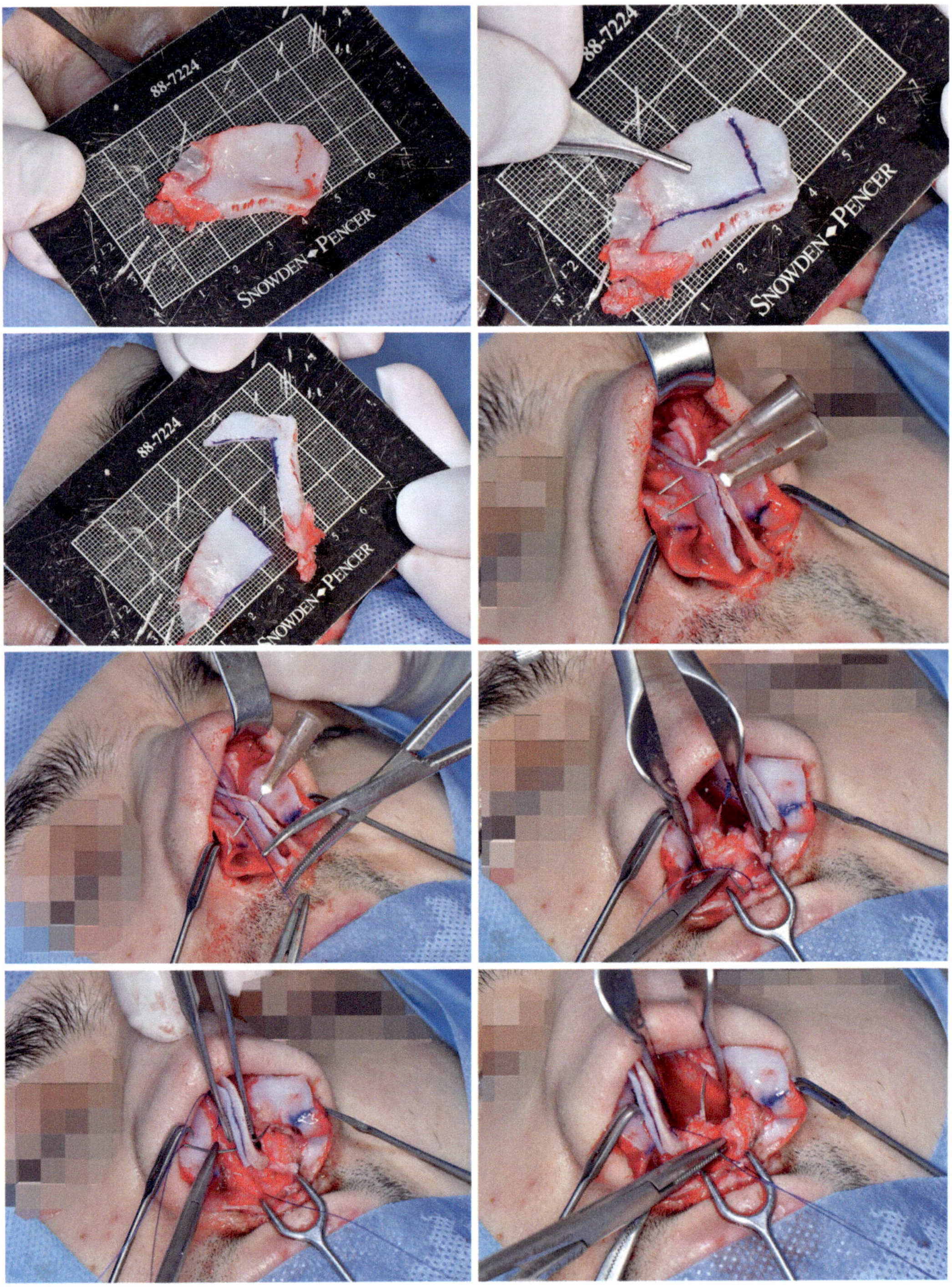

Fig. 9.9 (continued)

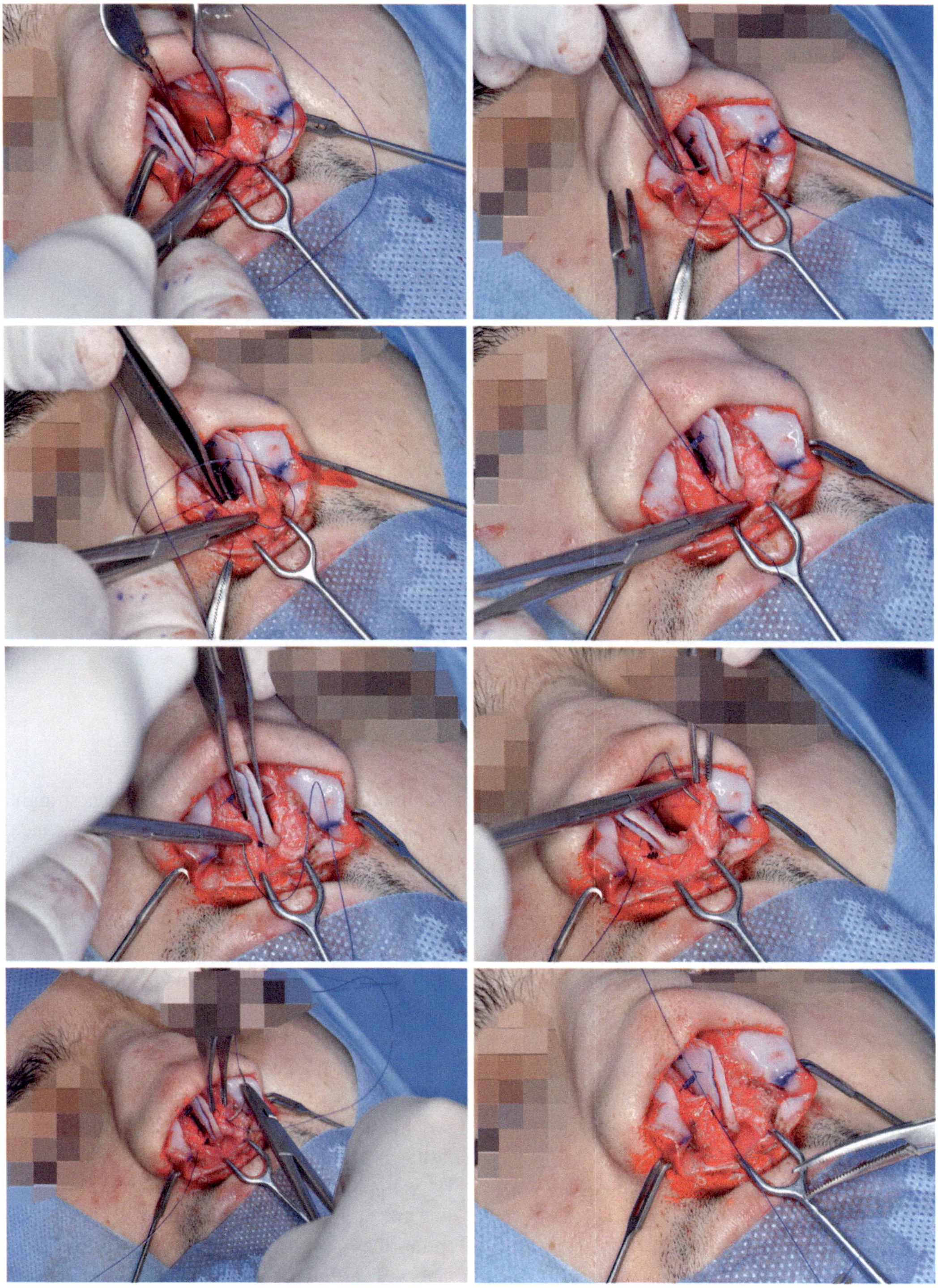

Fig. 9.9 (continued)

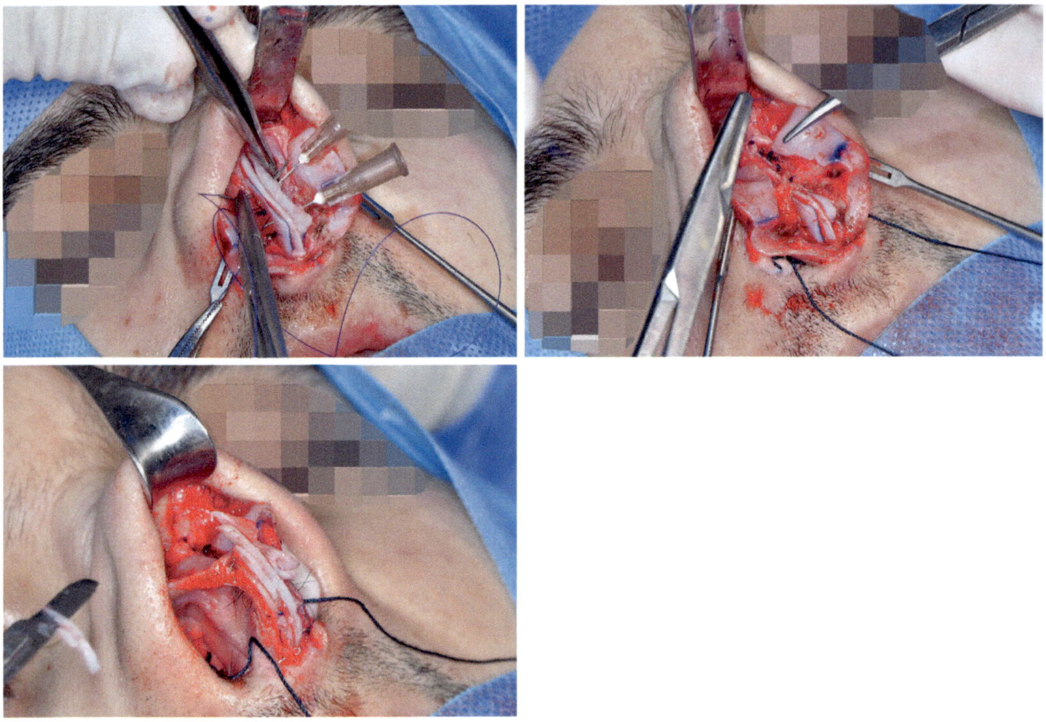

Fig. 9.9 (continued)

9.3 Concave

In 1896, Watson reported that many septal operations had been unsuccessful because they forgot that a deviated septum was larger than a straight one [6]. This statement should always be kept in mind when dealing with septal deviation. Concavity of the caudal segment is one of the biggest challenges in septal surgery because it narrows the internal nasal valve, which is the narrowest portion of the respiratory tract. In these cases, I prefer to dissect the mucoperichondrial flaps on both sides to diagnose the existing problem. When the caudal septum is longer than normal on the vertical plane, concavity can occur. If this is the case, the junction with the ANS of the caudal septum is detached, and the concavity is examined. If the caudal septum becomes straight, gradual shaving of the lower margin of the caudal septum is performed, and then it is sutured back to the anterior nasal spine (Fig. 9.10).

A second treatment option in cases of persistent concavity is cross-hatching of the concave surface of the caudal septum. Murakami et al. published an excellent article on the biomechanical behavior of septal cartilage [7]. They proposed applying full-thickness cuts to the concave surface of the cartilage while keeping the perichondrium intact on the convex side of the cartilage to straighten the convexity (Fig. 9.11a). They emphasized that partial cuts were not reliable for straightening the cartilage. The second option they suggested was to remove triangular slivers of cartilage from the convex part of the car-

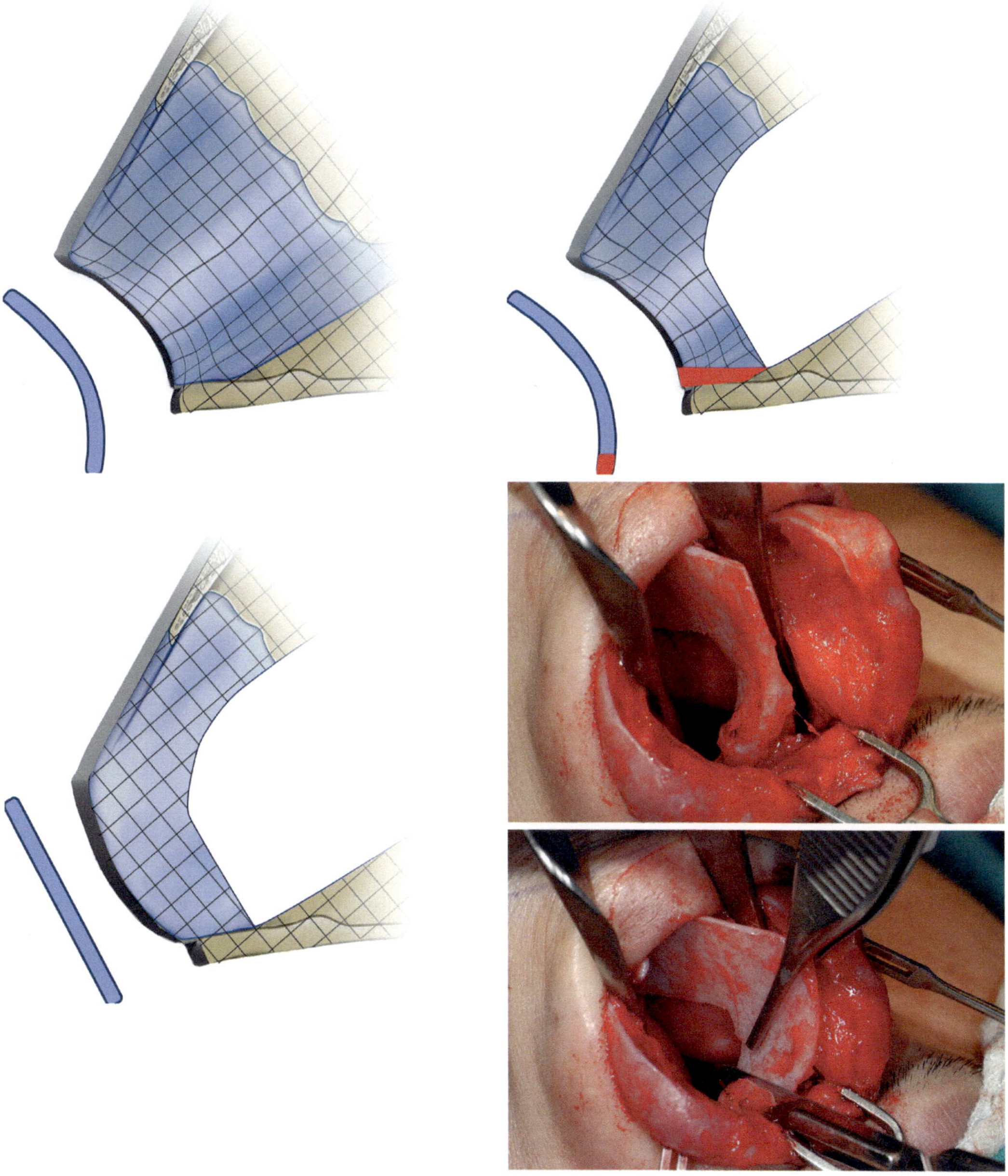

Fig. 9.10 Concavity of the caudal segment can be corrected by releasing it from the anterior nasal spine and then incrementally shaving from the lower portion of the caudal segment, and then it is sutured back to the anterior nasal spine

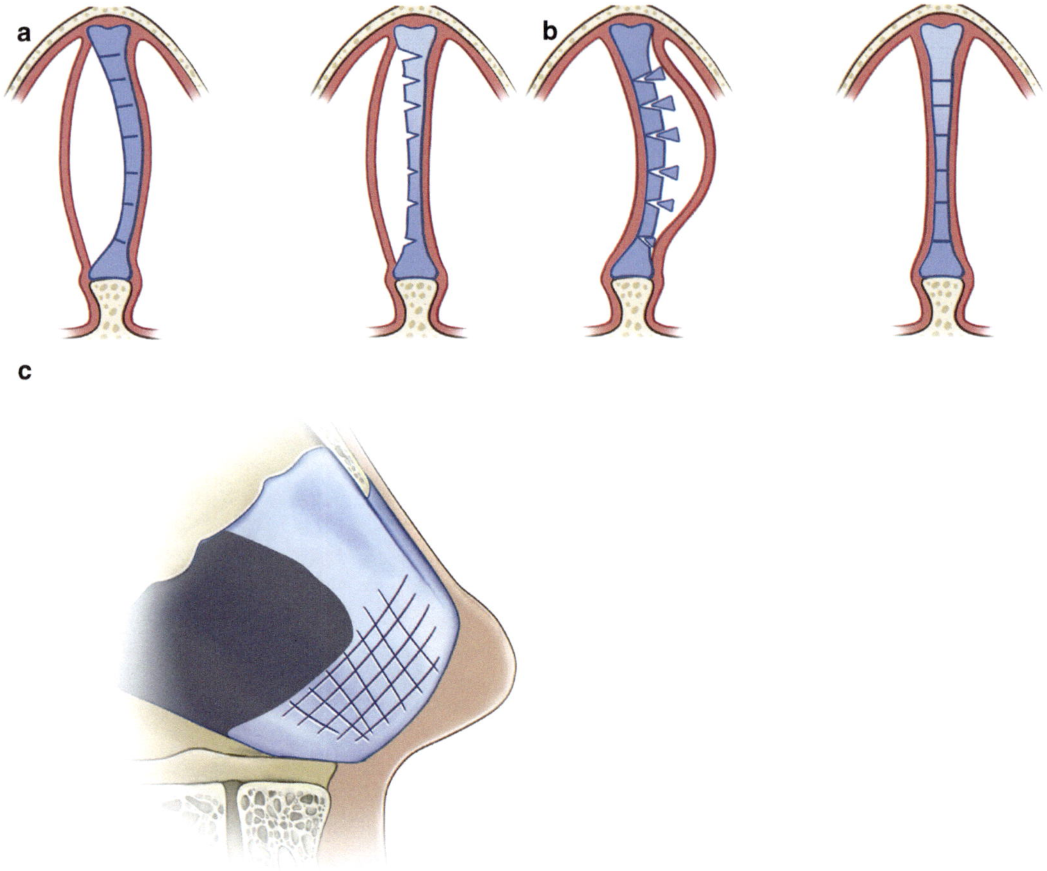

Fig. 9.11 Cross-hatching of the caudal septum. It can be performed in the shape of deep partial cuts to break the memory of the cartilage to prevent recurrent deviations (**a**). It can also be done on the convex surface by removing triangular slivers of cartilage from the convex part of the cartilage while keeping the perichondrium intact on the concave side (**b**). It is usually performed by horizontal and vertical cuts (**c**)

tilage while keeping the perichondrium intact on the concave side (Fig. 9.11b). I used them in the past, but I did not find them reliable. I faced two problems: recurrence of deviation and weakening of the caudal segment. Therefore, I have been using splinting batten grafts, usually grafts on the concave side after deep cross-hatching. These grafts are obtained from the bony or cartilaginous septum (Fig. 9.12). The reason I like bony grafts more is their width. They are much thinner than the cartilaginous grafts, although they can stiffen the nasal tip [4, 8] (Fig. 9.13). However, cartilage is found in ample amounts, and I like using cartilage batten grafts more. Sometimes, a caudal septal extension or L-strut graft can be used for the same purpose (Figs. 9.14 and 9.15).

A third option is to use the swinging door technique [2]. In this technique, the long caudal septum is dislocated from the anterior nasal spine, which is not in the midline and is crooked. Then, the caudal septum is placed on the contralateral side of the deviated anterior nasal spine, using it like a doorstop to stay in the midline. Sometimes, the deviated wing of the anterior nasal spine should be resected to widen the nasal airway (Fig. 9.16).

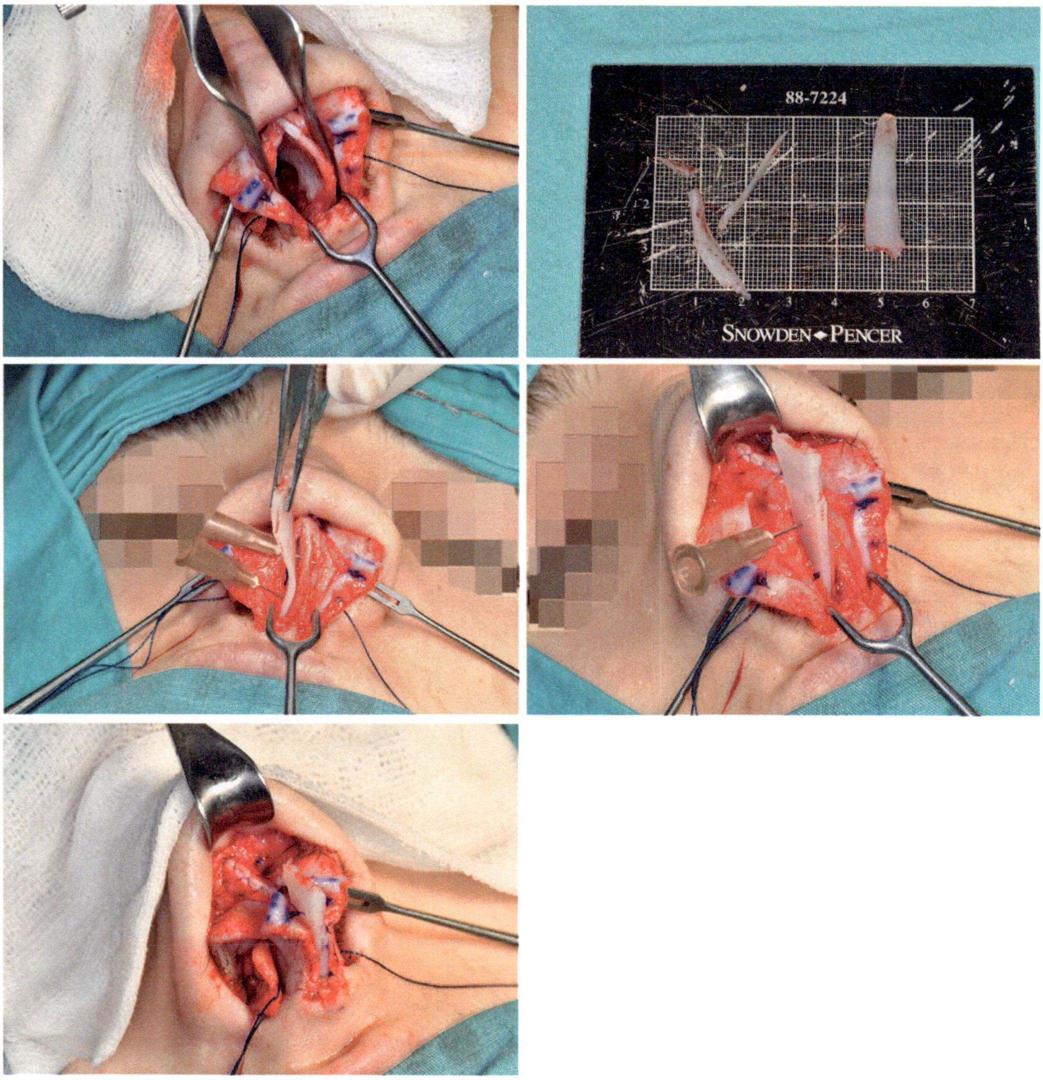

Fig. 9.12 Splinting batten grafts, usually grafts on the concave side after deep cross-hatching. These grafts are obtained from the bony or cartilaginous septum

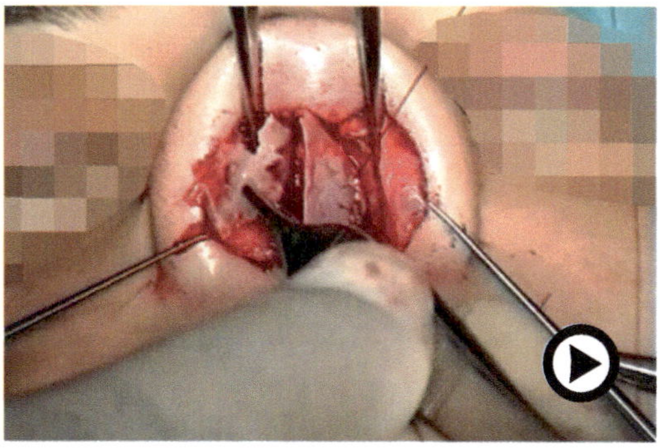

Fig. 9.13 Two pieces of ethmoid bone are used to splint the crooked septum like a sandwich (▶ https://doi.org/10.1007/000-dyh)

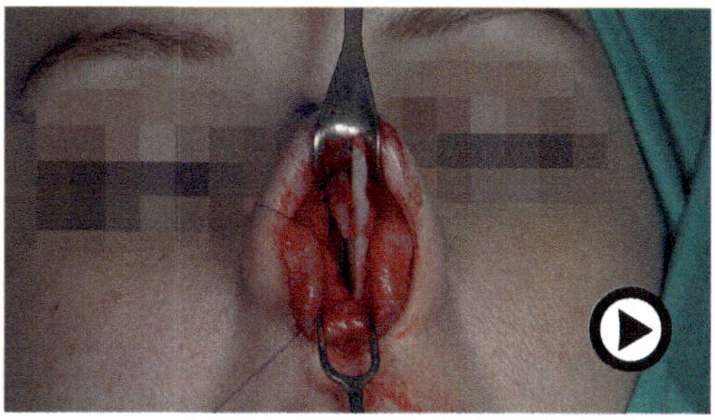

Fig. 9.14 Septal cartilage is used to reconstruct the L-strut framework (▶ https://doi.org/10.1007/000-dyj)

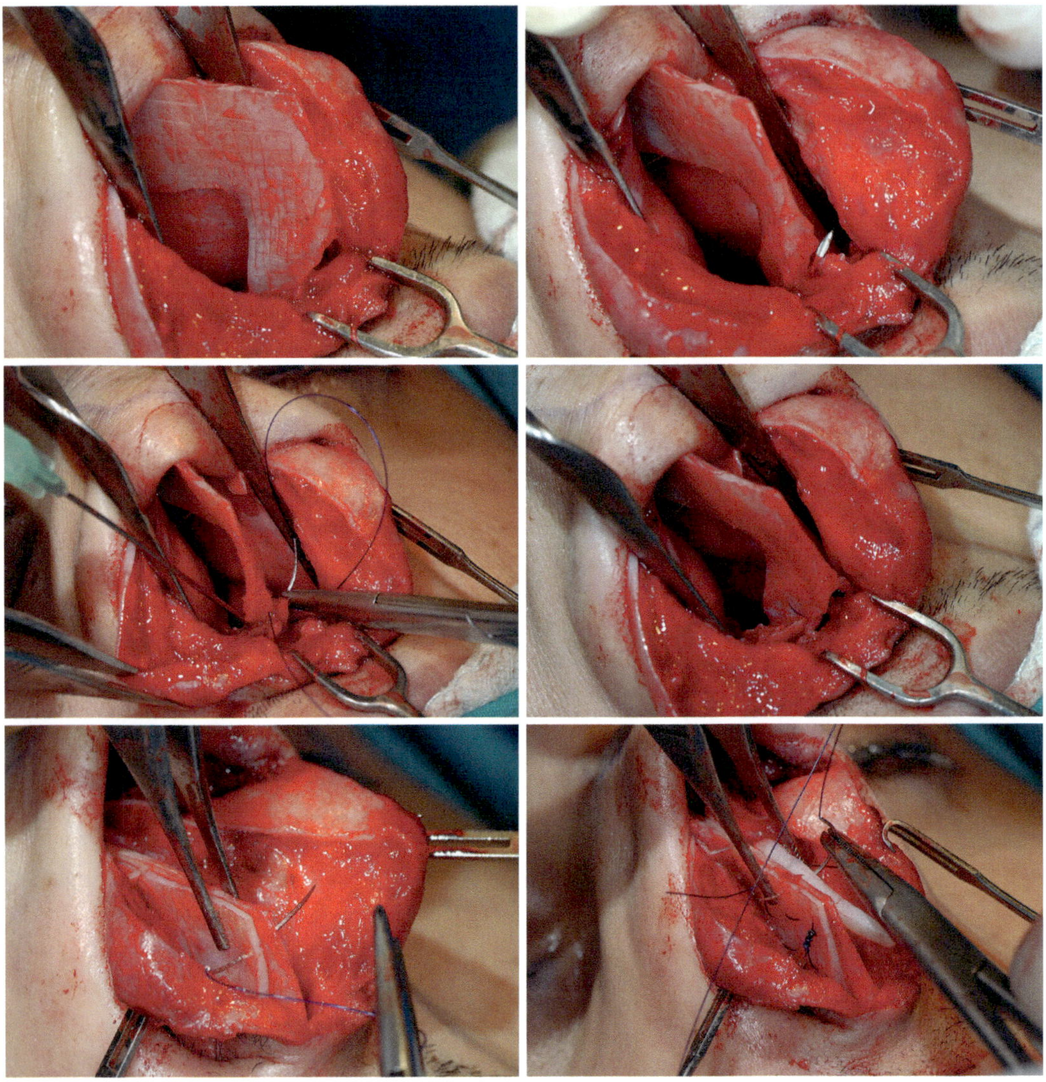

Fig. 9.15 An L-strut graft can be used to splint the cross-hatched caudal septum

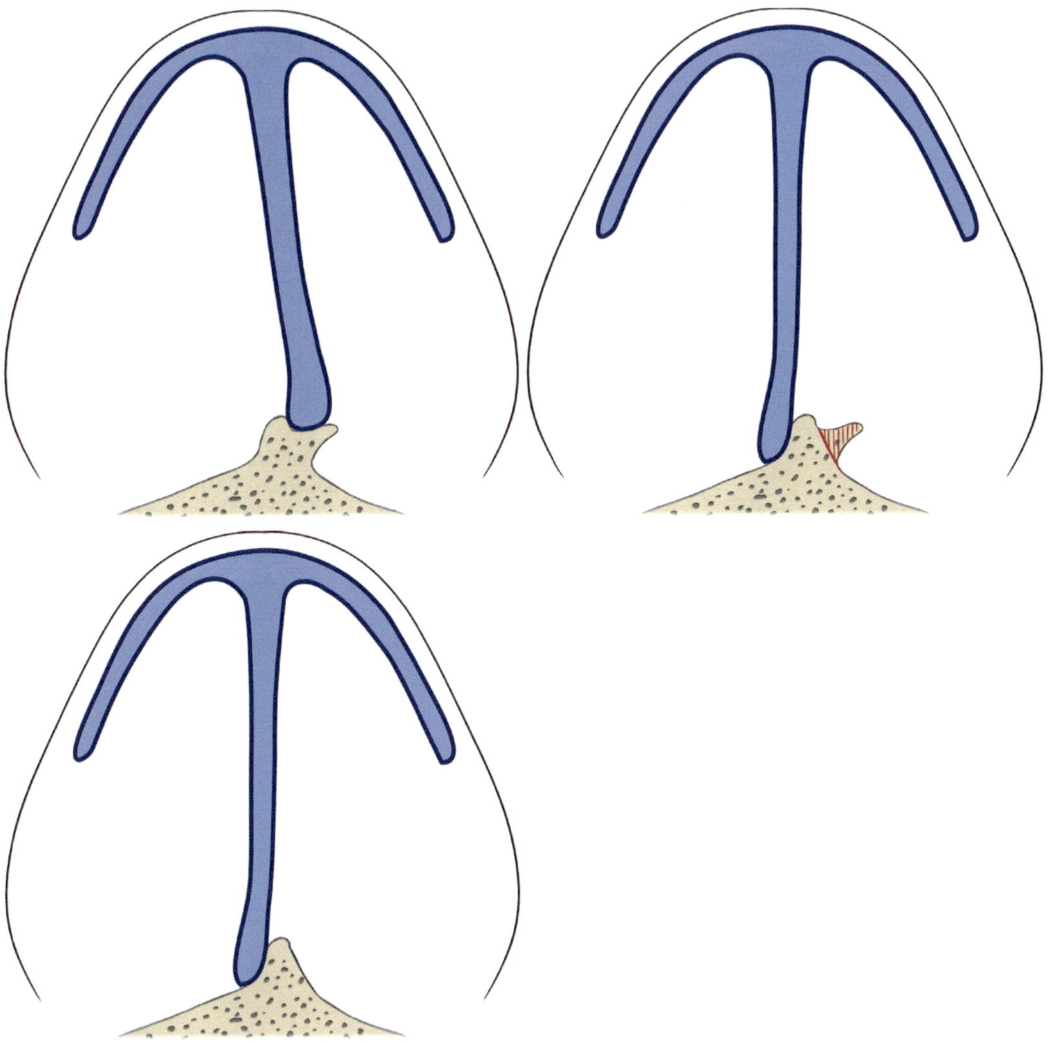

Fig. 9.16 Swinging door technique is a powerful technique to medialize the caudal septum by using the anterior nasal spine like a door stop. Sometimes the deviated wing of the anterior nasal spine should be resected to widen the nasal airway

9.4 Retracted

The caudal segment can be retracted because of previous nasal trauma, septal surgery, or rhinoplasty (Fig. 9.17). When the caudal septum is retracted, the tip is usually droopy because of losing an important supporting structure in the midline. The solution is to lengthen the caudal septum by using a septal extension graft (Fig. 9.18). There are many surgical alternatives to solve this problem. Byrd et al. described three forms of septal extension grafts: paired spreader grafts, paired batten grafts, and direct extension grafts [9] (Fig. 9.19). In crooked noses, paired spreader grafts work fine because the crooked dorsal segment is splinted and corrected, and the tip posi-

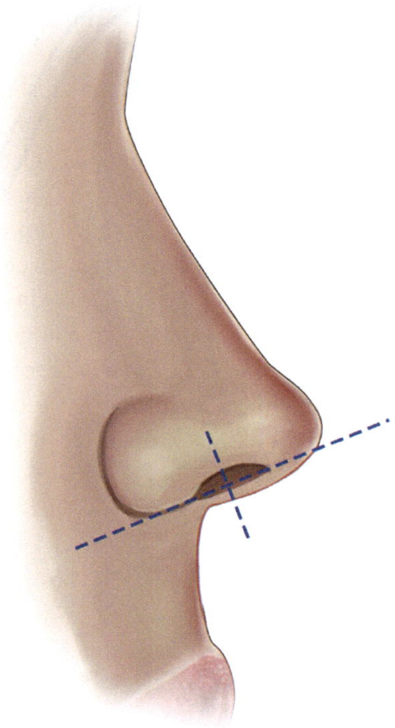

Fig. 9.17 Retracted columella can be due to a retracted caudal septum because of previous nasal trauma, septal surgery, or rhinoplasty

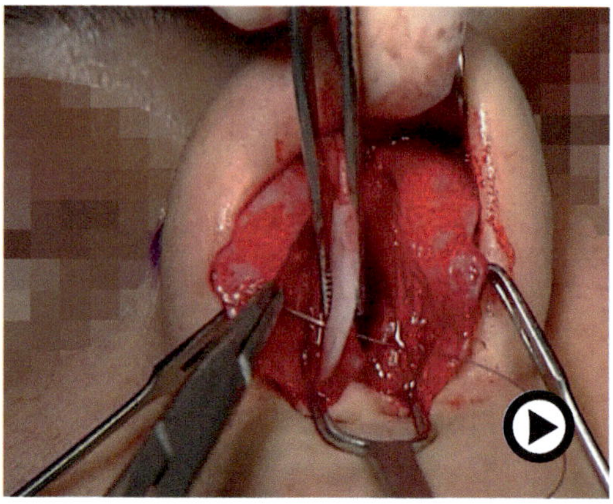

Fig. 9.18 Caudal Septal Extension Graft is designed and sutured (▶ https://doi.org/10.1007/000-dyk)

Fig. 9.19 Byrd described paired spreader grafts, paired batten grafts, and direct extension grafts as three forms of septal extension grafts

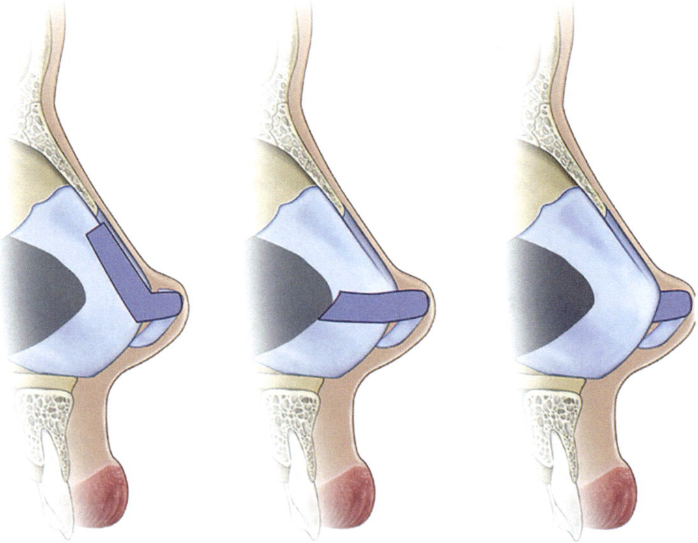

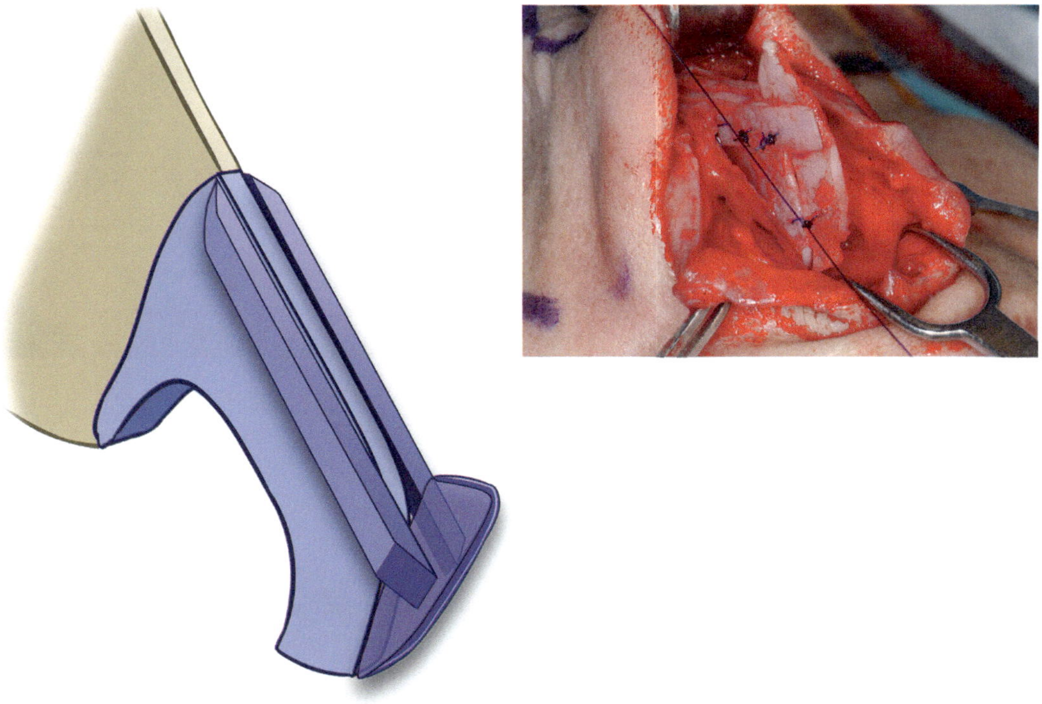

Fig. 9.20 Guyuron reported suturing the spreader grafts in place and suturing a septal extension graft to the spreader grafts and to the caudal septum.

tion can be adjusted on the longer end of these grafts. There is a need to obtain big septal cartilage from the nasal septum, which is not always easy. Guyuron reported a technique to lengthen the short nose, which can also be easily used in the case of a retracted columella. After suturing the spreader grafts in place with three sutures, a septal extension graft is sutured to the spreader grafts and to the caudal septum [10] (Fig. 9.20). In my opinion, this is the best technique for primary and revision cases to get rid of the retracted columella and to lengthen the nose. Toriumi used the same technique and added small slivers of cartilage for better fixation between the midportion of the caudal septum and septal extension graft [11] (Fig. 9.21).

In fact, all other techniques on the septal extension grafts are slight modifications of the three kinds of septal extension grafts described by Byrd. Paired batten grafts of Byrd have become more popular in the following years until now. Seyhan claimed that the Byrd techniques could cause nasal tip stiffness and thickening of the septum in the nasal valve area and proposed single batten grafts or bilateral asymmetric batten graft applications to overcome these problems [12] (Fig. 9.22). A one-sided overlapping caudal septal extension graft was described and became very popular, especially in Latin America and the Far East [13] (Fig. 9.23). I had a chance to witness the reasons for this technique by myself after lecturing and operating in these countries. The tip usually has weak cartilages and thick skin and needs strong midline support. Unfortunately, the caudal septum is also weak, and the septal cartilage is small. So, my colleagues have been using the main harvested cartilage as an overlapping septal extension graft to give the best possible projection and rotation to the tip [14–16] (Fig. 9.24).

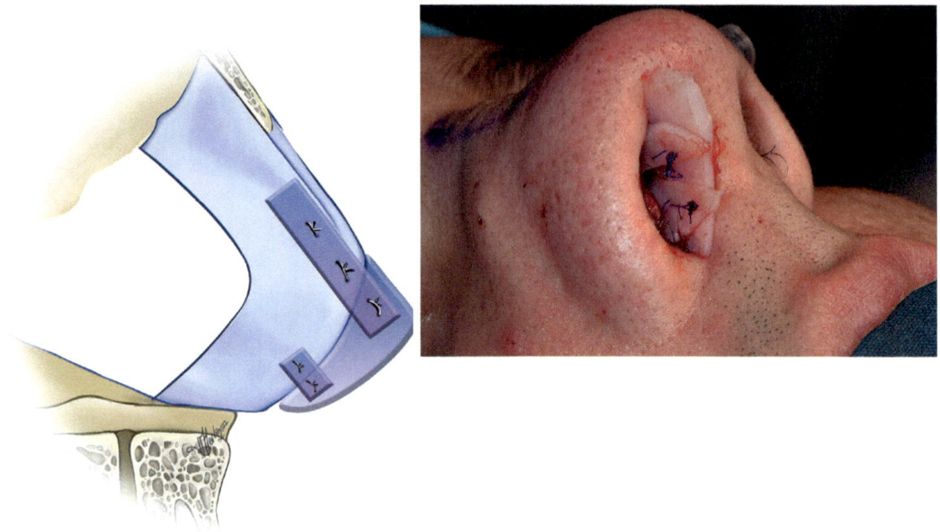

Fig. 9.21 Toriumi added small slivers of cartilage for better fixation between the midportion of the caudal septum and the septal extension graft. Illustration çiz

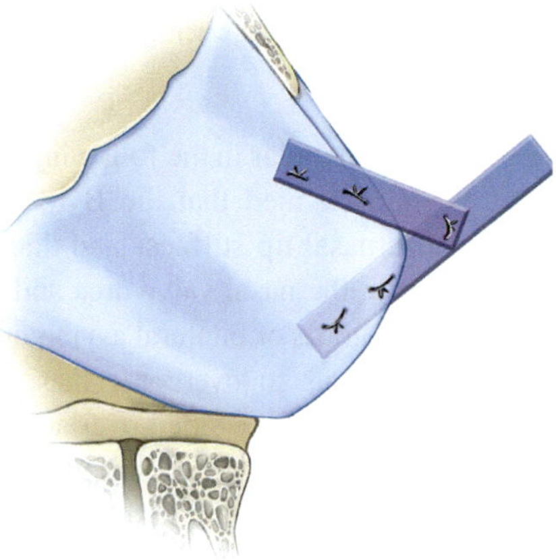

Fig. 9.22 Seyhan proposed single batten grafts or bilateral asymmetric batten graft applications to overcome nasal tip stiffness and thickening of the septum in the nasal valve area

In cases where there is not enough cartilage available, Byrd suggested the use of a direct extension graft. It was proposed before by Dibbell in 1976 as a cartilaginous columellar strut in cleft lip rhinoplasty patients [17]. I have also been using this technique in some cases by using "shoelace" type of suturing for the strut (Figs. 9.25 and 9.26). In this technique, a curved extended columellar strut is prepared to sit on the caudal end. Dimensions are customized according to the needs. Then, starting from below, continuous suturing using a mixture of sutures of eight and simple sutures is performed between the caudal segment and the back portion of the strut all the way up, and then down using 5-0 PDS. When the loose loops are tightened and tied, the extended columellar strut acts like a new caudal segment. There is one prerequisite for this technique: the caudal septum must be straight and strong enough to create a strong base for the graft. Davis published a modification of this graft, making it big to sit on the caudal end and the first 5–6 mm of the caudal portion of the dorsal segment of the septal cartilage [18] (Fig. 9.27). This is a smart idea because one of the main problems of using an end-to-end SEG is the possibility of twisting. When this graft is sutured to the nasal dorsum and caudal septum, it is less likely that it can twist. Although Davis reported successful results with this technique, I have two reservations: (1) a big piece of cartilage is needed to create this graft, and (2) the caudal septum is

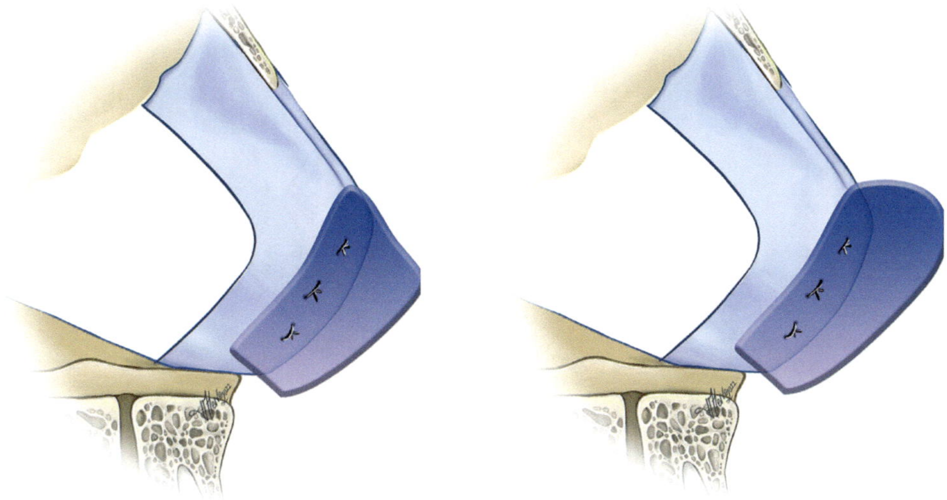

Fig. 9.23 One-sided overlapping caudal septal extension grafts can be of different sizes

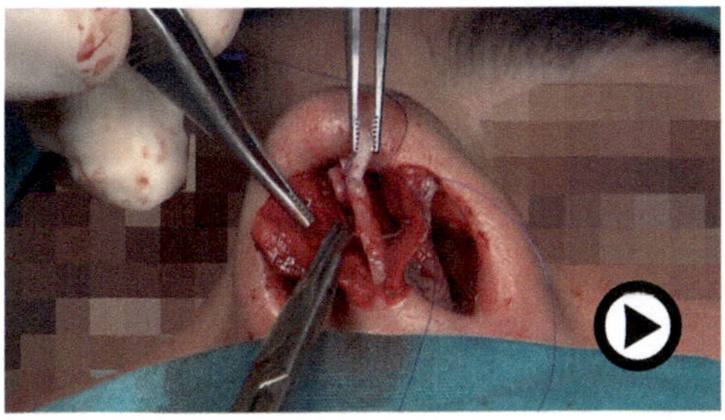

Fig. 9.24 A big size Caudal Septal Extension Graft is designed and sutured (▶ https://doi.org/10.1007/000-dym)

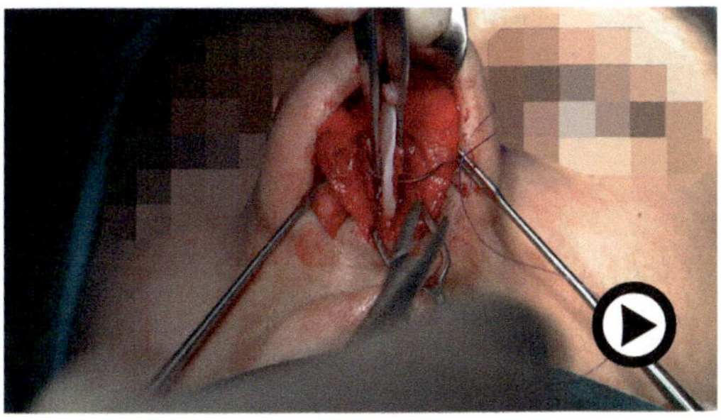

Fig. 9.25 Shoelace Suturing of Direct Septal Extension Graft (▶ https://doi.org/10.1007/000-dyf)

usually the weakest portion of the septal cartilage, and a big mass of cartilage is sutured on it to carry the tip. This can cause a collapse or twisting of the tip, which I have observed in a few cases by myself. Therefore, I do not use this technique.

My preference in retracted columella is to use an SEG coupled with one or two spreader grafts to secure the graft's position in the midline, as described by Guyuron and Toriumi. In cases where the caudal septum is deviated or weak, the extension graft overlaps the caudal septum and acts like a batten graft as well (Fig. 9.28). In these cases, it is important to overlap the extension graft on the wider side of the nasal airway. Otherwise, the graft itself can cause narrowing of the nasal valve area. Besides, a contralateral supporting spreader graft is of utmost importance to keep the septal extension graft in the midline (Fig. 9.29).

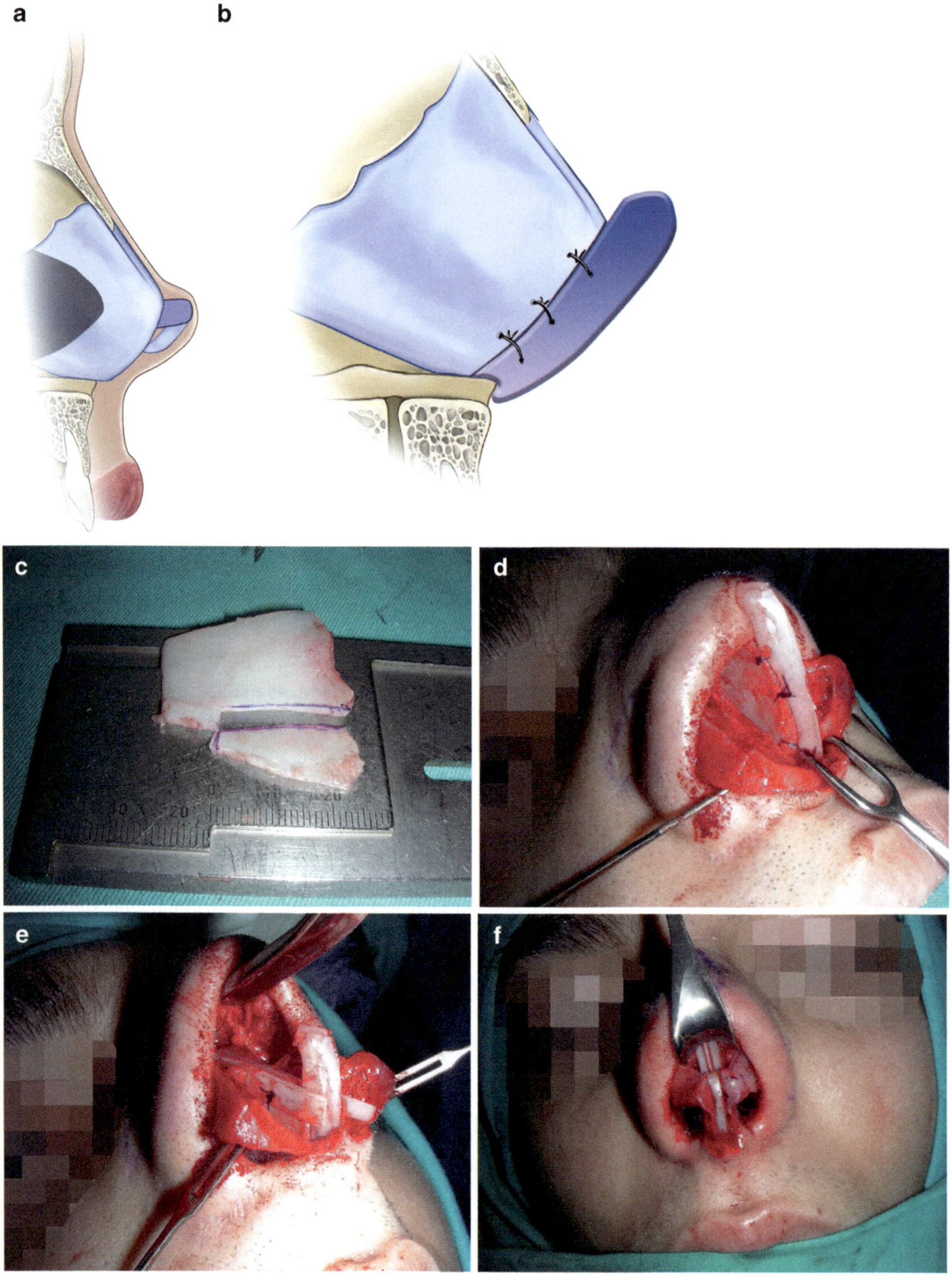

Fig. 9.26 Direct extension grafts can be used when there is not enough cartilage available. Byrd (**a**), Dibbell (**b**–**f**), and shoelace-type suturing of the strut (**g**) can be used

g

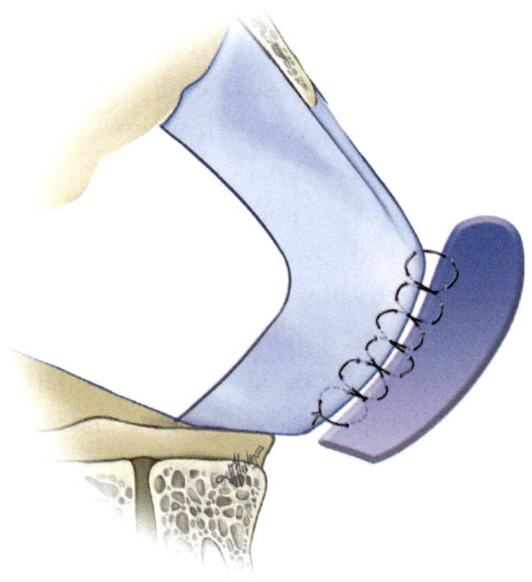

Fig. 9.26 (continued)

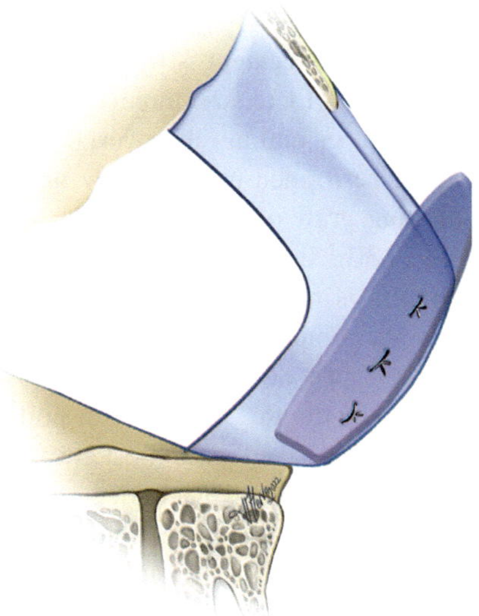

Fig. 9.28 In cases where the caudal septum is deviated or weak, the extension graft overlaps the caudal septum and acts like a batten graft

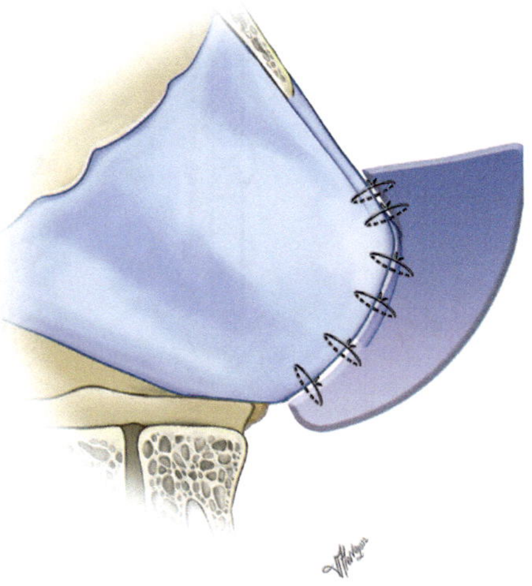

Fig. 9.27 Davis reported a big direct extension graft sitting on the caudal end and the first 5–6 mm of the caudal portion of the dorsal segment of the septal cartilage

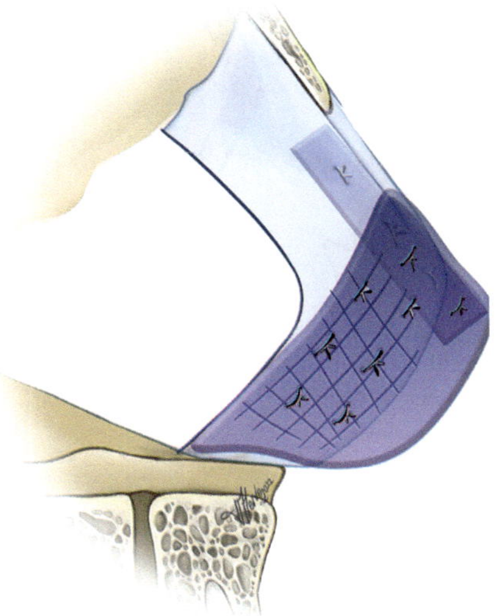

Fig. 9.29 A contralateral supporting spreader graft is of utmost importance to keep the septal extension graft in the midline

9.5 Fractured

If the caudal segment is fractured and causes an obstruction, there are three options: splinting, replacing, or cutting and overlapping. Splinting can be performed using a bony or cartilaginous splinting graft obtained from the nasal septum (Fig. 9.30). If there are multiple fractures and splinting is not possible, the caudal segment is removed completely. In my experience, although the anterior one-third of the nasal septum is affected by trauma, the posterior portions are not affected much, and it is almost always possible to obtain straight, large pieces of cartilage and bone. These fragments can be used for splinting or replacement (Figs. 9.31 and 9.32).

To obtain bony implants from the ethmoid and vomer, I have been using Heyman and Kaplan-Meyer scissors for decades. Recently, Piezo ultrasonic devices with longer tips have also been very helpful. The special difficulty is always cutting the bony fragments from their posterior ends. In these cases, the use of endoscopes and the long tips of Piezo are very helpful.

On rare occasions, a horizontal fracture line on the deviated caudal segment can be cut, and the upper and lower segments can be overlapped and sutured; thus, the deviation is corrected. Although I used this method in a couple of cases, I still felt the necessity of adding a batten graft to stay on the safe side (Figs. 9.33 and 9.34). A similar technique was described by Kim by adding an interposition batten graft between the divided fractured fragments [19] (Fig. 9.35). It is also possible to excise a triangular piece of cartilage at the fracture line and rejoin the fractured and folded caudal nasal septum by sutures and/or batten graft [20] (Fig. 9.30).

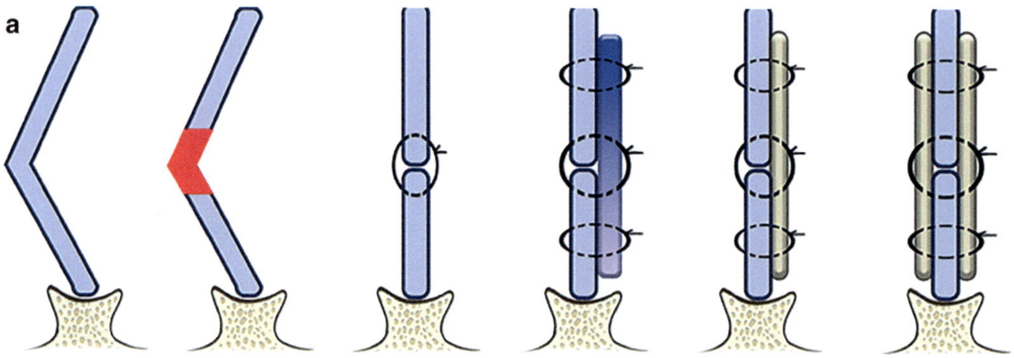

Fig. 9.30 If the caudal segment is fractured, the fracture line can be resected, sutured end-to-end, and splinted by cartilage or bone (**a–f**)

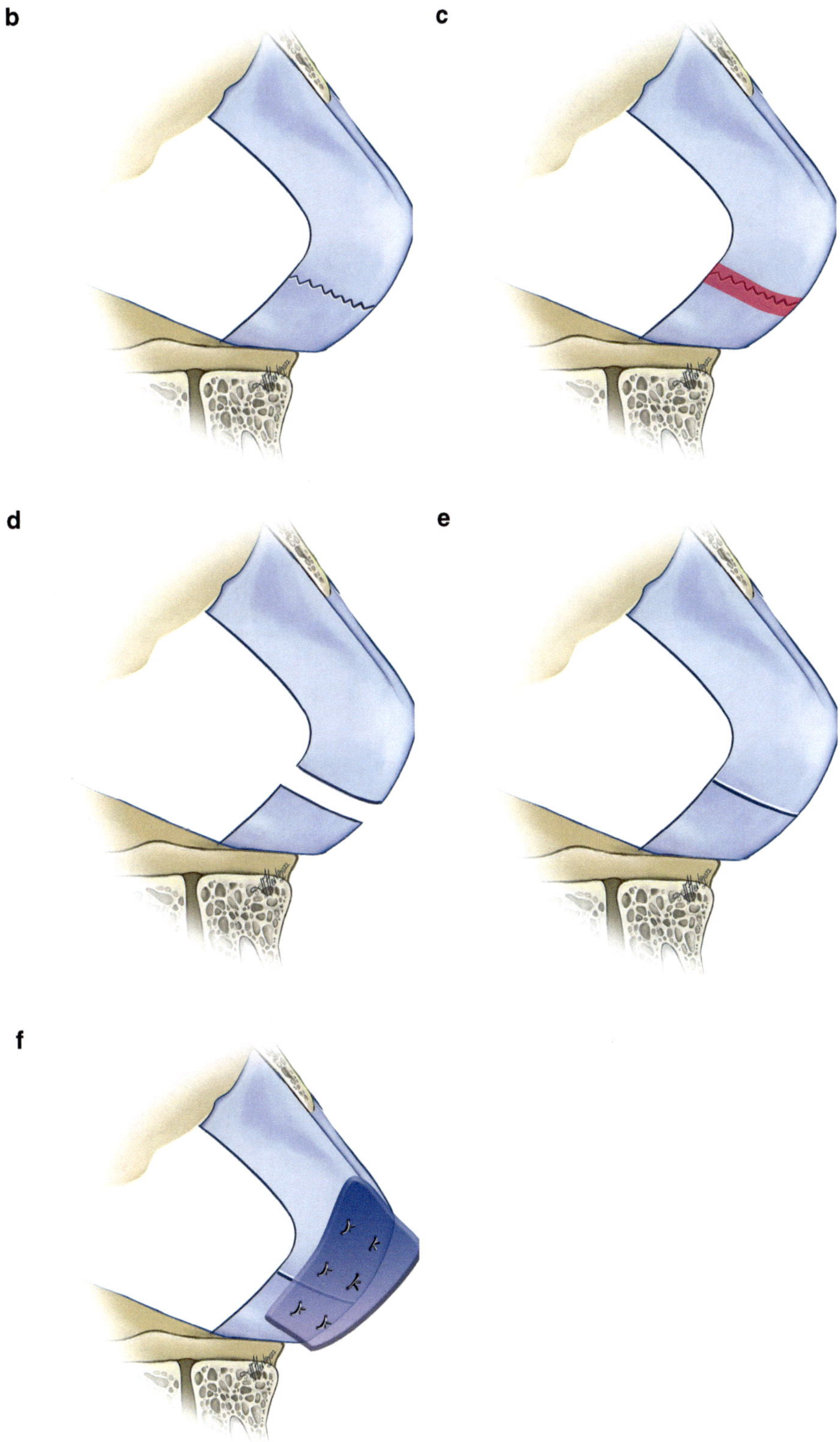

Fig. 9.30 (continued)

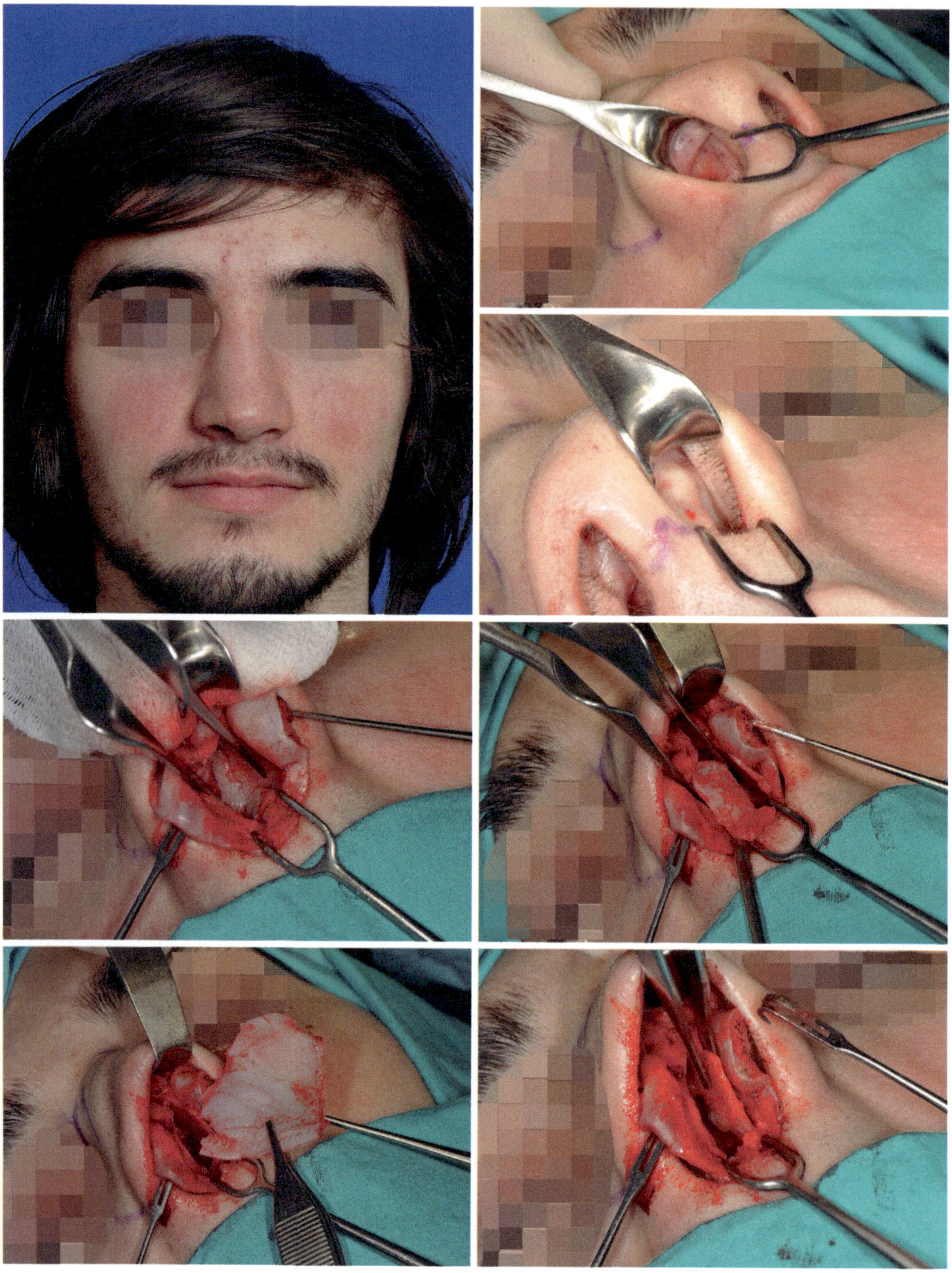

Fig. 9.31 In this case, there are multiple fracture lines on the caudal segment. They were resected, and a caudal septal replacement graft was used. Besides, the right wing of the anterior nasal spine was removed. The postoperative pictures were taken in the first year

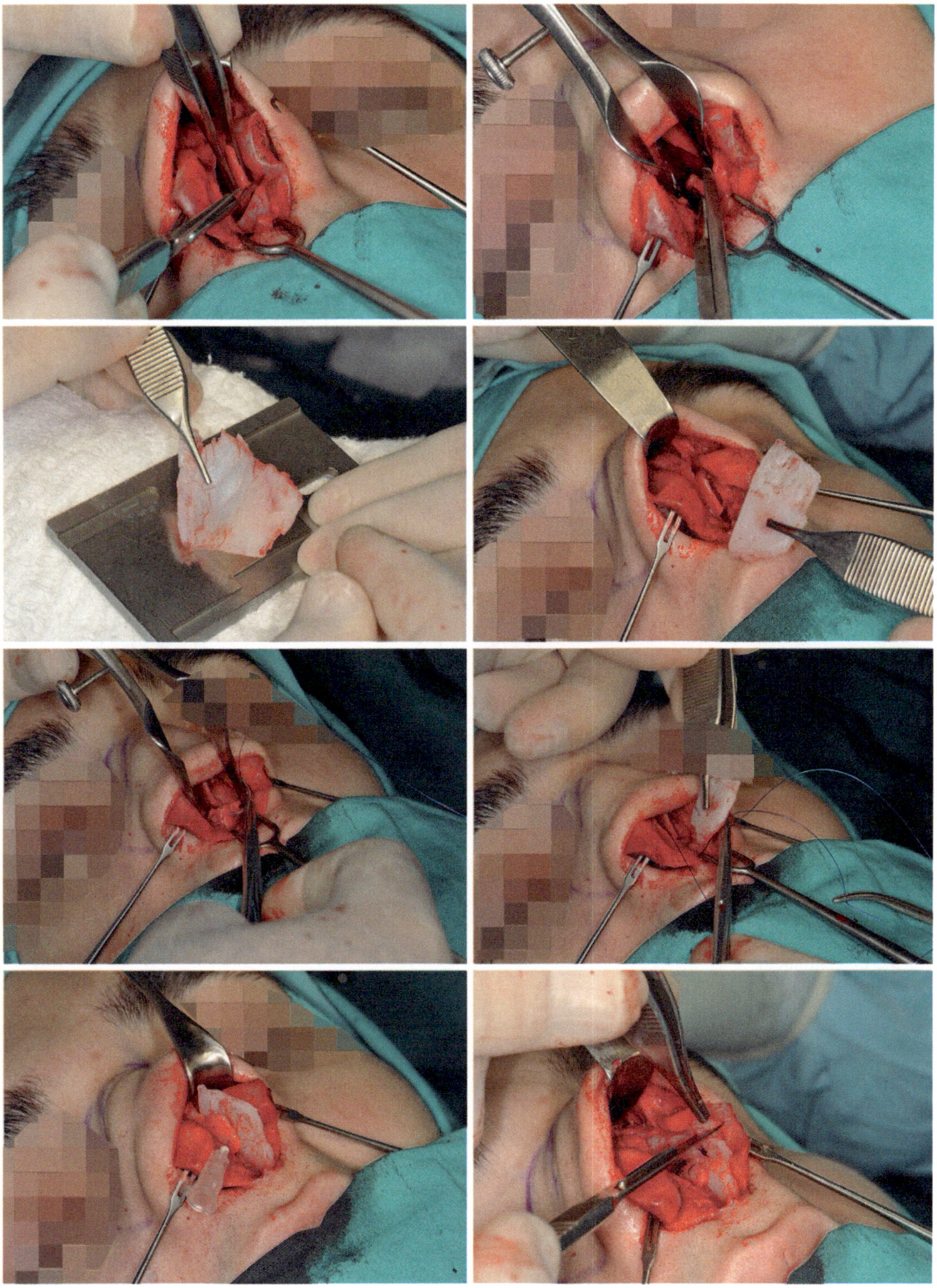

Fig. 9.31 (continued)

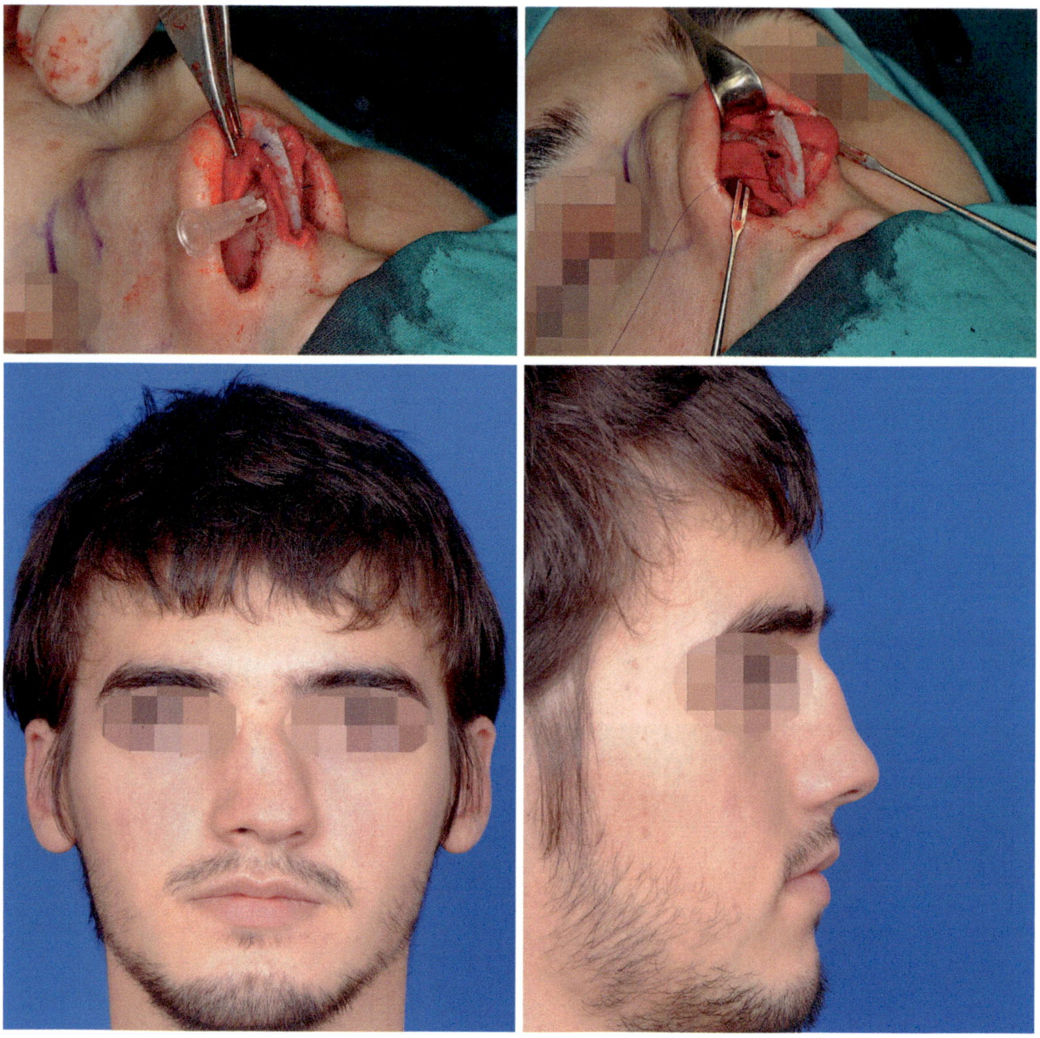

Fig. 9.31 (continued)

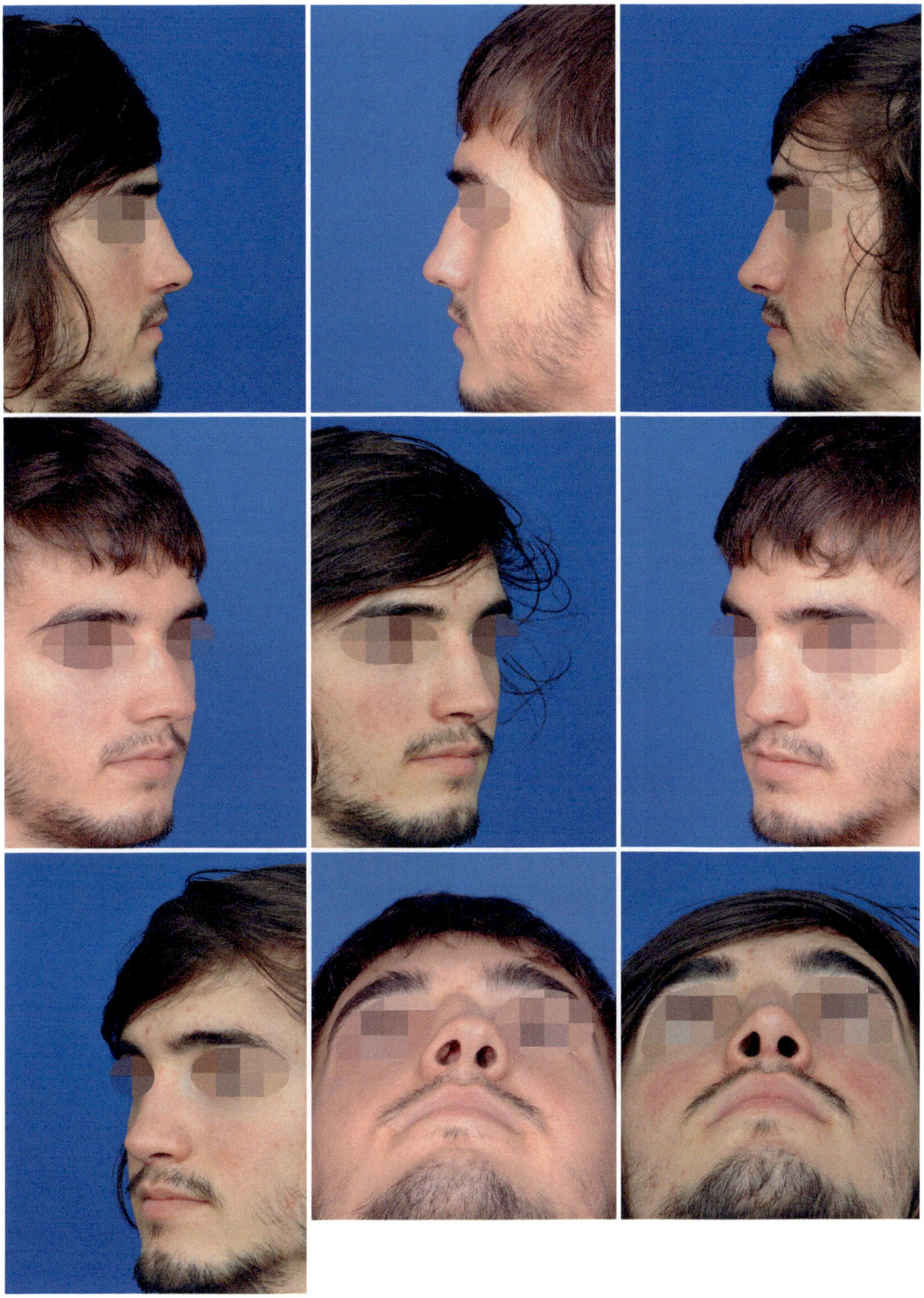

Fig. 9.31 (continued)

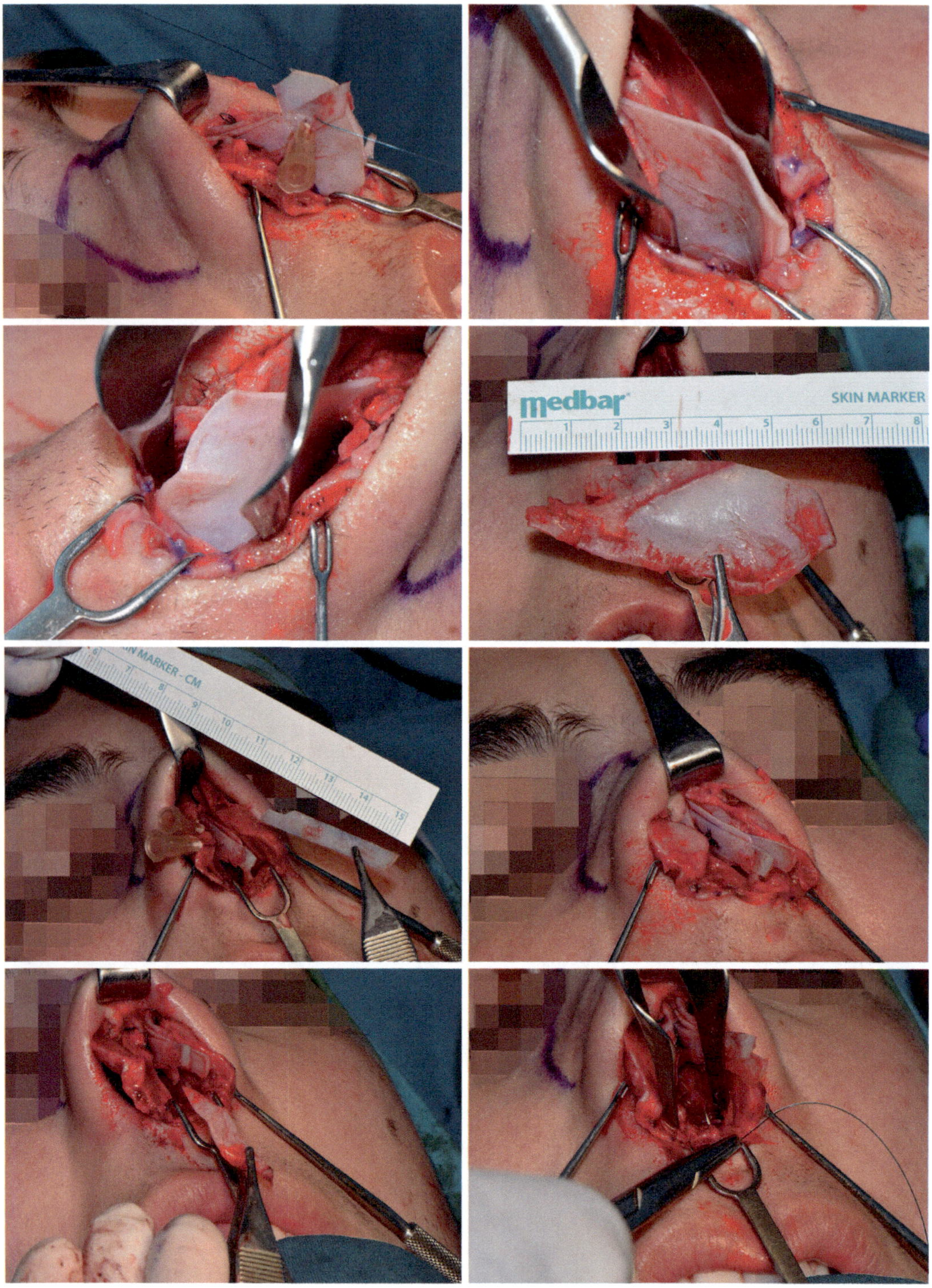

Fig. 9.32 In this case, the lower part of the fractured segment was resected. Two spreader grafts and a caudal septal replacement graft were used to reconstruct the L-strut framework

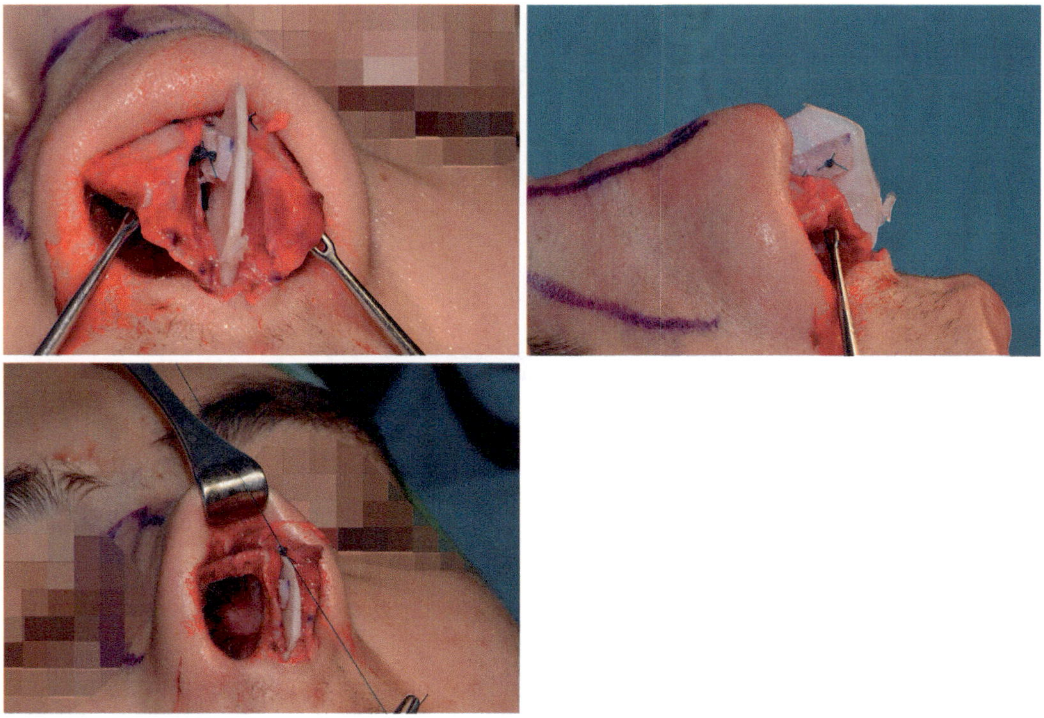

Fig. 9.32 (continued)

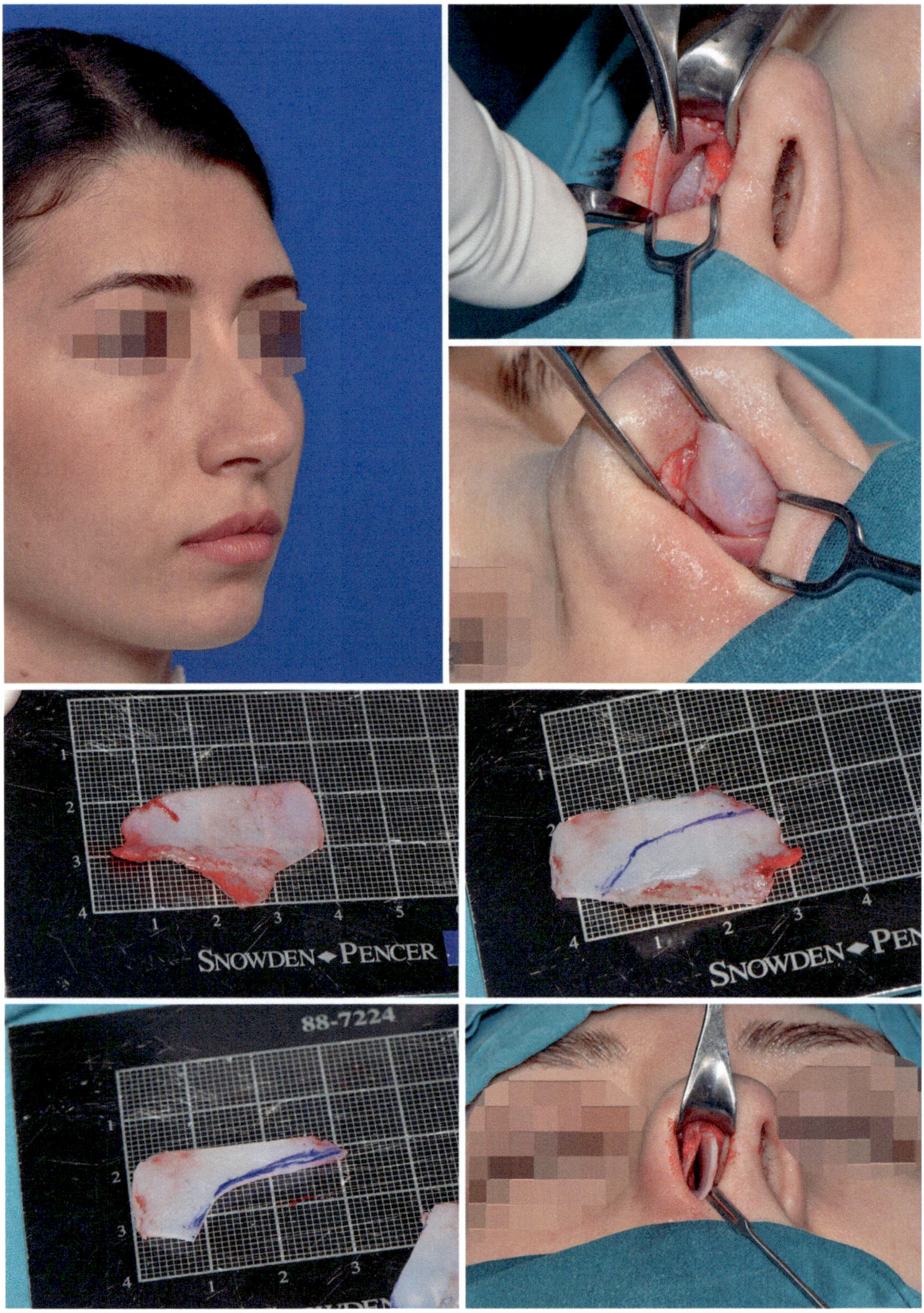

Fig. 9.33 There is a fracture line on the caudal segment. It was splinted with an L-strut graft. The caudal septum was long, so it was cut, and the cut ends were overlapped and sutured

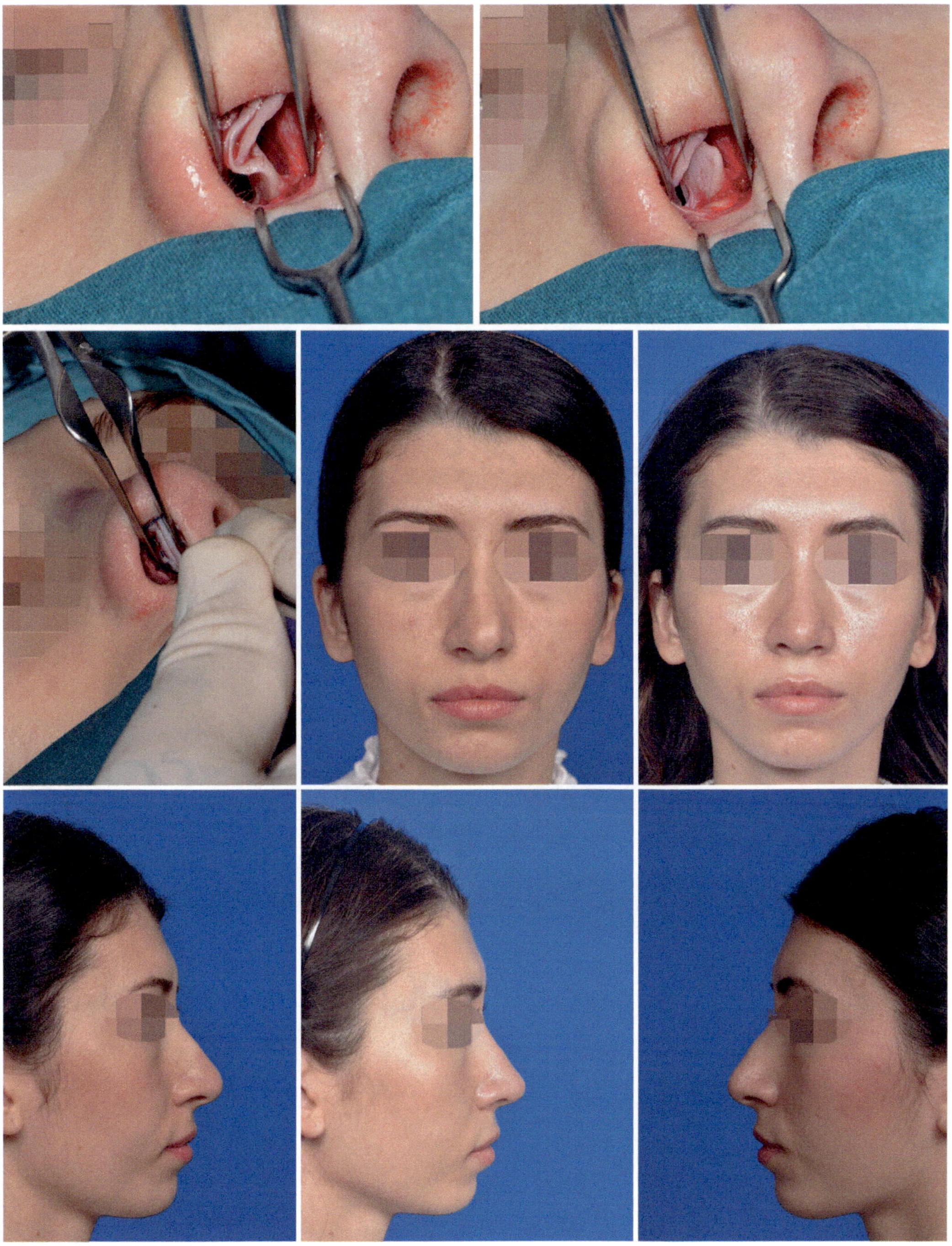

Fig. 9.33 (continued)

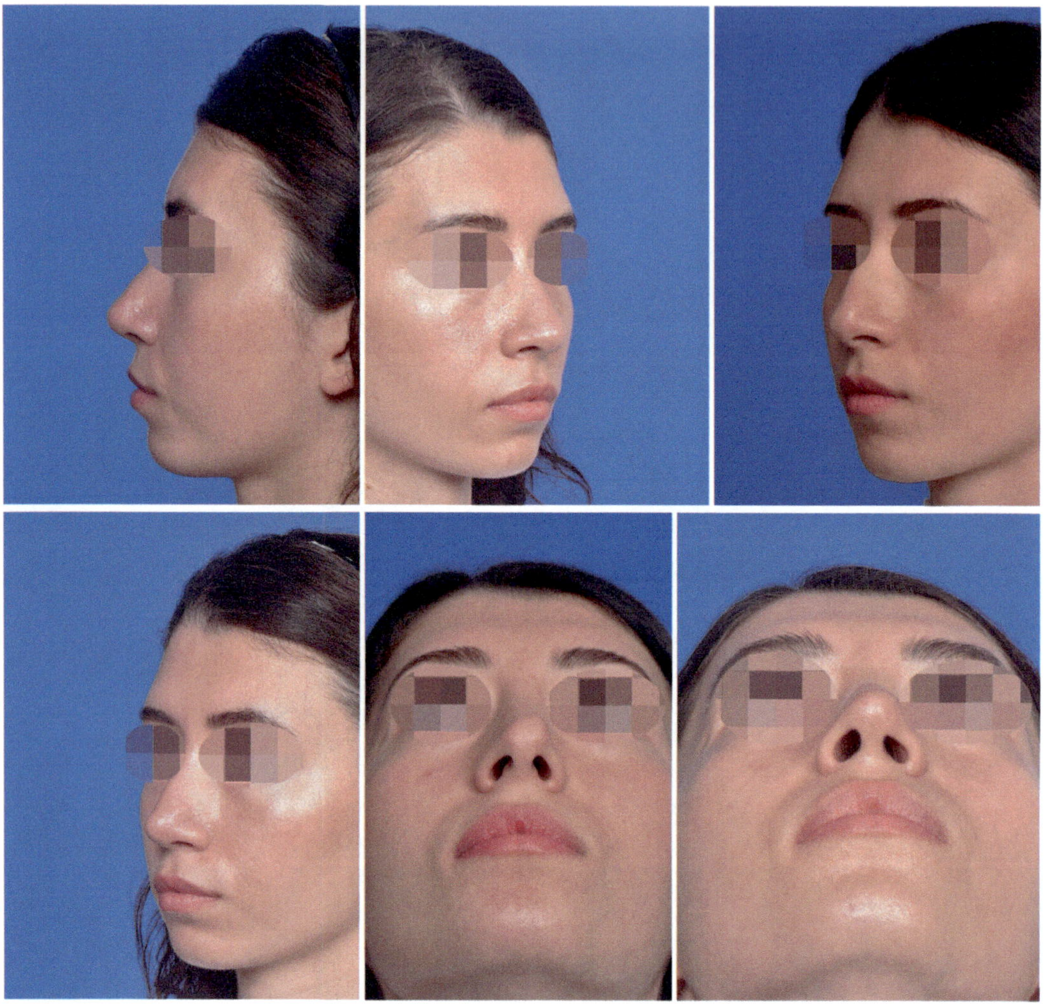

Fig. 9.33 (continued)

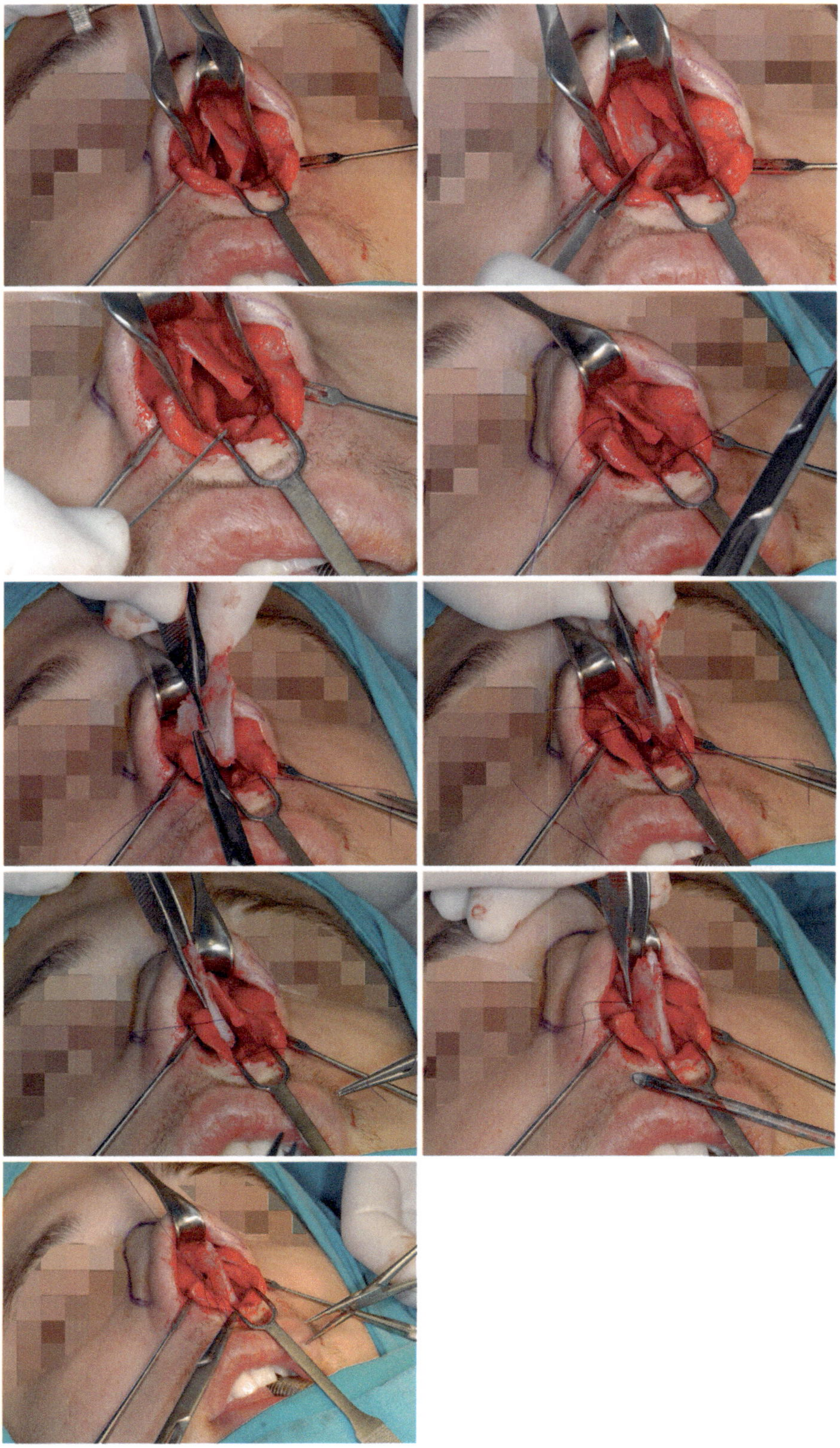

Fig. 9.34 In this case the lower part of the fractured segment was resected, and a caudal septal replacement graft was used to support the caudal septum.

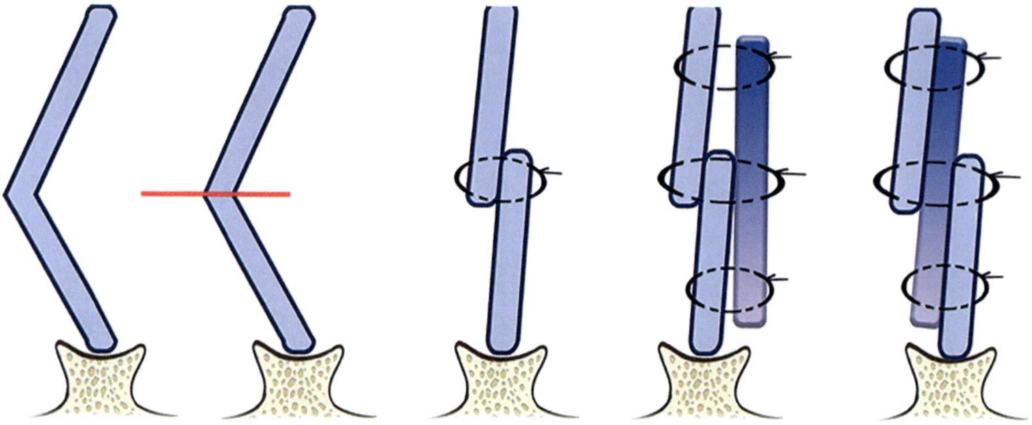

Fig. 9.35 A full cut on the fracture line can be done, and the edges can be overlapped and supported by a batten graft. A different technique is to add an interposition batten graft between the divided fractured fragments

9.6 Missing Caudal Segment

This situation may be due to previous trauma and surgery. It is the most difficult situation to correct (Fig. 9.36). If there is sufficient cartilage in the nasal septum, it is relatively easy to carve a caudal septal replacement graft (Figs. 9.35 and 9.37). If not, grafts from the conchal cartilage or costal cartilage should be used. Because conchal cartilage is like a bowl in shape, it should be reshaped by folding it over itself and sutured to straighten. Then, it can be used as the new caudal segment (Figs. 9.38, 9.39, 9.40, 9.41 and 9.42).

Peer was the first to describe caudal septal replacement graft in 1937 in the management of severely crooked noses [21]. The details of this technique were given in Chap. 2. The same terminology was later brought to our attention by Foda in 2008. He published his experience of using caudal septal replacement grafts obtained from septum, ear, and irradiated rib cartilage in 120 cases [22].

In cases where the septal cartilage and ear cartilage are not enough and more cartilaginous implants are necessary, the rib cartilage is the best option for me. I have been using rib cartilage for surgery for more than three decades. In my hands, the costal cartilages from 5 to 8 can be used during rhinoplasty. I have used two techniques to obtain caudal septal replacement grafts: (1) Davis and Gibson's method [23] and (2) the oblique split technique [24]. In the first technique, the middle portion of the rib cartilage is used. I have used these types of grafts for years, since 1999, mainly in revision cases, with success (Fig. 9.43). I did not have warping issues except in a few cases. I had two main issues with

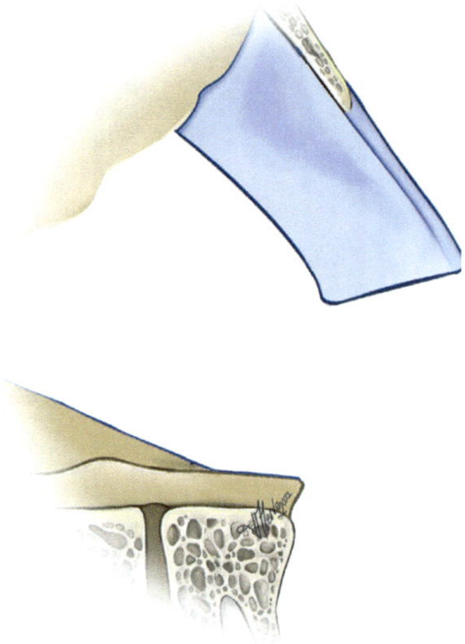

Fig. 9.36 The caudal segment of the nasal septum can be missing due to previous surgery or trauma

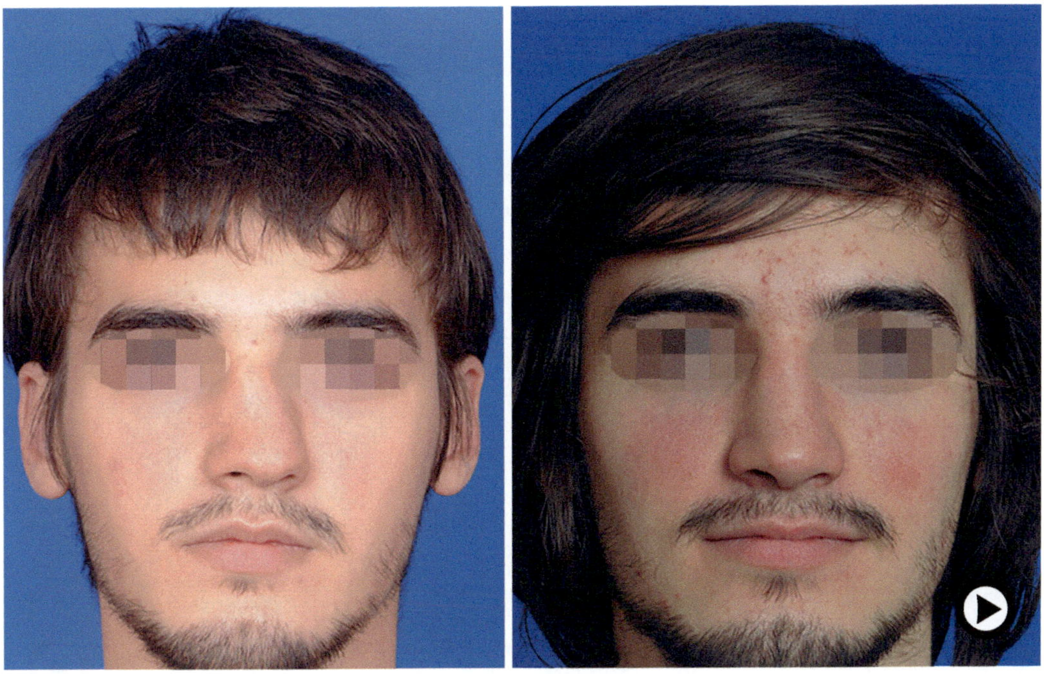

Fig. 9.37 Caudal Septal Replacement Graft in Crooked Nose (▶ https://doi.org/10.1007/000-dyp)

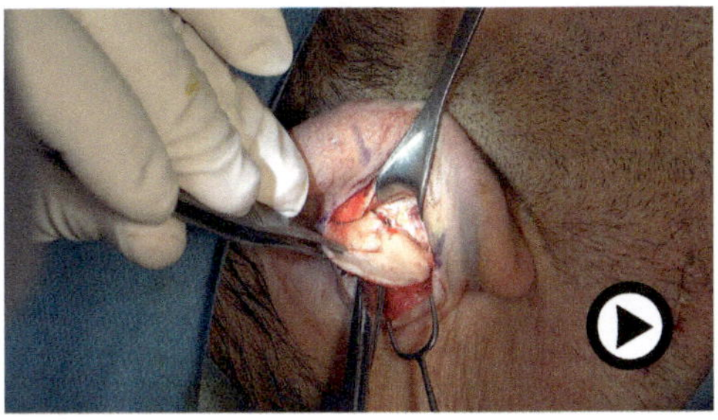

Fig. 9.38 Ear cartilage harvest from a postauricular approach (▶ https://doi.org/10.1007/000-dyq)

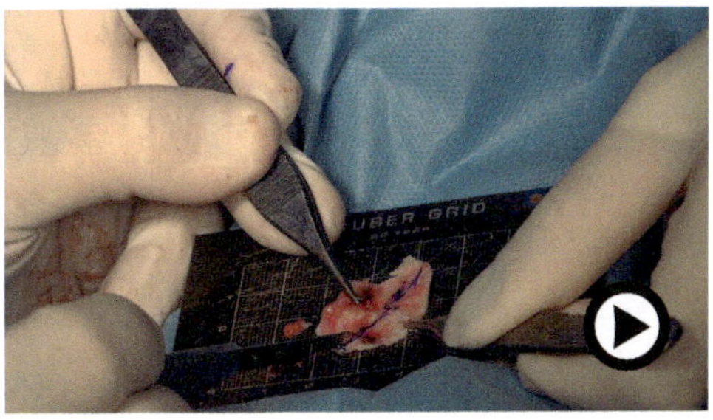

Fig. 9.39 A caudal septal extension graft is designed from ear cartilage and sutured in place (▶ https://doi.org/10.1007/000-dyr)

this method. I could not have enough implants for other grafts, and my grafts were bulky. I switched to the oblique split technique in 2011. In this technique, the costal cartilage is cut obliquely. With this method, I can obtain more grafts with variable thickness, and I observed that there was less chance of warping and resorption, as all layers of the inner and outer cortex of the costal cartilage were preserved in all the implants [25] (Figs. 9.44 and 9.45).

The caudal portion of the nasal septum is the most affected part of the nose in trauma and surgery. Besides, the lower third of the nose is mobile in comparison to semimobile middle third and fixed upper third. Surgery of this portion is always challenging for these two reasons. The surgeon should have most of the techniques presented in this chapter in his/her armamentarium to deal with the problems of the caudal septum (Fig. 9.46).

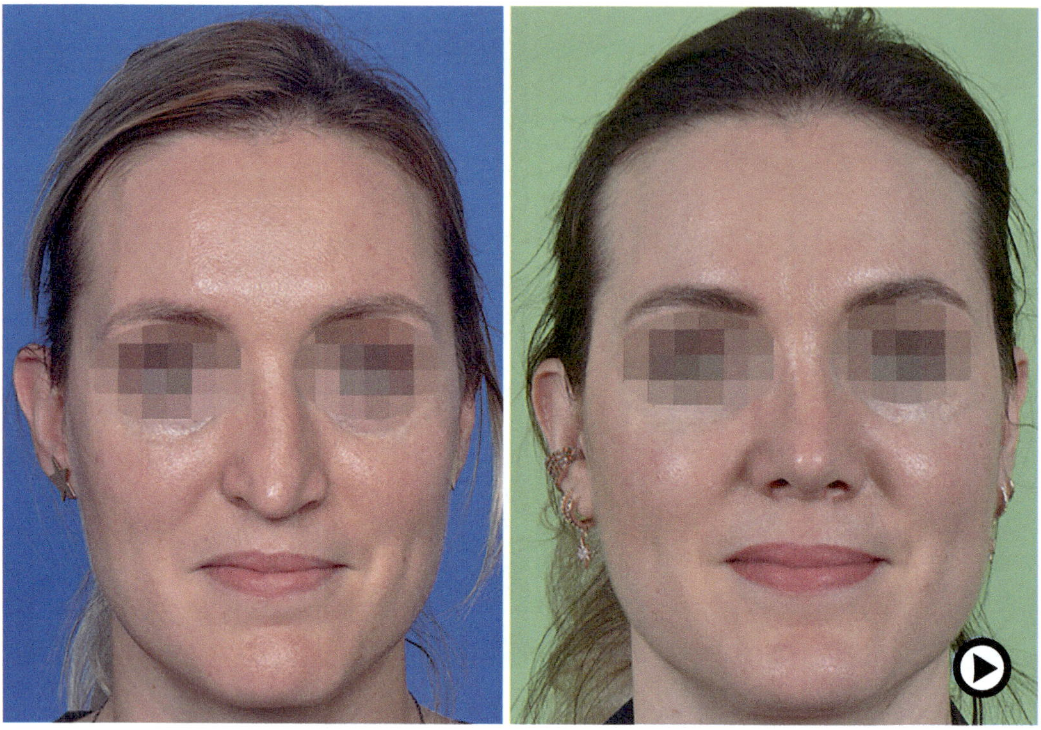

Fig. 9.40 After a septal abscess formation, the entire septal cartilage was disappeared resulting saddle nose. Ear cartilage is used to repair this deformity (▶ https://doi.org/10.1007/000-dys)

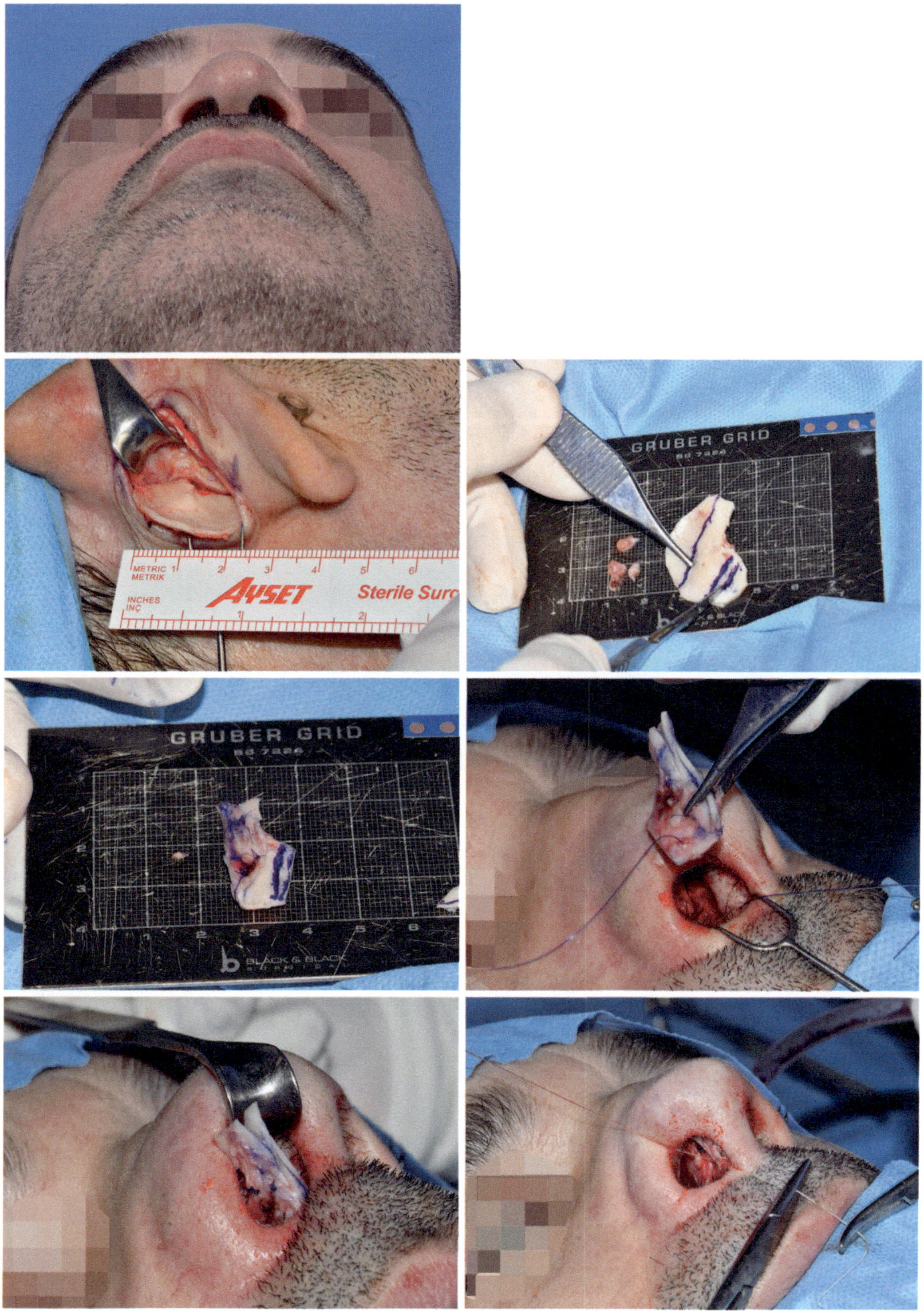

Fig. 9.41 The conchal cartilage is like a bowl in shape. It should be reshaped by folding over itself and sutured to straighten. In this case, it was used to support the nasal tip as a caudal septal extension graft because the original caudal septum was deep inside, probably because of previous submucous resection. The effect of this graft can be seen in the postoperative pictures

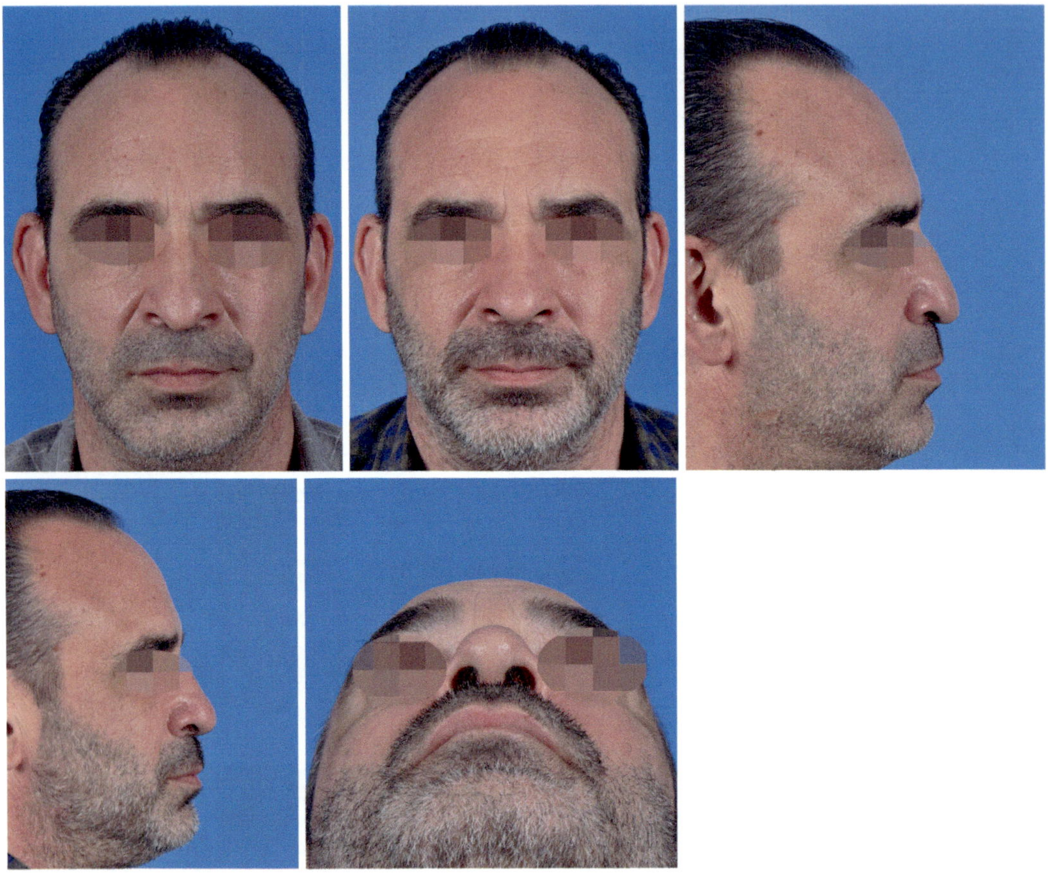

Fig. 9.41 (continued)

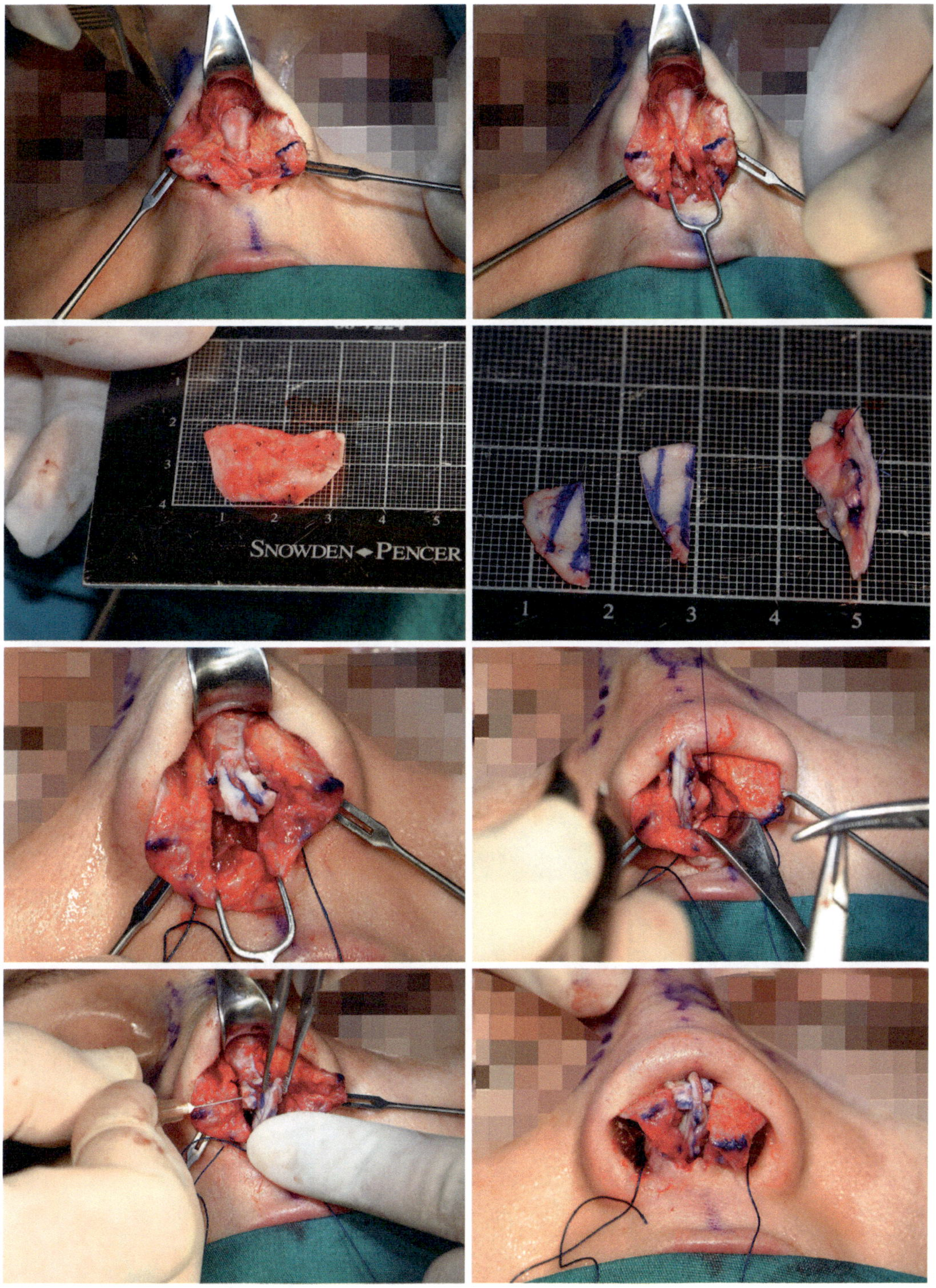

Fig. 9.42 In this revision case, the caudal segment was missing. The conchal cartilage was used as a double-layer caudal septal replacement graft and two short spreader grafts. I have been following this patient for 7 years, and the pictures presented here are after the second year. The nose is still keeping its shape. So the ear cartilage is also a very helpful source of grafts in revision surgeries

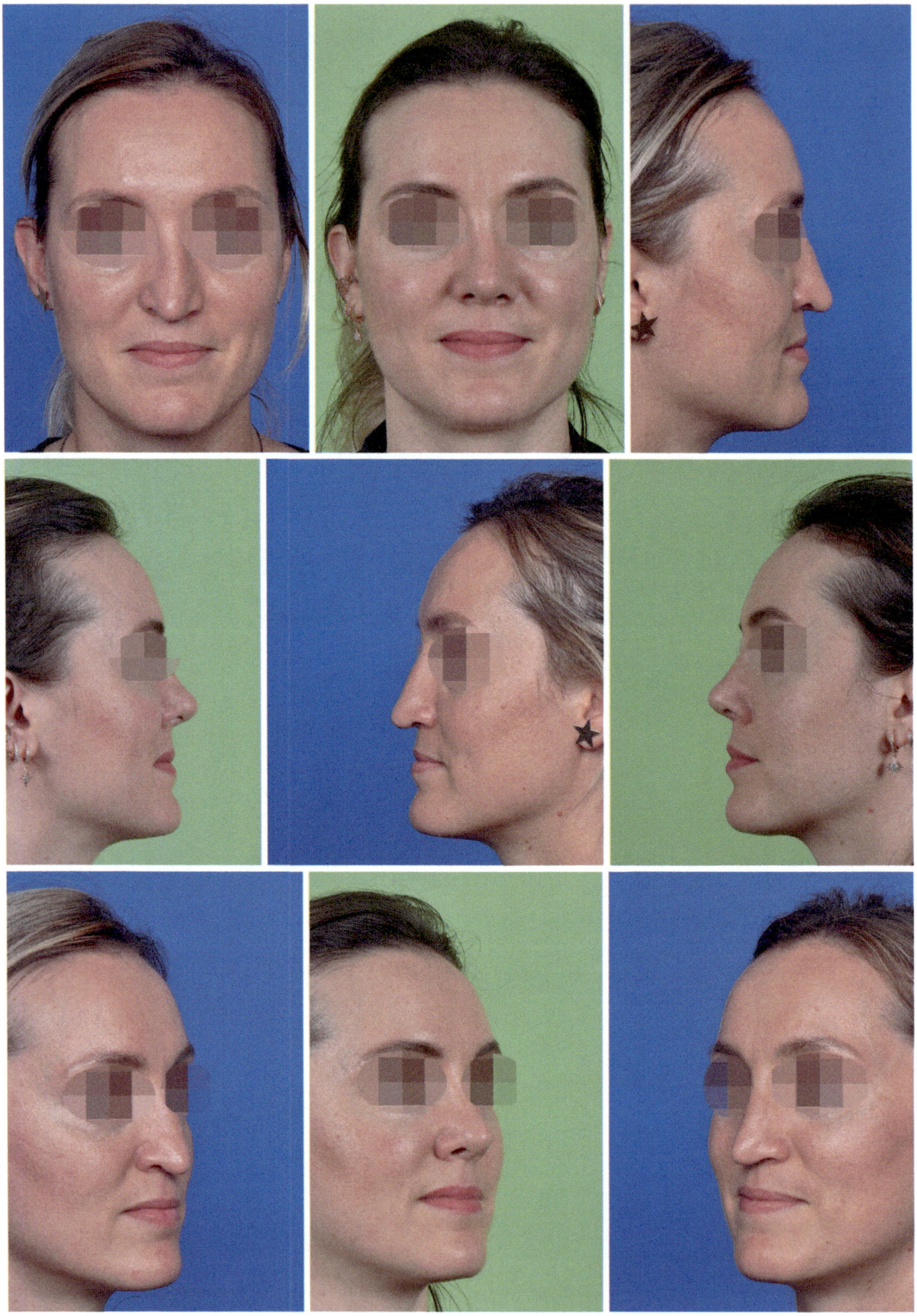

Fig. 9.42 (continued)

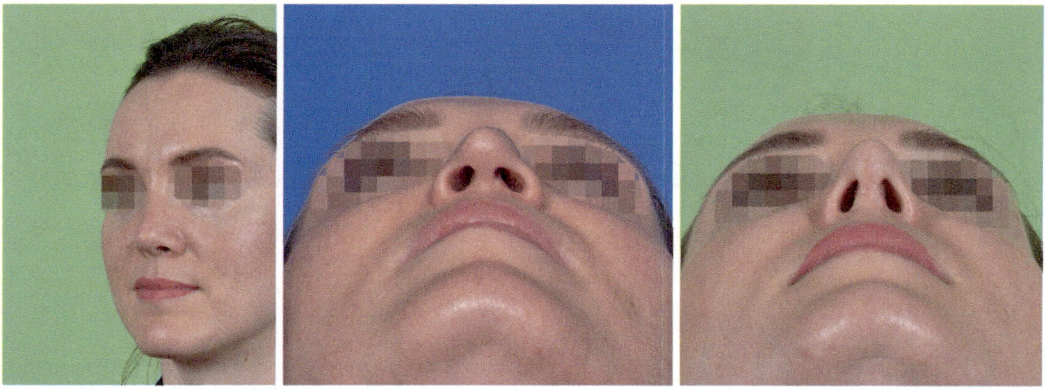

Fig. 9.42 (continued)

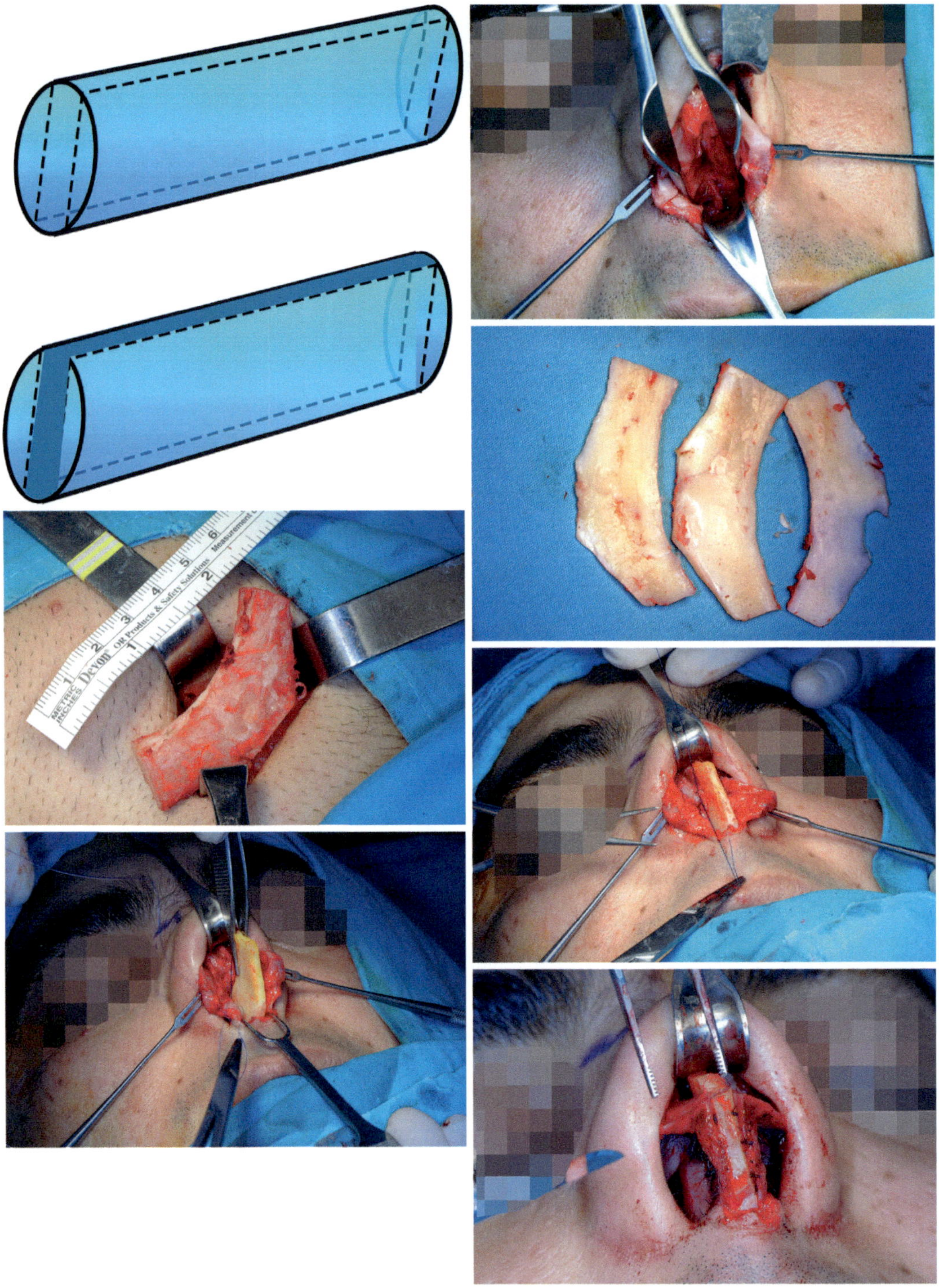

Fig. 9.43 In Davis and Gibson's method, the middle portion of the rib cartilage is used to prevent warping. In this case, the sixth rib was harvested, and the graft sculpted from the middle portion was used as an L-strut graft for subtotal septal reconstruction

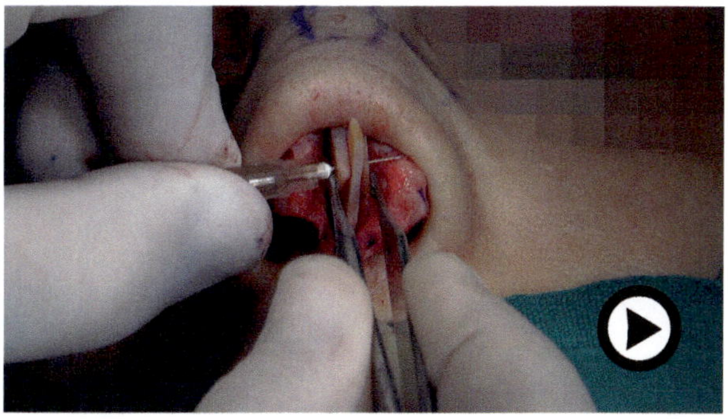

Fig. 9.44 Ear cartilage is used to make a partial reconstruction of the septum (▶ https://doi.org/10.1007/000-dyt)

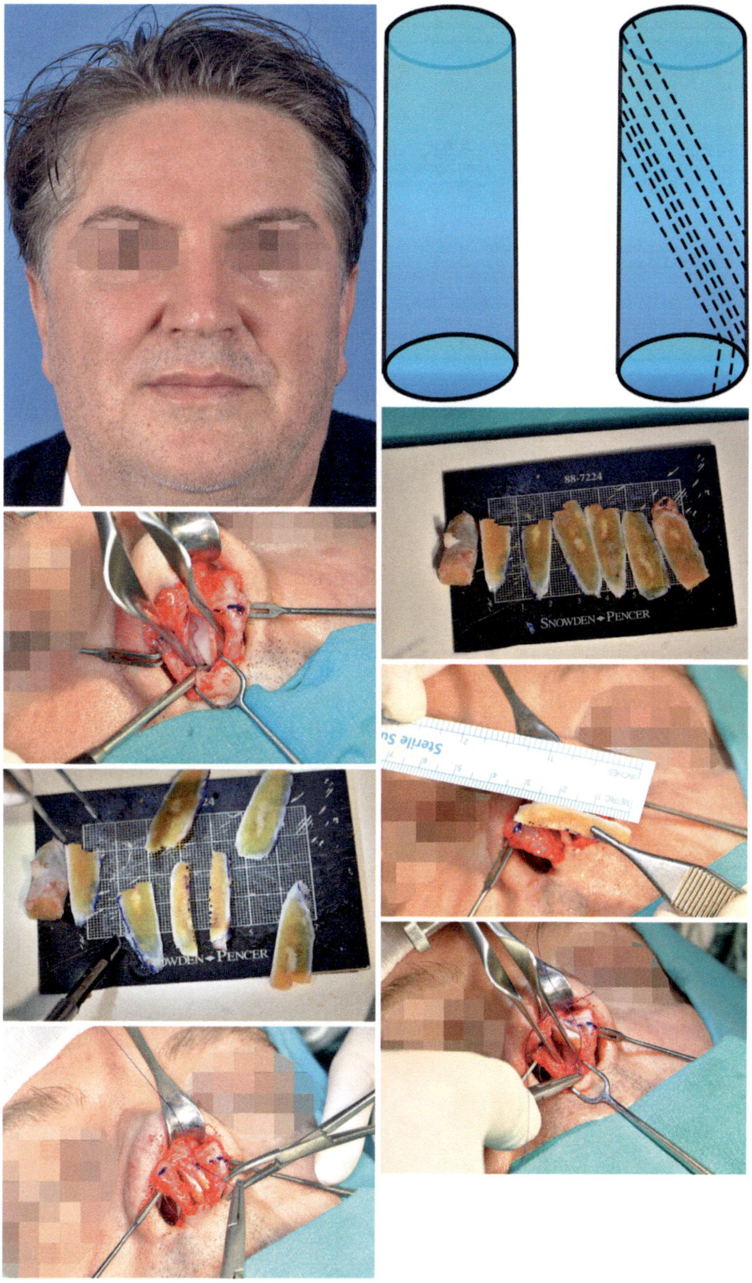

Fig. 9.45 In the oblique split technique, the costal cartilage is cut obliquely to obtain more grafts with variable thickness and length. In this revision rhinoplasty case, the deformed caudal septum was replaced by a caudal septal replacement graft supported by two spreader grafts

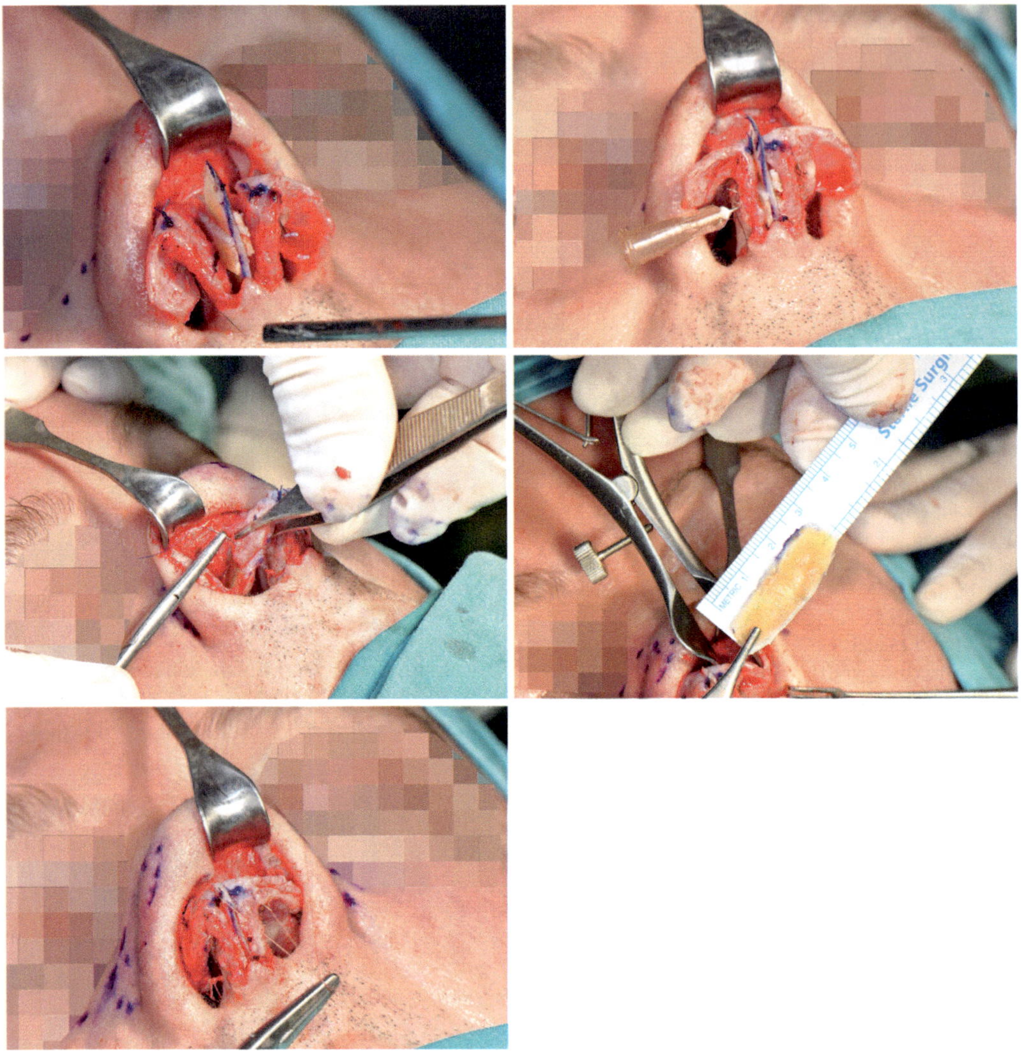

Fig. 9.45 (continued)

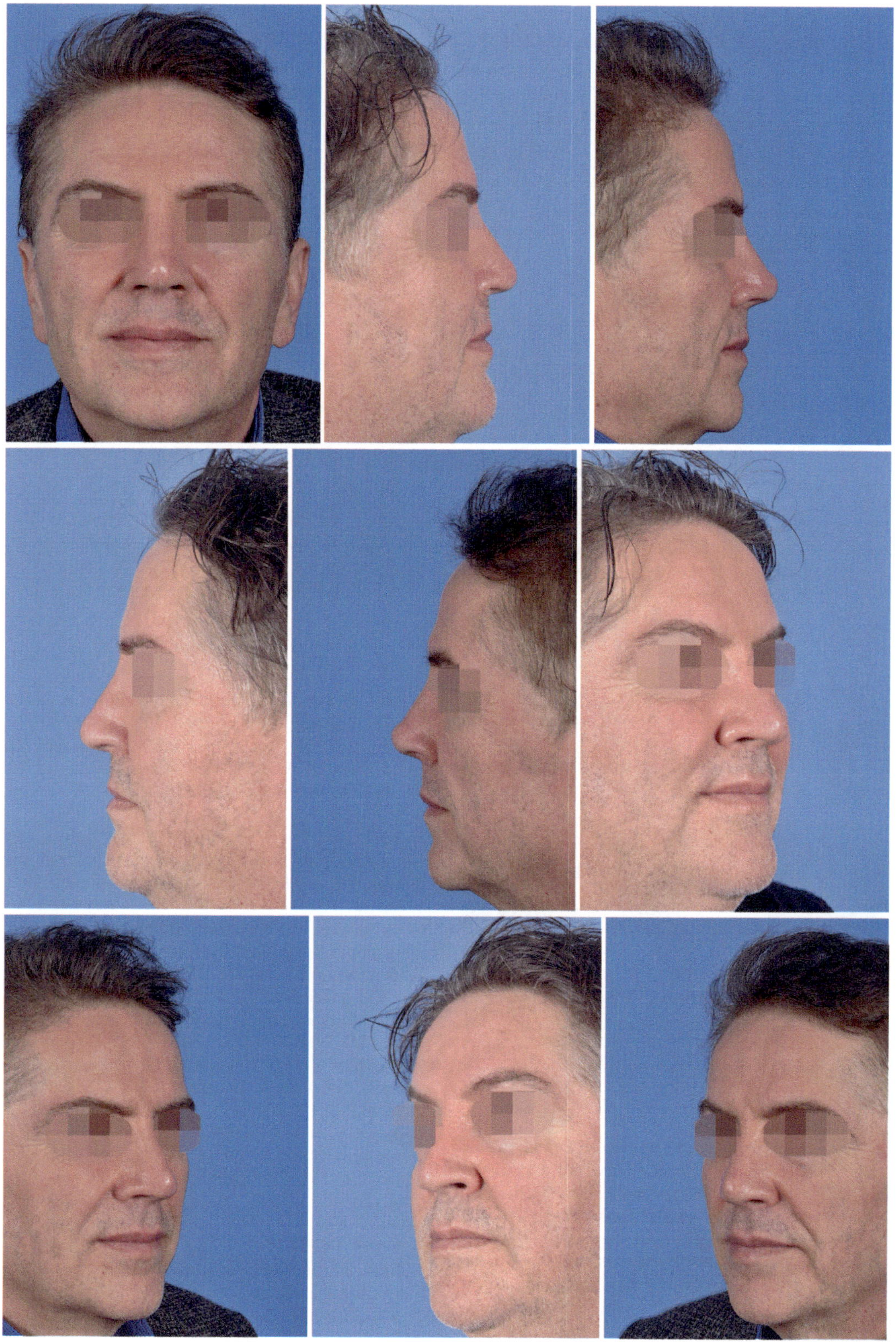

Fig. 9.45 (continued)

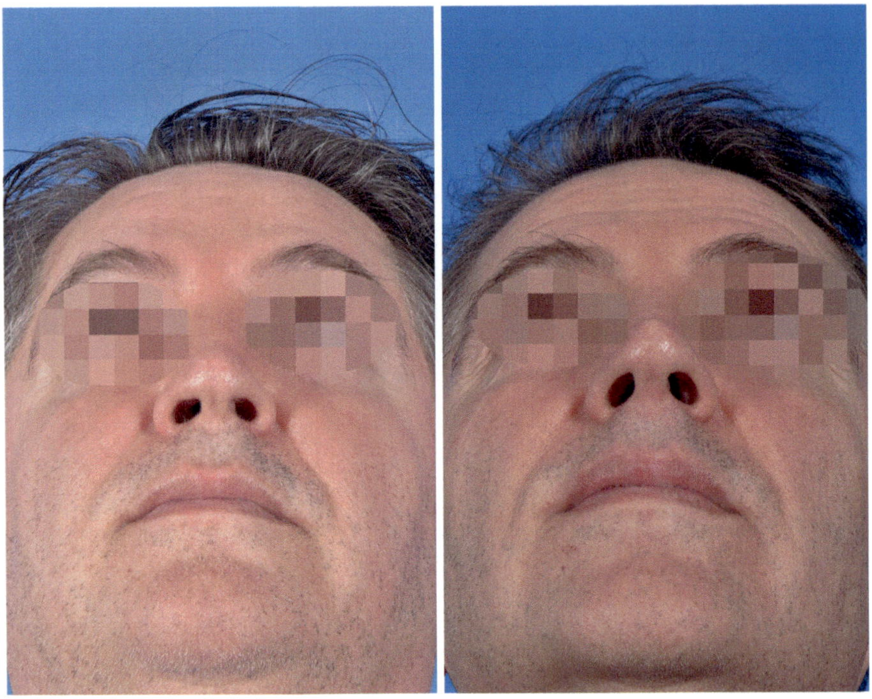

Fig. 9.45 (continued)

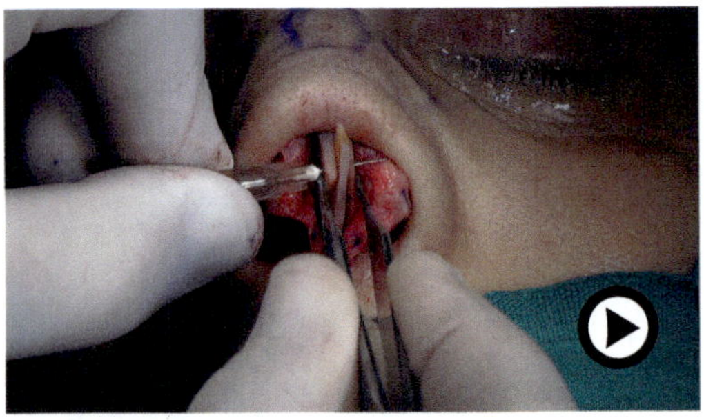

Fig. 9.46 Caudal septal replacement graft in revision rhinoplasty (▶ https://doi.org/10.1007/000-dyv)

References

1. Van Loosen J, Yiang J, Howard CV, Van Zanten GA, Verwoerd-Verhoef HL, Verwoerd CDA, Van Velzen D. Nasal cartilage maturation assessed by automated computer-assisted image analysis. Adv Otorhinolaryngol. 1997;51:51–60.
2. Metzenbaum M. Replacement of the lower end of the dislocated septal cartilage versus submucous resection of the dislocated end of the septal cartilage. Arch Otolaryngol. 1929;9:282–96.
3. Byrd HS, Salomon J, Flood J. Correction of the crooked nose. Plast Reconstr Surg. 1998;102:2148–57.
4. Metzinger SE, Boyce RG, Rigby PL, Joseph JJ, Anderson JR. Ethmoid bone sandwich grafting for caudal septal defects. Arch Otolaryngol Head Neck Surg. 1994;120:1121–5.
5. Apaydin F, Garcia RFF, Tas V. L-strut graft: a very versatile graft in the management of crooked and traumatic noses. Facial Plast Surg Aesthet Med. 2021;23:110–7.
6. Watson AW. The operation for deviation of the nasal septum. N Y Med J. 1896;1–6.
7. Murakami WT, Wong LW, Davidson TM. Applications of the biomechanical behavior of cartilage to nasal septoplastic surgery. Laryngoscope. 1982;92:300–9.
8. Kim DY, Nam SH, Alharethy SE, Jang YJ. Surgical outcomes of bony batten grafting to correct caudal septal deviation in septoplasty. JAMA Facial Plast Surg. 2017;19:470–5.
9. Byrd HS, Andochick S, Copit S, Walton KG. Septal extension grafts: a method of controlling tip projection shape. Plast Reconstr Surg. 1997;100:999–1010.
10. Guyuron B, Varghai A. Lengthening the nose with a tongue-and-groove technique. Plast Reconstr Surg. 2003;111:1533–9.
11. Toriumi DM. Nasal tip contouring: anatomic basis for management. Facial Plast Surg Aesthet Med. 2020;22:10–24.

12. Seyhan A, Ozden S, Ozaslan U, Sir E. A simplified use of septal extension graft to control nasal tip location. Aesthetic Plast Surg. 2007;31:506–11.
13. Toriumi DM. Caudal septal extension graft for correction of the retracted columella. Oper Tech Otolaryngol Head Neck Surg. 1995;6:311–8.
14. Jang YJ, Yu MS. Rhinoplasty for the Asian nose. Facial Plast Surg. 2010;26:93–101.
15. Hwang NH, Dhong ES. Septal extension graft in Asian rhinoplasty. Facial Plast Surg Clin North Am. 2018;26:331–41.
16. Cobo R. Rhinoplasty in Latino patients. Clin Plast Surg. 2016;43:237–54.
17. Dibbell DG. A cartilaginous columellar strut in cleft lip rhinoplasties. Br J Plast Surg. 1976;29:247–50.
18. Davis RE. Lateral crural tensioning for refinement of the wide and underprojected nasal tip: rethinking the lateral crural steal. Facial Plast Surg Clin North Am. 2015;23:23–53.
19. Kim SA, Jang YJ. Caudal septal division and interposition batten graft: a novel technique to correct caudal septal deviation in septoplasty. Ann Otol Rhinol Laryngol. 2019;128:1158–64.
20. Jeon YJ, Seo JH, Joo YH, Cho HJ, Jeon SY, Kim SW. Triangular excision and submucosal rejoining to correct horizontally folded caudal nasal septum. Int Forum Allergy Rhinol. 2019;9:1381–6.
21. Peer LA. An operation to repair lateral displacement of the lower border of the septal cartilage. Arch Otolaryngol. 1937;25:475–7.
22. Foda HM. The caudal septum replacement graft. Arch Facial Plast Surg. 2008;10:152.
23. Gibson T, Davis WB. The distortion of autogenous cartilage grafts: its cause and prevention. Br J Plast Surg. 1958;10:257–73.
24. Taştan E, Yücel ÖT, Aydin E, Aydoğan F, Beriat K, Ulusoy MG. The oblique split method: a novel technique for carving costal cartilage grafts. JAMA Facial Plast Surg. 2013;15:198–203.
25. Apaydin F. Oblique split technique: a game changer in costal cartilage sculpting. Plast Aesthet Res. 2019;6:9.

Dorsal Deviations of the Septum 10

10.1 Introduction

The deviations of the dorsal segment of the nasal septum are usually part of a crooked nose, which creates a big challenge for the rhinoplasty surgeon (Fig. 10.1). The dorsal deviations can be classified as linear, C-shaped, or S-shaped [1] (Fig. 10.2).

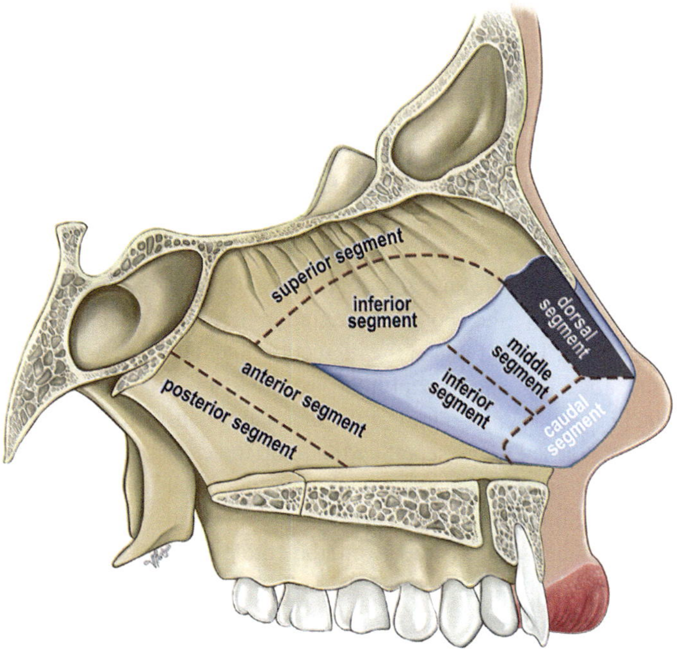

Fig. 10.1 The dorsal segment of the nasal septum joins with the upper lateral cartilages, making an important part of the middle vault

Supplementary Information The online version contains supplementary material available at https://doi.org/10.1007/978-3-031-74734-2_10. The videos can be accessed individually by clicking the DOI link in the accompanying figure caption or by scanning this link with the SN More Media App.

© The Author(s), under exclusive license to Springer Nature Switzerland AG 2025
F. Apaydın, *Septal Surgery Challenges in Rhinoplasty*,
https://doi.org/10.1007/978-3-031-74734-2_10

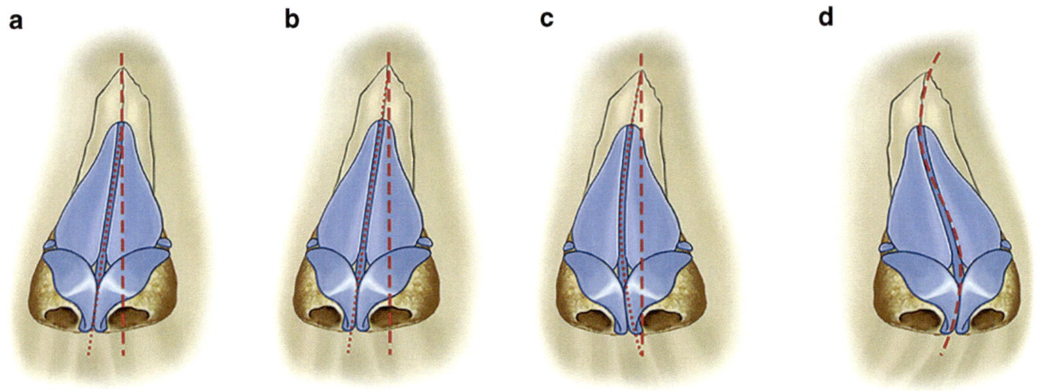

Fig. 10.2 There are four types of deviations of the dorsal segment of the nasal septum: (**a**) Linear-cartilaginous, (**b**) linear-bony-cartilaginous, (**c**) C-shaped, (**d**) S-shaped

10.2 Linear

The linear deviations can include the lower two-thirds or all thirds of the nose. In the latter, osteotomies are surely needed to bring the entire nose into the midline in addition to septoplasty. If the deviation includes the lower two-thirds, the challenge is when the deviation is at the junction where the septal cartilage meets the ethmoid. In these cases, there may be a need for partial or full mobilization of this joint and fixation with spreader grafts (Fig. 10.3). I have a critical trick in these situations. I usually open two subdorsal tunnels under the bony-cartilaginous dorsum (Fig. 10.4). Then, I widen the dissection to determine the entire nasal septum from the convex side. I try to keep 4–6 mm of the mucoperichondrium attached to the septal cartilage on the contralateral side. This attachment prevents total mobilization of the septal cartilage even though the cartilage is totally freed from the ethmoid, as in extracorporeal septoplasty.

A second option is to cut the dorsal segment of the septal cartilage in the midline or at the angle of deflection or fracture line, and sometimes resect a sliver of cartilage at this level. The cartilage attached to the ethmoid loses its ability to push the splinting spreader grafts. Therefore, two splinting spreader grafts can be used to couple the cephalic and caudal portions of the dorsal segment (Fig. 10.5). The cephalic end of the splinting spreader grafts should bypass the ethmoidocartilaginous junction by 5–6 mm on both sides to effectively straighten the deviation (Fig. 10.6a–c).

A third option is to use the push-down or let-down method with Cottle-type dorsum preservation and totally release the septal cartilage from the ethmoid [2]. According to my experience, this technique is technically much easier than the previous techniques but sometimes more difficult to obtain predictable profiles (Fig. 10.7).

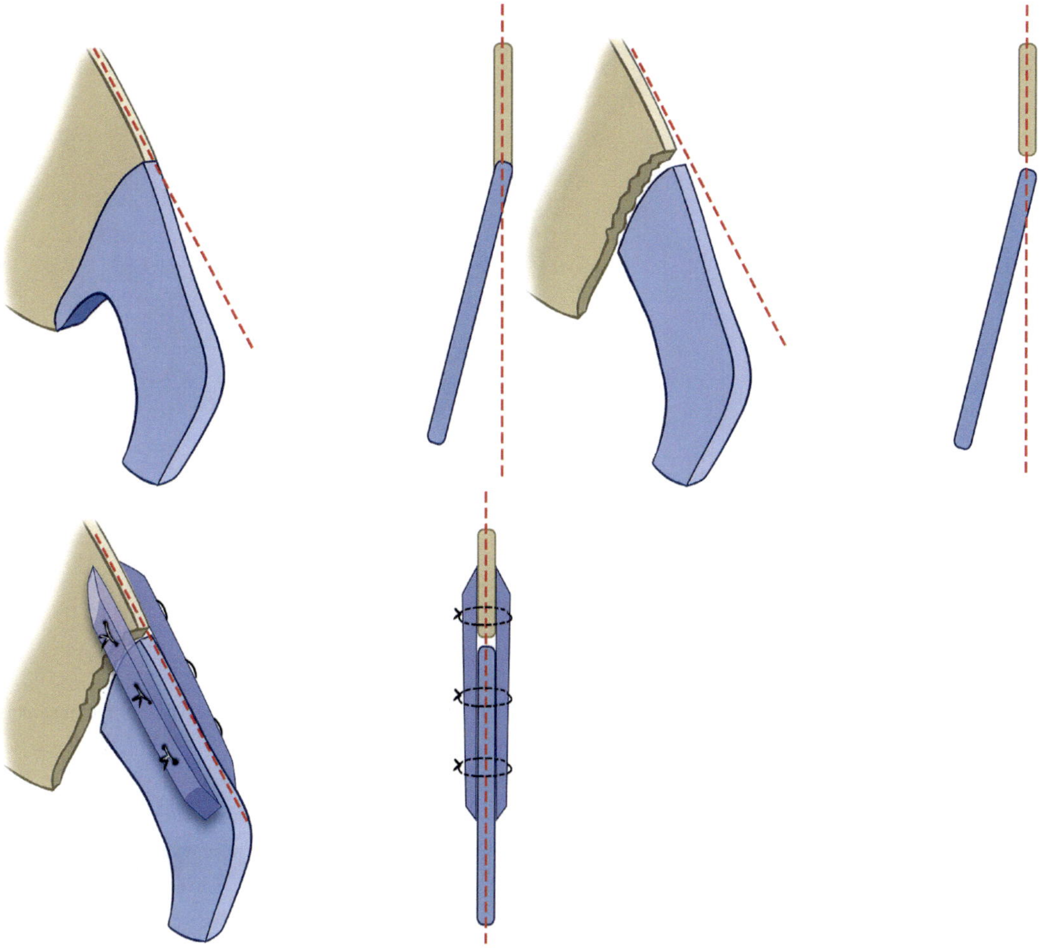

Fig. 10.3 High septal deviation creates a challenge for the surgeon. Partial or full mobilization of the joint between the septal cartilage and ethmoid at the keystone may be necessary. The fixation of the detached septal cartilage can be done with spreader grafts. Besides, opening holes in the nasal bones is required for more secure fixation

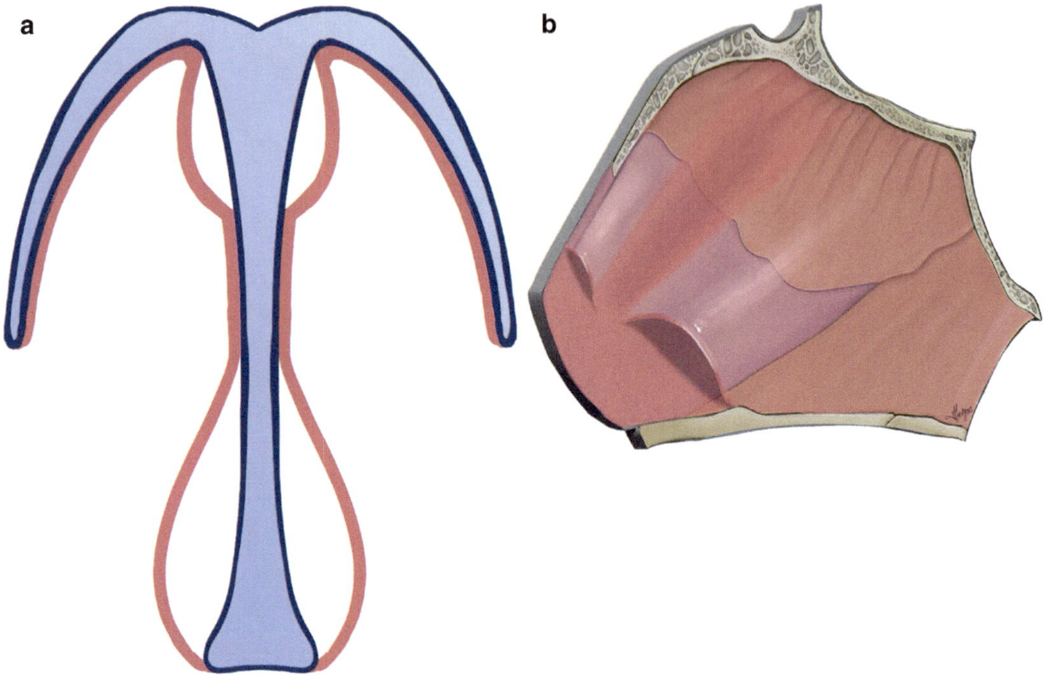

Fig. 10.4 Subdorsal tunnels are opened under the bony-cartilaginous dorsum. After keeping 4–6 mm of the mucoperichondrium attached to the septal cartilage under the tunnels, inferior tunnels are opened for septoplasty

Fig. 10.5 Bilateral spreader grafts are designed from septal cartilage and sutured in place (▶ https://doi.org/10.1007/000-dz0)

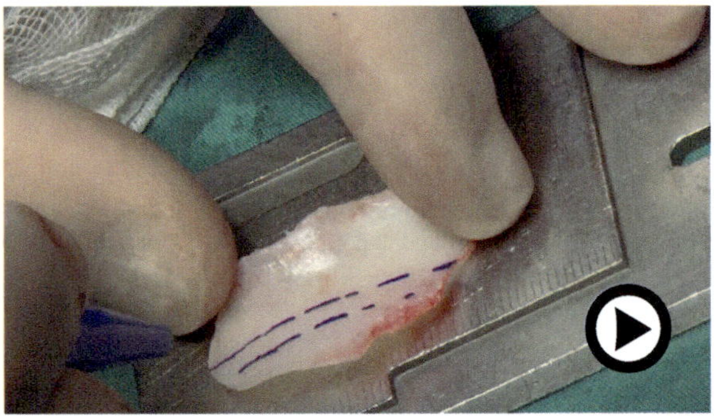

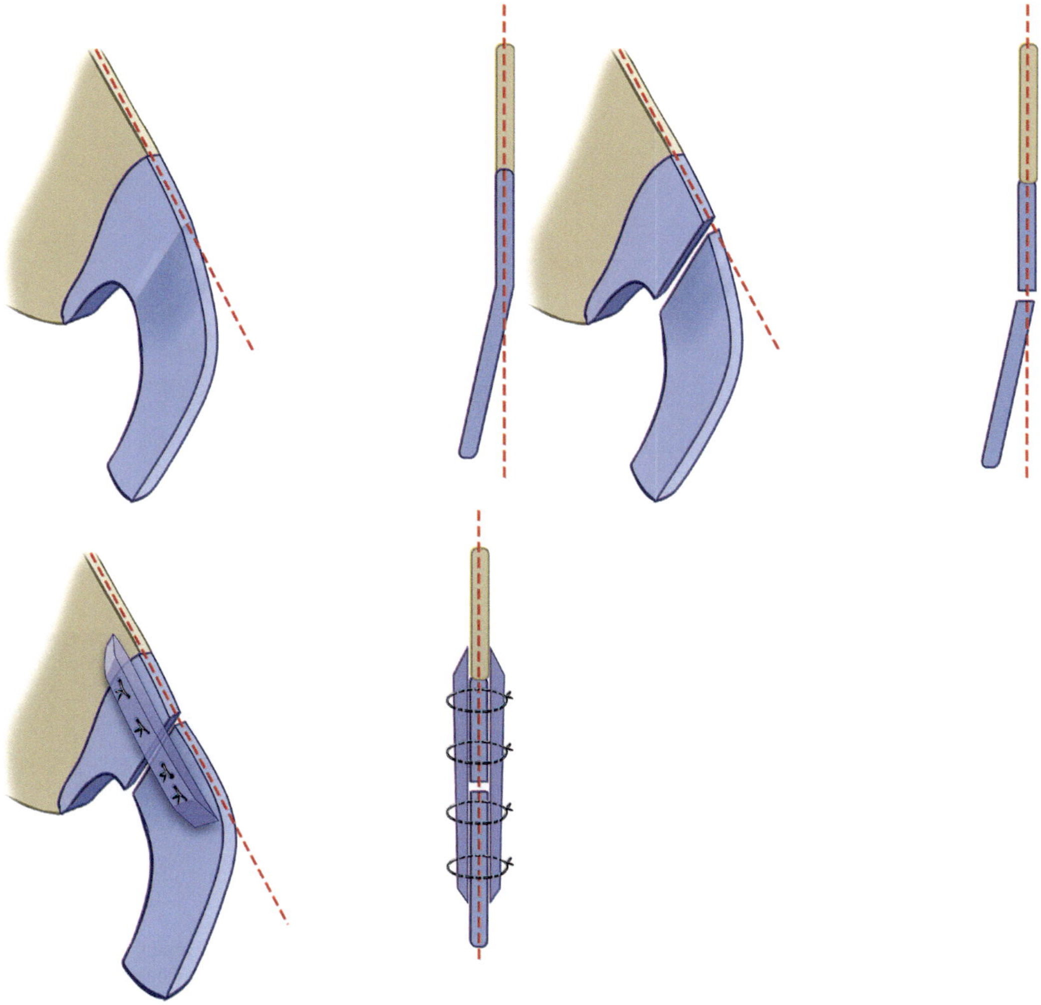

Fig. 10.6 A second option is to cut the dorsal segment of the septal cartilage at the level of the deviation and splint both sides with spreader grafts

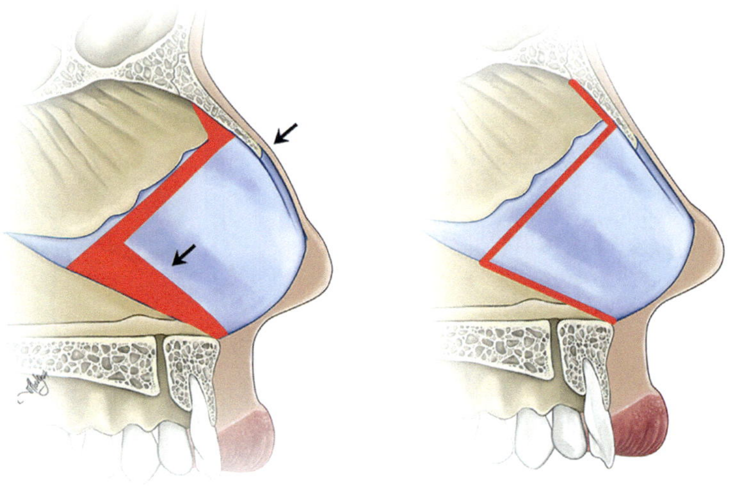

Fig. 10.7 A third option is to use the push-down or let-down method with Cottle-type dorsum preservation and total release of the septal cartilage from the ethmoid

10.3 C-Shaped

This type is the most often encountered in my practice. In these cases, the deviation is usually due to a fracture of the septal cartilage, which is curvilinear, starting close to the anterior nasal spine or maxillary crest and extending close to the middle vault or keystone area. The reconstruction methods of these cases create a special challenge for the surgeon, and spreader grafts are my workhorse in the correction of the dorsal deflections in such cases.

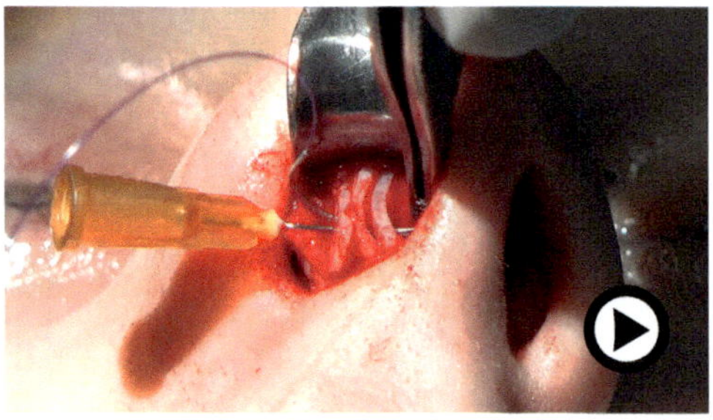

Fig. 10.8 Spreader grafts are designed from septal cartilage and sutured by endonasal approach (▶ https://doi.org/10.1007/000-dyx)

10.3.1 Spreader Grafts

Sheen [3] described the use of endonasal placement of spreader grafts in primary rhinoplasty patients with thin skin and weak ULCs, in those with short nasal bones and narrow middle vaults, and in revision cases (Fig. 10.8).

The external approach to rhinoplasty has expanded the indications and use of spreader grafts. These include [4]:

1. Maintenance and reconstruction of the dorsal nasal roof
2. Restoration or maintenance of the internal valve
3. Straightening and buttressing a high dorsally deviated septum
4. Recreation of the dorsal esthetic lines

I have been using spreader grafts since 1999, and I am very happy to use them in primary and revision rhinoplasty. I strongly believe and have experienced in my daily routine that spreader grafts are very helpful in restoring or maintaining the internal nasal valve. In my routine, there are different ways to use spreader grafts (Table 10.1).

When the dorsal segment is deviated, and in case it is weak, strong and thick splinting spreader grafts are usually sufficient (Fig. 10.9). However, in the majority of cases, deep scoring is usually necessary to relieve tension on the deflected car-

Table 10.1 Different ways of using spreader grafts

1. Traditional (Bilateral)
• Rectangular in shape
• Beveled
2. Modified
• One-sided
• Asymmetric (thickness)
• Two layers
3. Splinting material
• Cartilaginous
• Bony-cartilaginous
• Bony

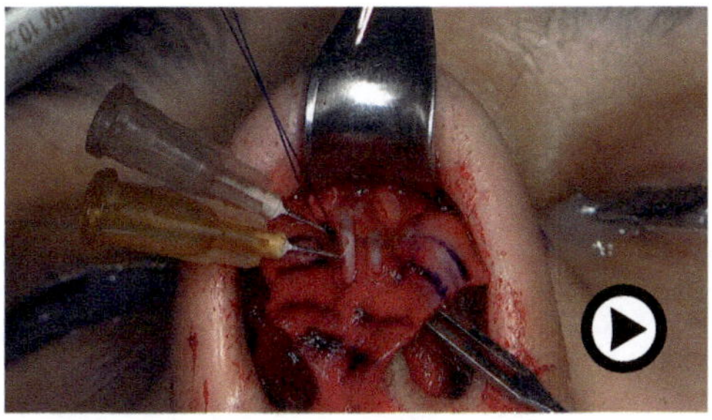

Fig. 10.9 Spreader graft fixation by external approach (▶ https://doi.org/10.1007/000-dyy)

tilage and splint it with spreader grafts to straighten the dorsal segment (Fig. 10.10a–c). In some rare cases, the tension between the dorsal and caudal segments is not relieved; therefore, a deviated strip of cartilage or angle of deflection may need to be removed using the splinting spreader grafts as columns holding these two segments in the proper position (Fig. 10.11).

I have been using spreader grafts for 24 years, and in my daily routine, they can be used in many ways depending on the individual situation [5].

10.3.1.1 Traditional

10.3.1.1.1 Rectangular

This is the classical shape described by Sheen in 1984, who inserted them into the subperichondrial pockets [3]. If the dorsum is intact and there is no need to dissect the upper lateral cartilages from the nasal septum, spreader grafts can be inserted into these pockets to straighten the deviation and open the nasal valve (Fig. 10.12). This situation is less likely and is applicable only when there is a fracture line close to the anterior septal angle. More often, the upper lateral cartilages need to be dissected away from the nasal septum to identify the cause of the deviation and to determine the condition of the nasal septum without any distortion. The spreader grafts are sutured to the septal cartilage caudally and cephalically by mattress sutures (Fig. 10.13). If there is a fracture line that needs to be resected, I recommend suturing one spreader graft to the nasal septum and then resecting the fracture line. In this way, the position of the L-strut framework does not change, and the second spreader graft is then sutured to further support the dorsal segment. The superior margin of the spreader grafts is positioned at the same level as the superior margin of the dorsal segment of the septal cartilage.

The superior edges of the spreader grafts must be placed caudal to the nasal bones to prevent open roof deformity, and the caudal edges are placed 2–3 mm behind the anterior septal angle. In addition, the cephalic portion should be 2–3 mm thick, and the caudal portion should be 1.5–2 mm thick to facilitate spreading and splinting. This thickness can sometimes cause widening of the middle vault. To prevent this situation, it is better to place the spreader grafts 1–2 mm below the superior margin of the dorsal segment of the septal cartilage (Fig. 10.14).

10.3.1.1.2 Beveled

I prefer beveling the caudal and cephalic edges of the spreader grafts. I think that it does two things: (1) the supportive length of the graft becomes longer, and (2) it does not create a bulk at the internal valve angle (Fig. 10.14).

In addition to the abovementioned types, there are two different types of spreader grafts that I use. One of them is thinner at the internal valve area and thicker at the keystone area. The idea is to mimic the original dorsum anatomy. The second one is a longer spreader graft to support the whole nasal septum. The portion going under the bony dorsum should be 2 mm lower than the portion sitting at the middle vault. I use this kind mostly in revision rhinoplasties and obtain them from rib cartilages (Fig. 10.15).

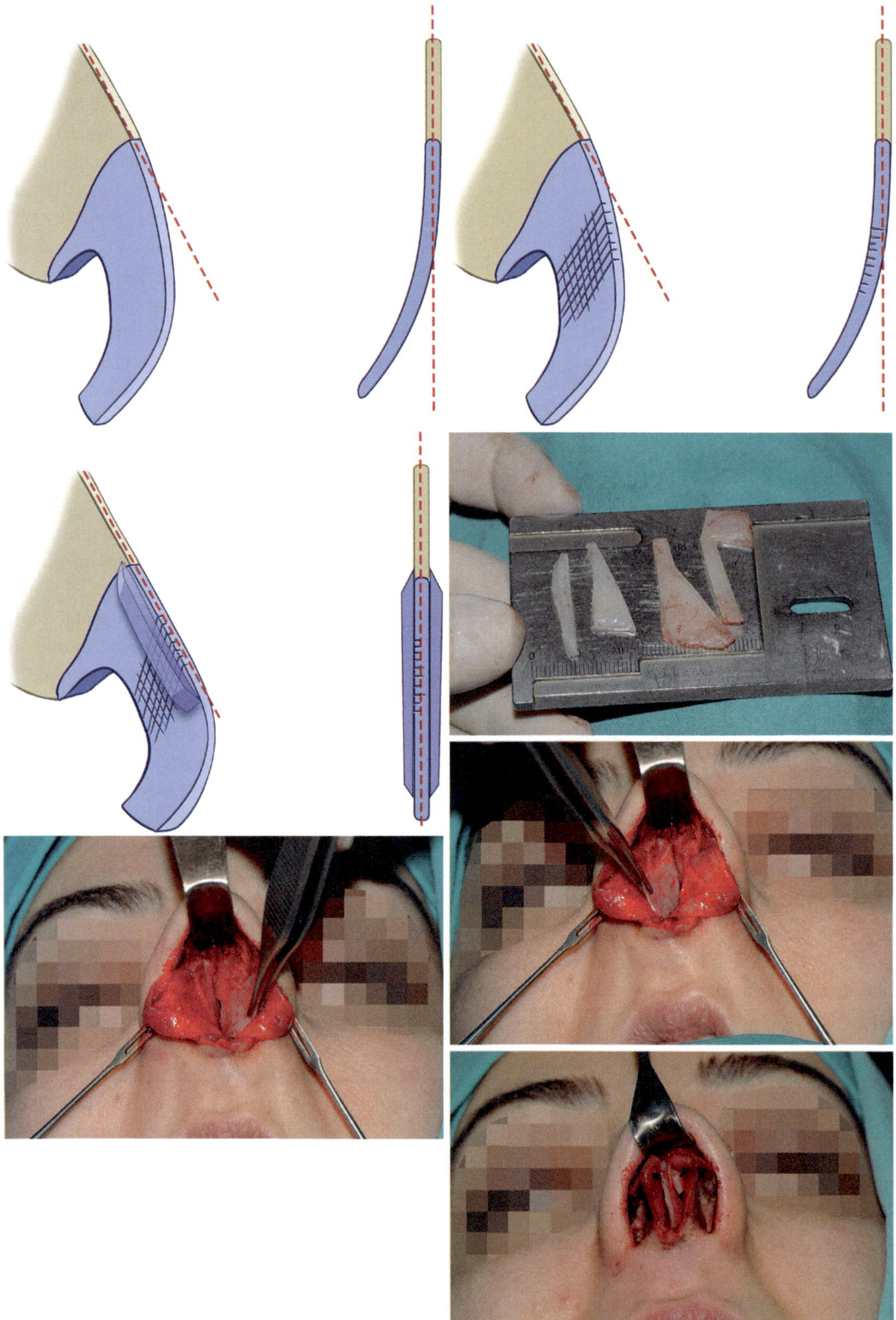

Fig. 10.10 Deep scoring on the deflected cartilage and splint with spreader grafts

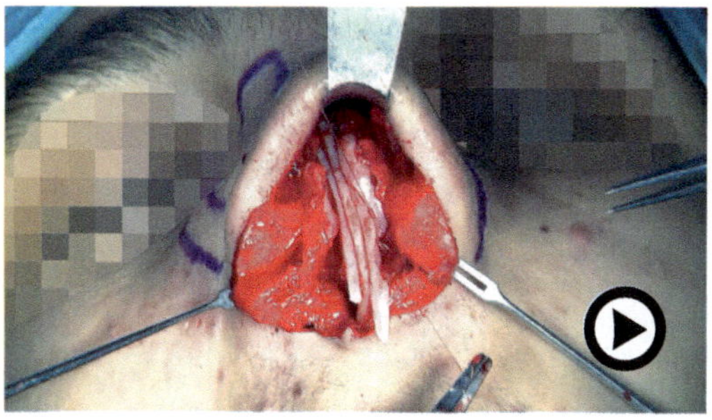

Fig. 10.11 Septal cartilage spreader grafts are used tu splint the dorsal segment and a dog ear is resected from the septum (▶ https://doi.org/10.1007/000-dyz)

10.3.1.2 Modified

10.3.1.2.1 One-Sided

In crooked noses where there is a concave deformity of the dorsal segment causing one-sided depression or crookedness, a one-sided spreader graft can be successfully used [6, 7] (Fig. 10.16). I do not agree with this suggestion because I found that this was not the case all the time. I have seen cases where a one-sided graft was pushing the septal cartilage more laterally, making the problem worse. Therefore, I do like using spreader grafts always bilaterally, using the contralateral spreader graft as a counterbalance graft to keep the septal cartilage in the middle.

10.3.1.2.2 Asymmetric (thickness)

When there is marked asymmetry of the nose in C-shaped noses, spreader grafts of varying thicknesses can be used [7] (Fig. 10.16). The idea is to achieve the best possible symmetry through the entire axis of the nose.

10.3.1.2.3 Two Layers

When the spreader graft is not thick enough, it does not serve its purpose of spreading and splinting. The thicker portion of the septal cartilage is the portion adjacent to the maxillary crest and in the midhorizontal region. If spreader grafts are carved from these portions, they are usually ideal in width. However, this is not always the case. Therefore, in these cases, two layers of cartilage can be sutured together to reach the desired thickness (Fig. 10.16). When cartilage is obtained from the ear, it is not thick and straight enough to be used as a spreader graft. Two layers of conchal cartilage with opposing concave surfaces facing each other are sutured together to obtain more ideal spreader grafts (Fig. 10.17).

10.3.1.3 Splinting

There are two main approaches to correcting deviated septal cartilage: (1) Splinting and (2) resecting and reconstructing. I find resection and reconstruction techniques more aggressive and unnecessary in most cases. I favor splinting techniques. In segmental septal reconstruction, spreader grafts act as my workhorse in straightening the deviated dorsal segment of the nasal septum. For splinting purposes, spreader grafts must be strong and long enough. As a material, I prefer to use septal cartilage if possible. However, there are times when the cartilage is not big enough and/or a longer graft is needed. In these situations, I prefer to use bony-cartilaginous or bony grafts [8–10]. They can be inserted 1–2 mm below the superior margin of the nasal dorsum in order not to create middle vault widening (Figs. 10.18 and 10.19).

10.3.1.4 Reconstructive

In crooked noses or revision rhinoplasty, some parts of the dorsal segment can be deficient or need to be removed. Spreader grafts inserted in pockets under the bony vault or sutured to the remaining septal cartilage at the keystone area can be used to reconstruct the dorsal segment of the nasal septum [10, 14] (Figs. 10.20 and 10.21).

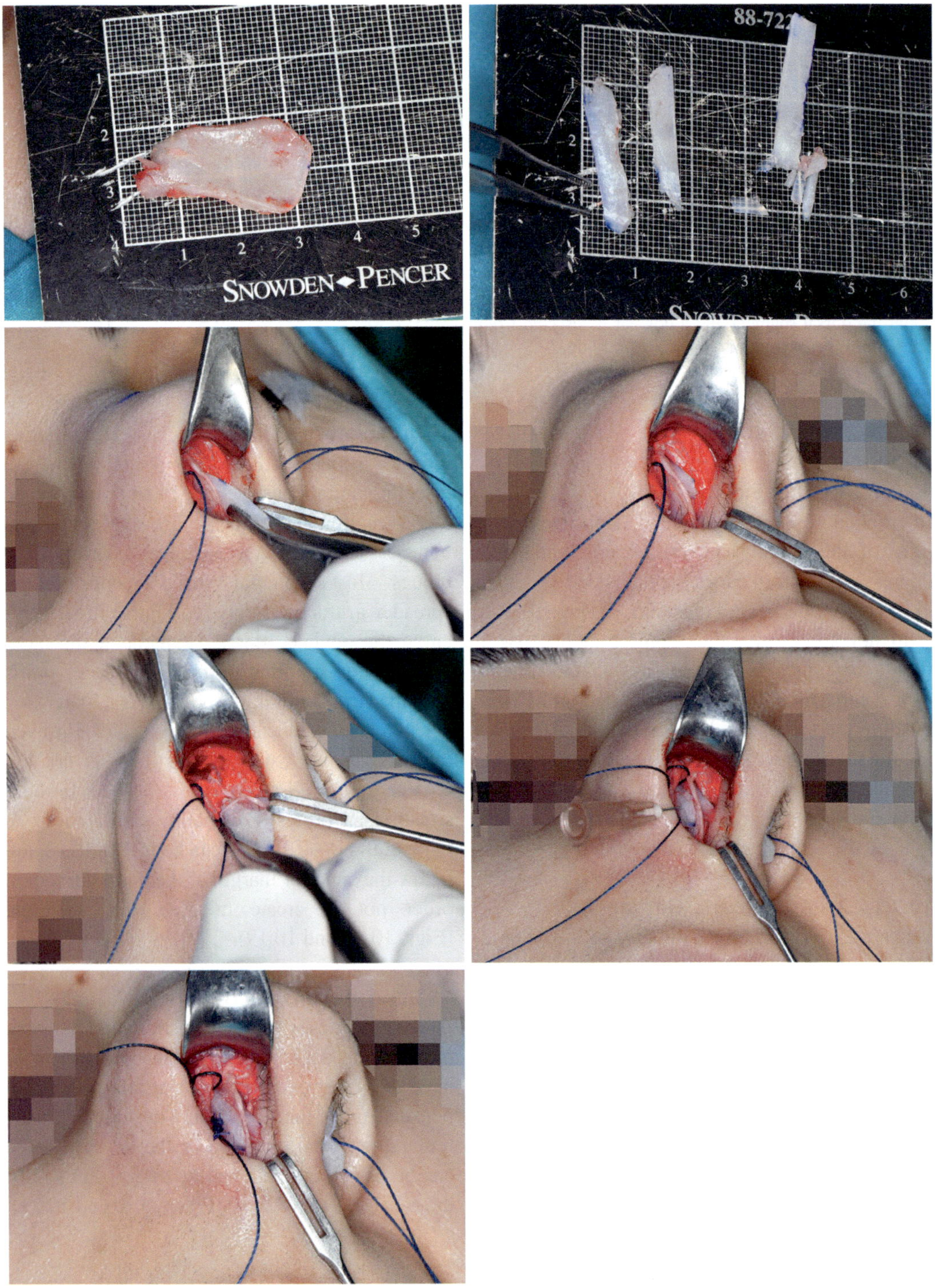

Fig. 10.12 Traditional spreader grafts are rectangular in shape. They can be inserted in subdorsal pockets and sutured to the anterior septal angle

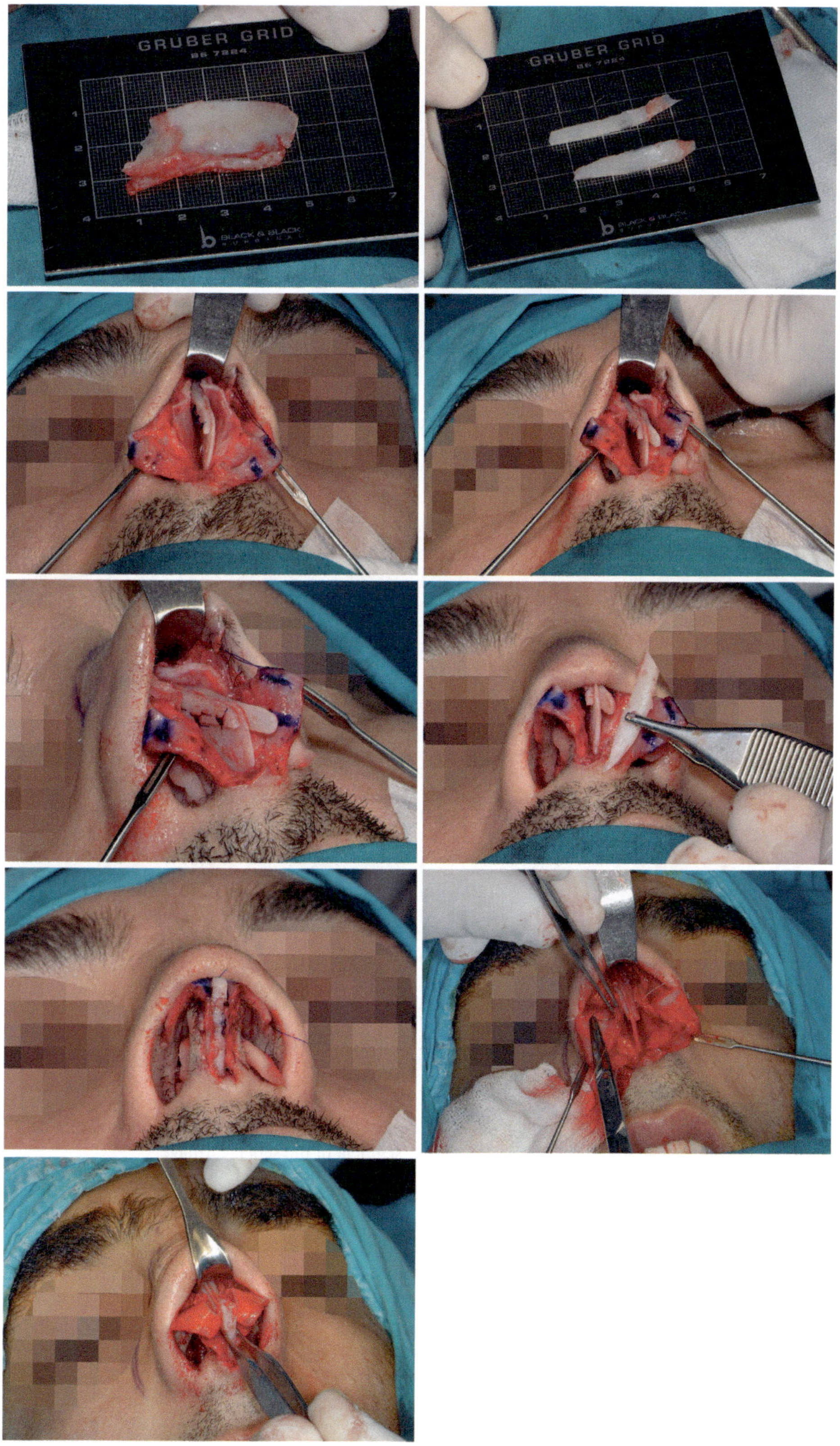

Fig. 10.13 The spreader grafts can be sutured to the dorsal segment after humpectomy. In this case, one of the left spreader grafts was longer than usual to suture the caudal septal extension graft to it

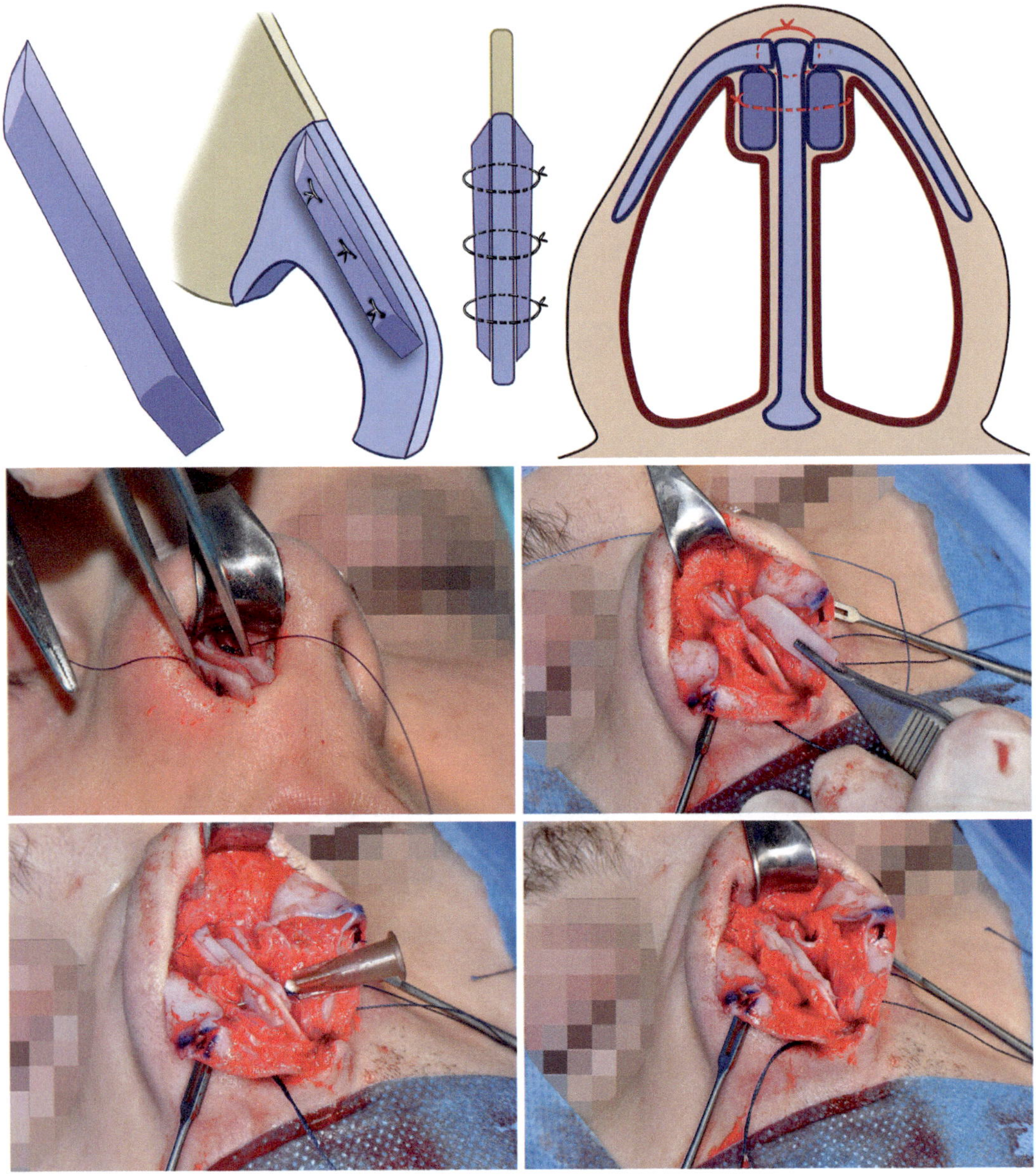

Fig. 10.14 The superior edges of the spreader grafts must be placed caudal to the nasal bones to prevent open roof deformity, and the caudal edges are placed 2–3 mm behind the anterior septal angle. Besides, they should be placed 1–2 mm below the superior margin of the dorsal segment of the septal cartilage

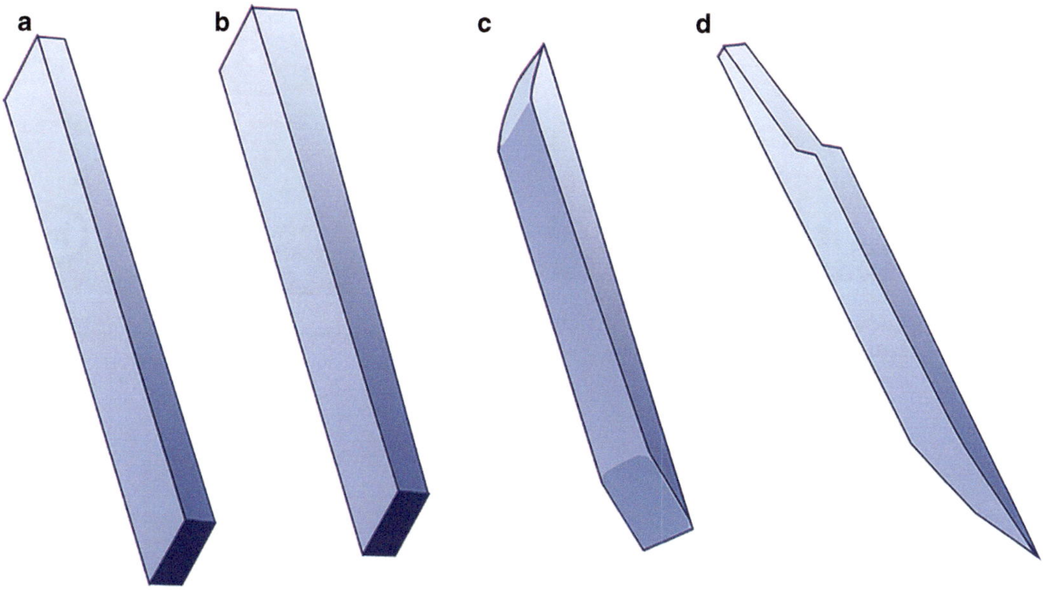

Fig. 10.15 In this illustration, four different types of spreader grafts are presented. The rectangular graft described by Sheen is presented in (**a**). Some surgeons prefer to use the thinner end close to the internal valve angle and thicker portion close to the keystone area (**b**). I like to use type b after beveling the edges to support the septal cartilage more and to give a smoother transition (**c**). In revision rhinoplasties, when I use longer spreader grafts to support all of septum, the portion of the graft under the bony pyramid is further sculpted in order not to create an open roof (**d**)

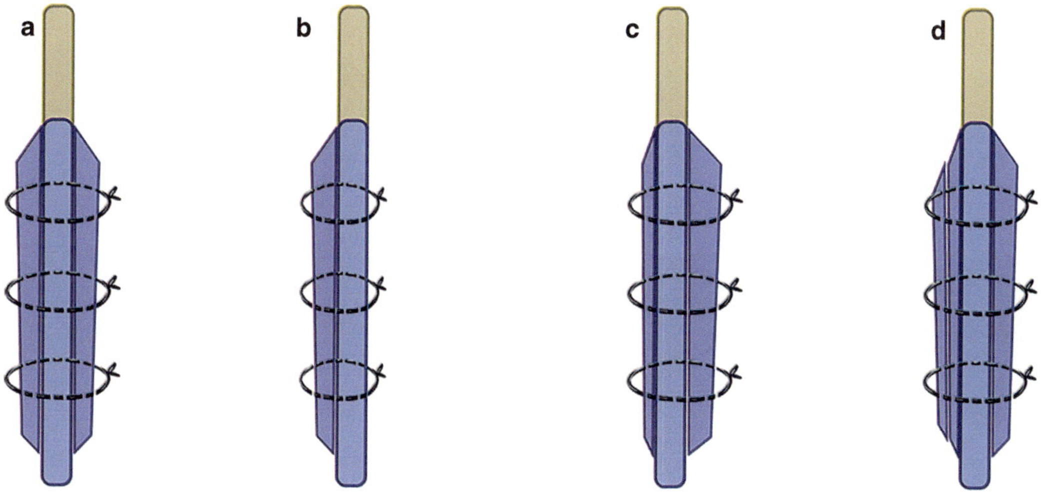

Fig. 10.16 Traditionally, the spreader grafts are carved as symmetric grafts to create symmetry in the frontal view (**a**). In C-shaped deviations and for splinting purposes, they can be used on one side (**b**). In cases of asymmetric dorsums, spreader grafts can be carved in different thicknesses to create symmetry on the dorsum (**c**). Sometimes, the grafts prepared as spreader grafts are so thin that they should be used in two layers to have a spreading and/or splinting effect (**d**)

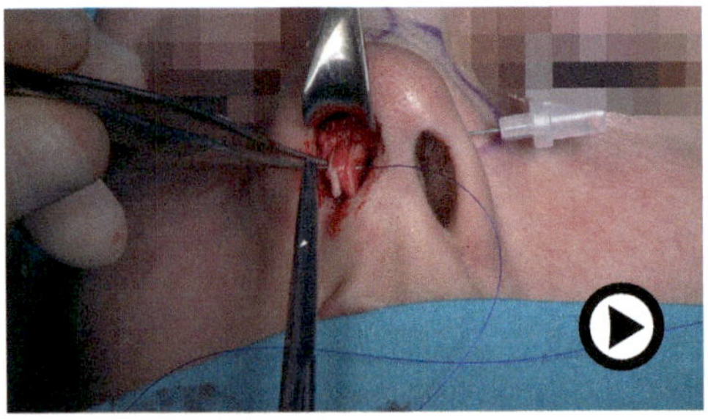

Fig. 10.17 Bilateral spreader grafts are designed from ear cartilage and sutured in place (▶ https://doi.org/10.1007/000-dyw)

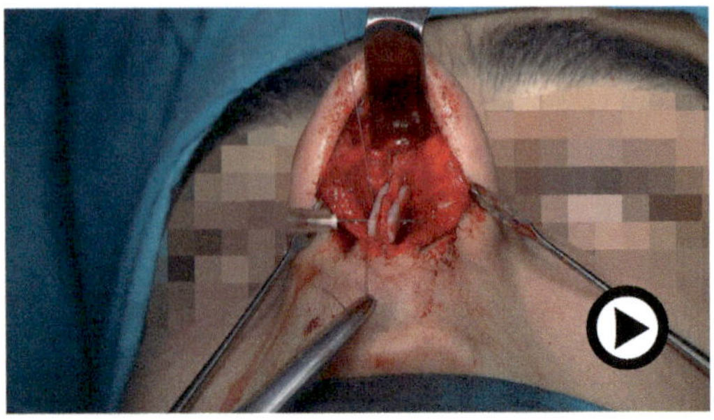

Fig. 10.18 Spreader grafts are fixated to splint a crooked dorsum (▶ https://doi.org/10.1007/000-dz1)

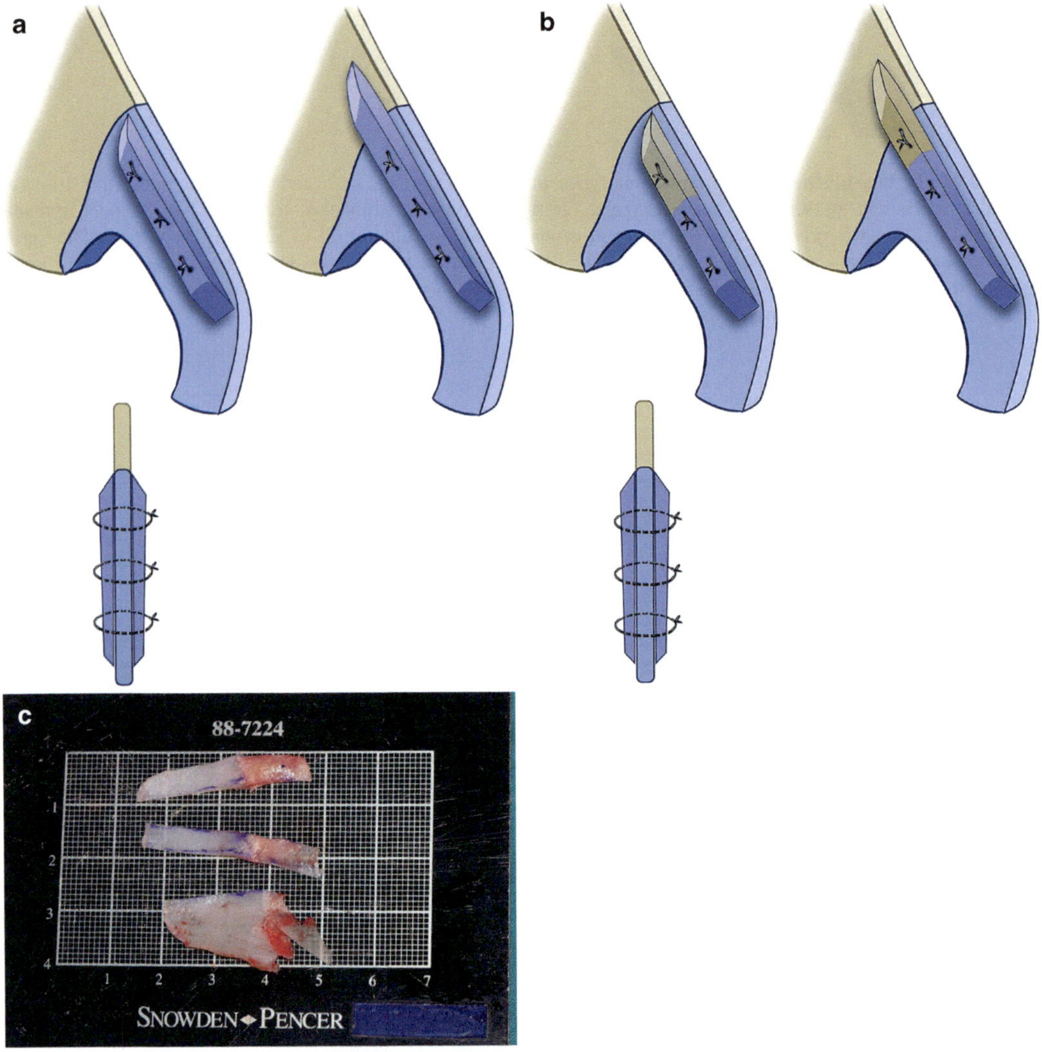

Fig. 10.19 Spreader grafts can be used for splinting the dorsal segment. They must be strong and long enough. They can be obtained from cartilaginous (**a**), bony-cartilaginous (**b**), or bony (**c**) grafts. They can be inserted 1–2 mm below the superior margin of the nasal dorsum in order not to create middle vault widening

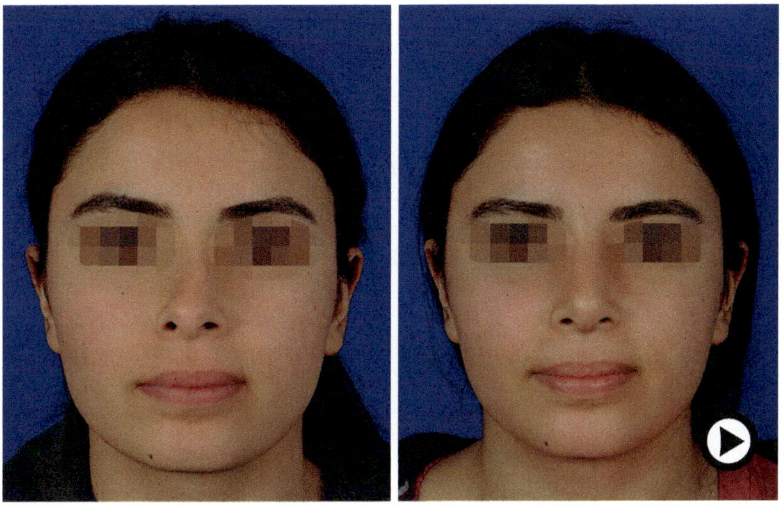

Fig. 10.20 Bilateral spreader grafts are designed and used to reconstruct the nasal dorsum (▶ https://doi.org/10.1007/000-dz2)

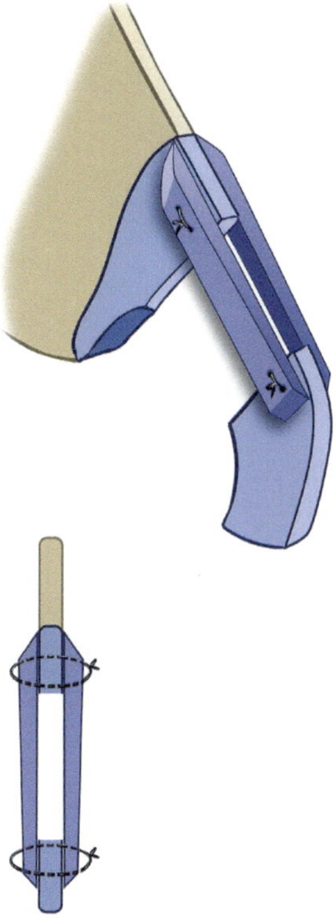

Fig. 10.21 The spreader grafts can be used to reconstruct the dorsal segment in some severe crooked noses or revision rhinoplasty cases

10.4 S-Shaped

This entity is more rarely seen in comparison with the previous two deformities. It is usually a more severe deformity, and the treatment will be discussed in the next chapter.

10.5 Revision Septoplasty

In rhinoplasty, one of the main reasons for revision is the deviated septum and deflections of the dorsal segment. When we find enough cartilage inside the nose, it is easier to solve the problems (Figs. 10.22 and 10.23). Unfortunately, while trying to correct these deformities, it is difficult to find sufficient septal cartilage for reconstruction. Therefore, the need to use grafts from the ear and, in the case of septal reconstruction, from the rib is higher. My preferred technique is to obtain cartilage from the sixth or seventh rib. I have been using rib cartilage to correct these deformities for 24 years. For the first 11 years, I have employed the Davis–Gibson principles to sculpt spreader grafts and

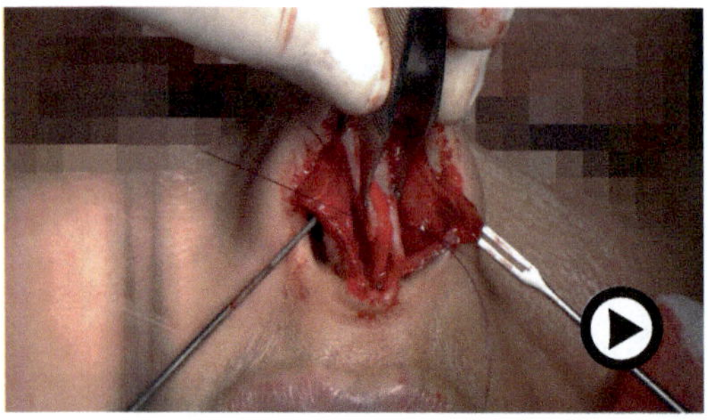

Fig. 10.22 A revision rhinoplasty was performed using septal cartilage grafts (▶ https://doi.org/10.1007/000-dz3)

caudal septal replacement grafts [11]. Although successful in many cases, the nose could be wide and stiff because the grafts were usually thick, rarely resulting in warping. Within the last 12 years, I switched to using the oblique split technique in sculpting the grafts, which has become a game changer for me [12, 13]. In this technique, the grafts are cut obliquely at 20–40 mm in length by keeping the outer cortex intact. The thickness can be adjusted from 0.5 to 3 mm without the fear of warping because eccentric cuts with the outer cortex intact have proven to be reliable in keeping the grafts straight (Fig. 10.24). As the grafts can be used thinner, the problem of widening of the middle vault disappeared, and the noses were less stiff. The obtained implants can be used to reconstruct a new dorsal segment using two splinting spreader grafts that are easily coupled with a caudal septal extension or replacement graft (Fig. 10.25). In addition, when these grafts can be sculpted thinner, they almost act like septal cartilage in shape and consistency [13].

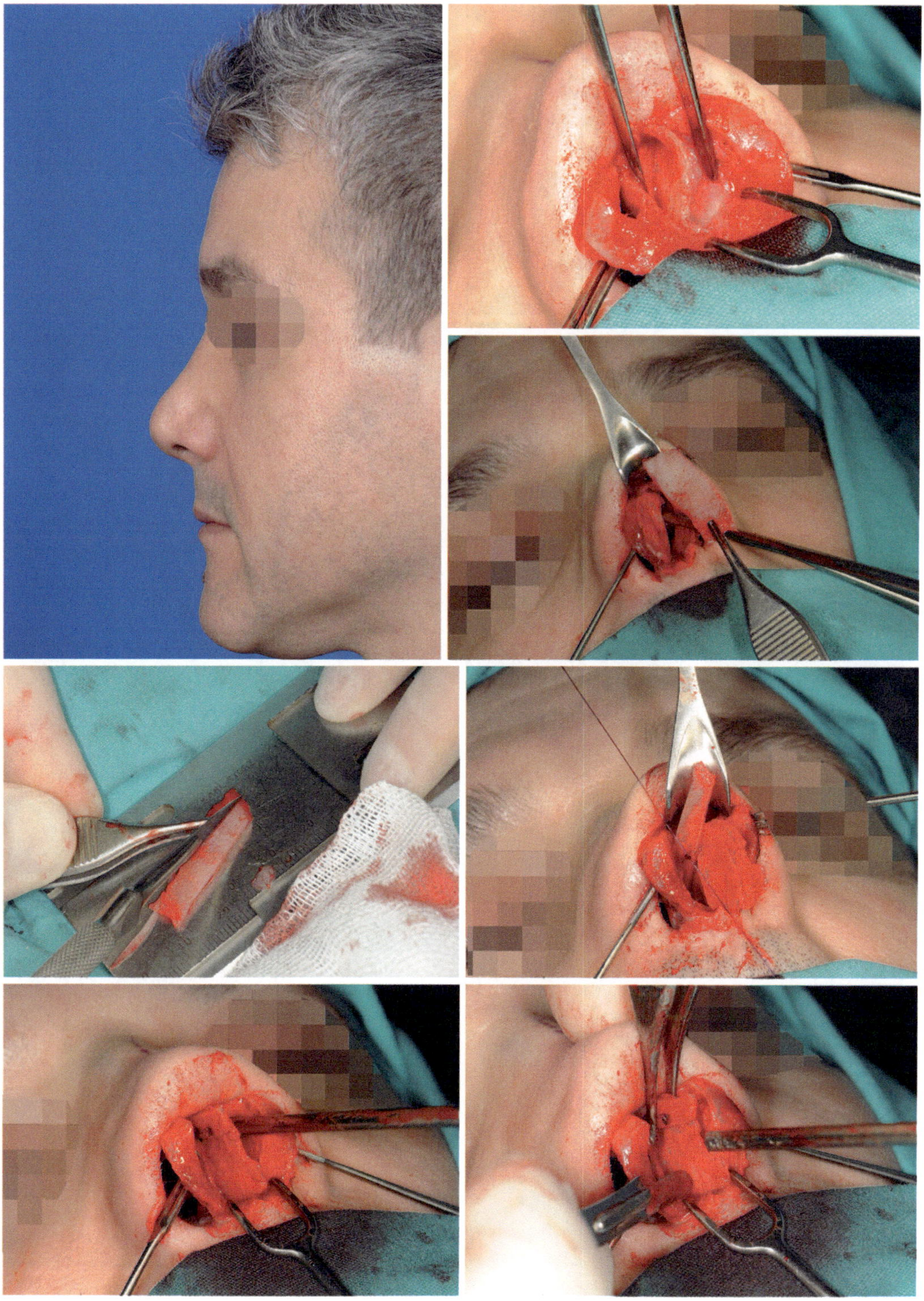

Fig. 10.23 This is a patient with a crooked nose after rhinoplasty. During surgery, enough cartilage could be found inside the nose. A unilateral spreader graft and a batten graft for the caudal septum were used. Besides, ear cartilage was harvested and used for columellar strut, alar battens, and rim grafts. The sixth year postoperative pictures can be seen here

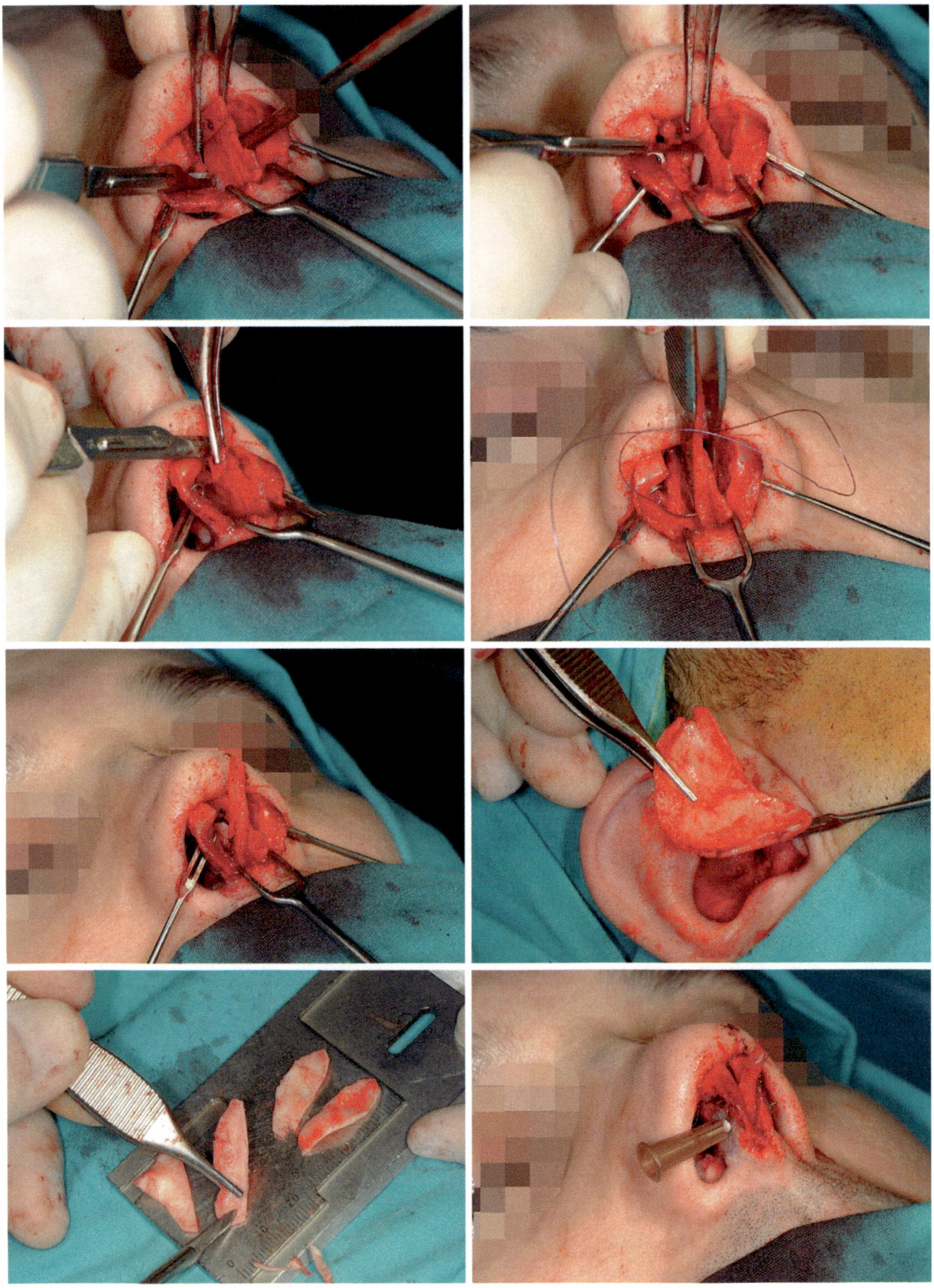

Fig. 10.23 (continued)

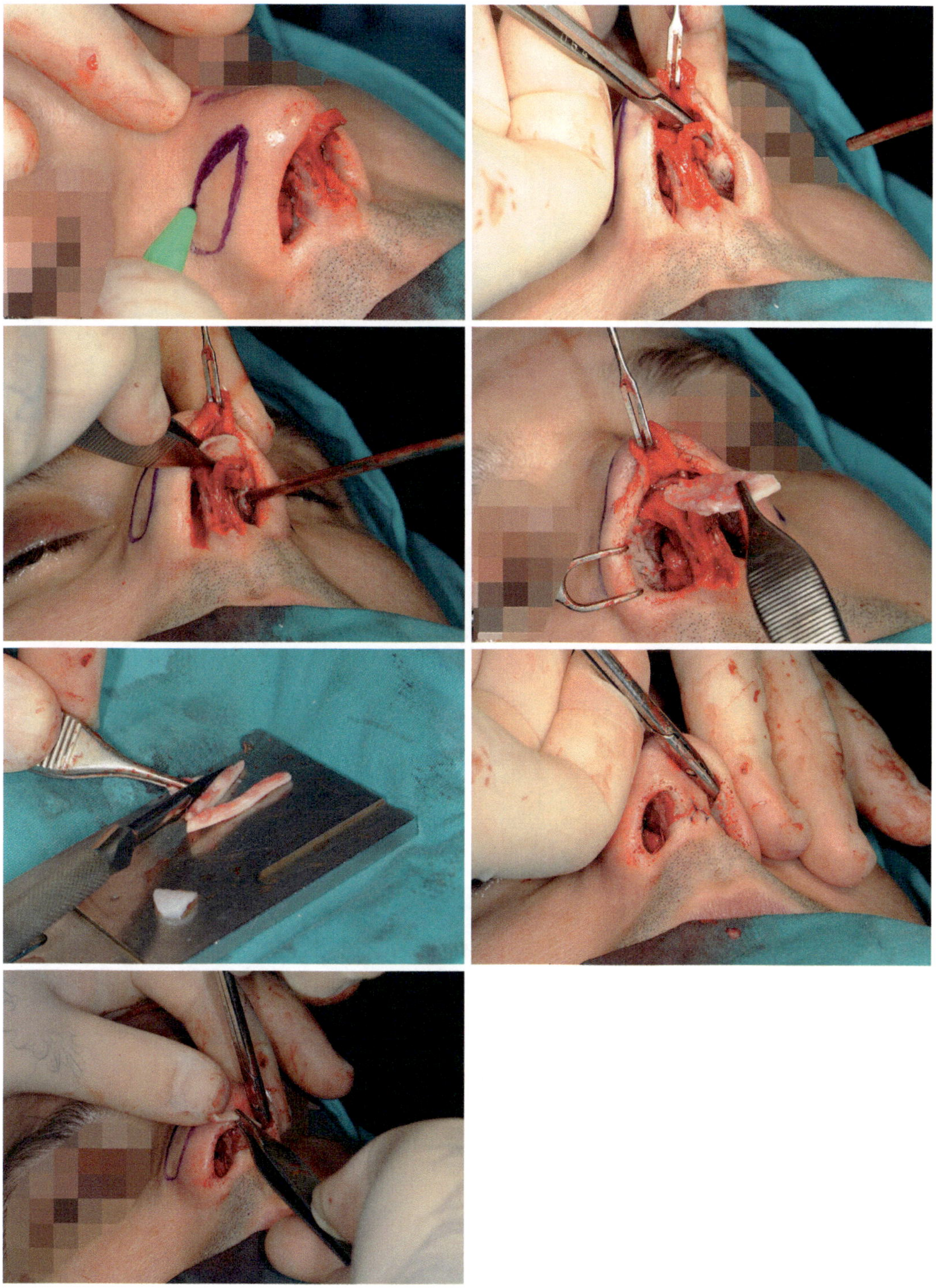

Fig. 10.23 (continued)

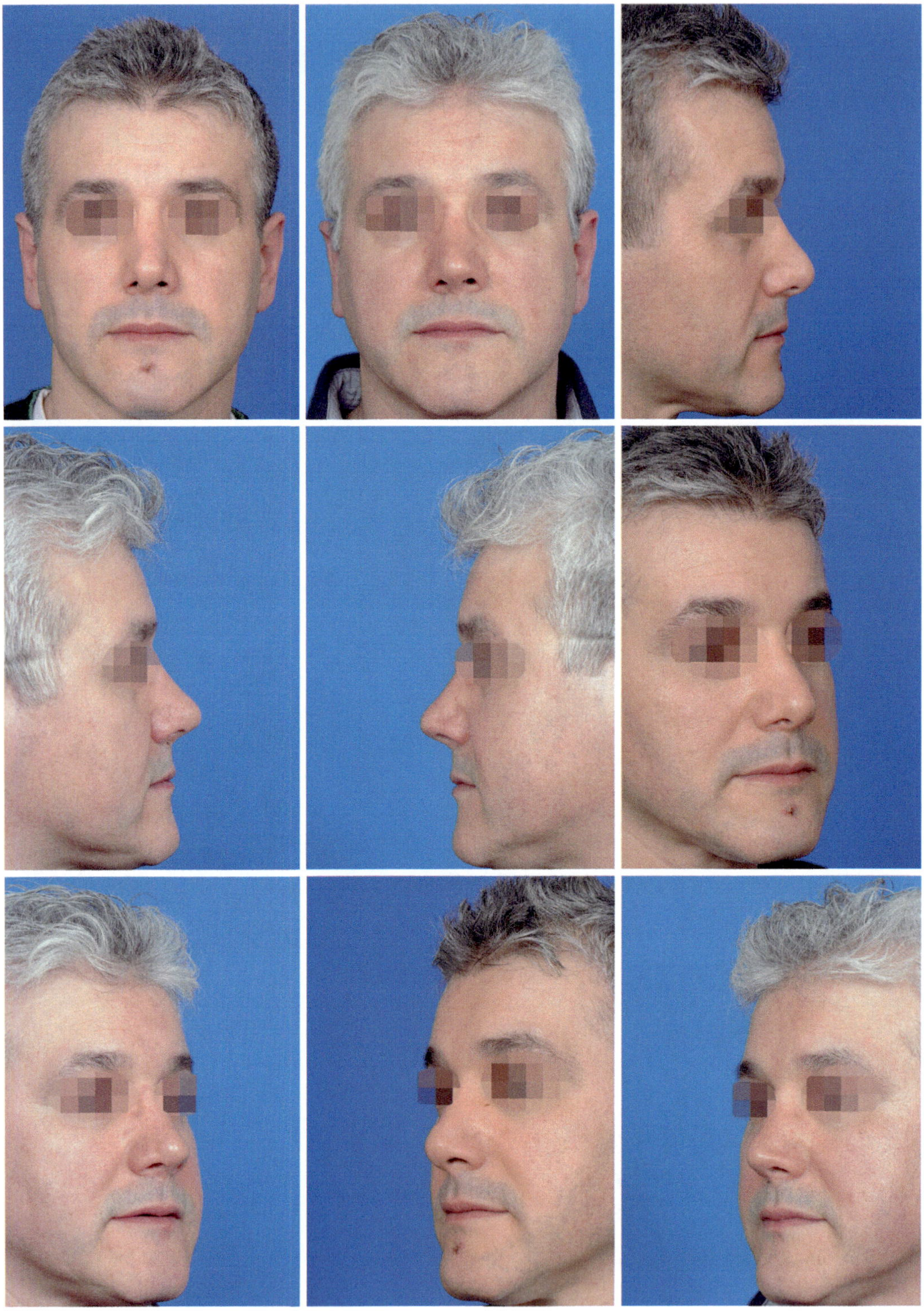

Fig. 10.23 (continued)

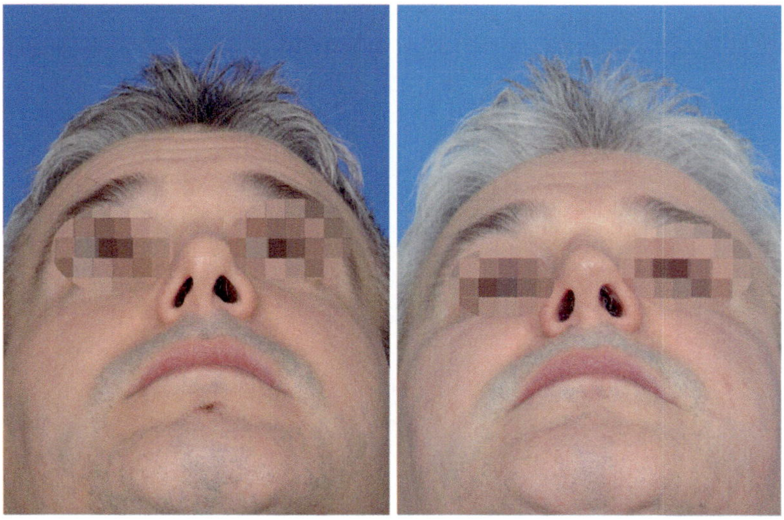

Fig. 10.23 (continued)

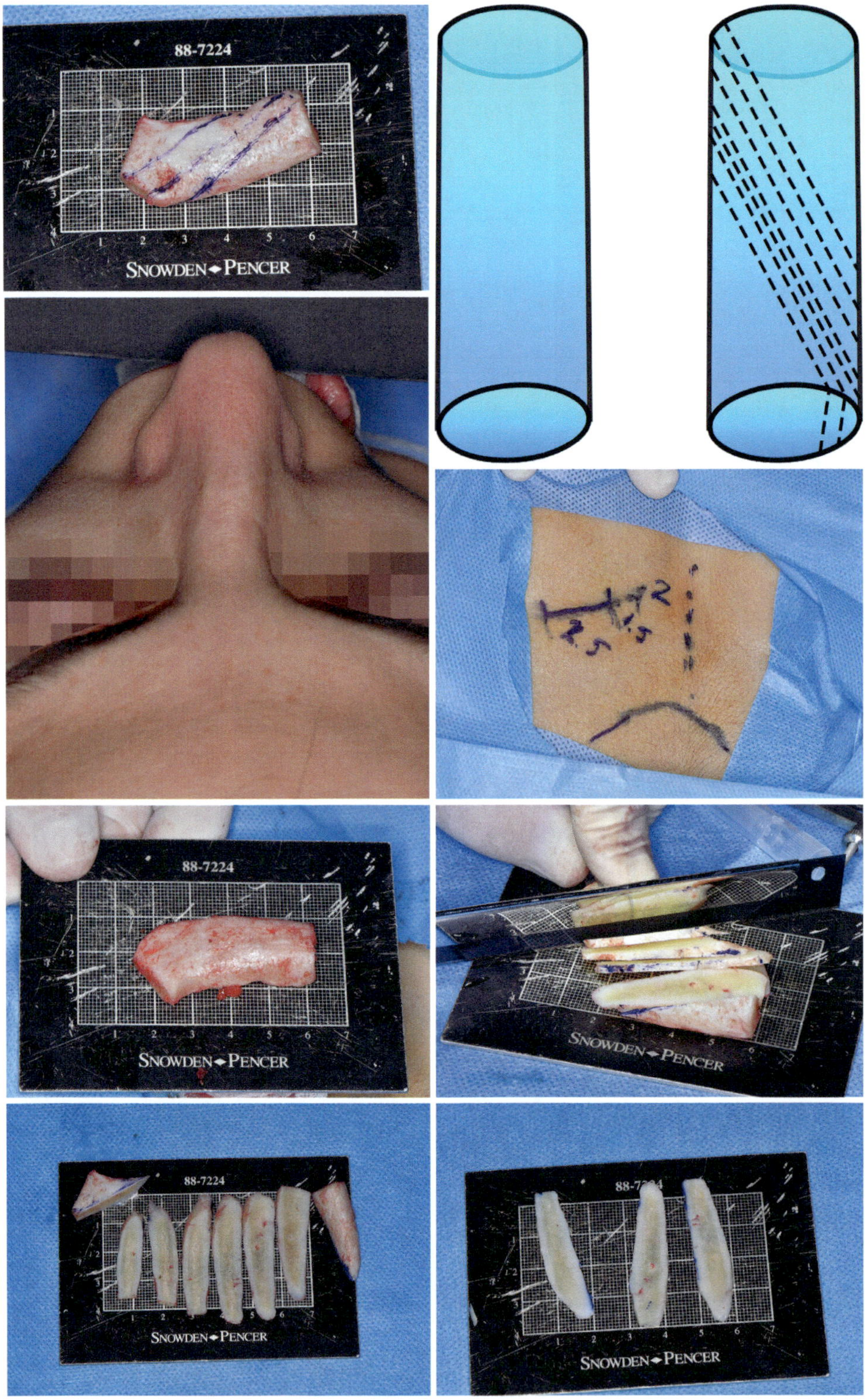

Fig. 10.24 Oblique split technique is a game changer for me in sculpting the implants that can be used during revision rhinoplasties. It is possible to obtain longer grafts of different thickness and size with less chance of warping. In this case, the crookedness was due to high septal deviation at the ethmoid junction. Stronger splinting grafts from rib cartilage easily helped us to correct the crookedness

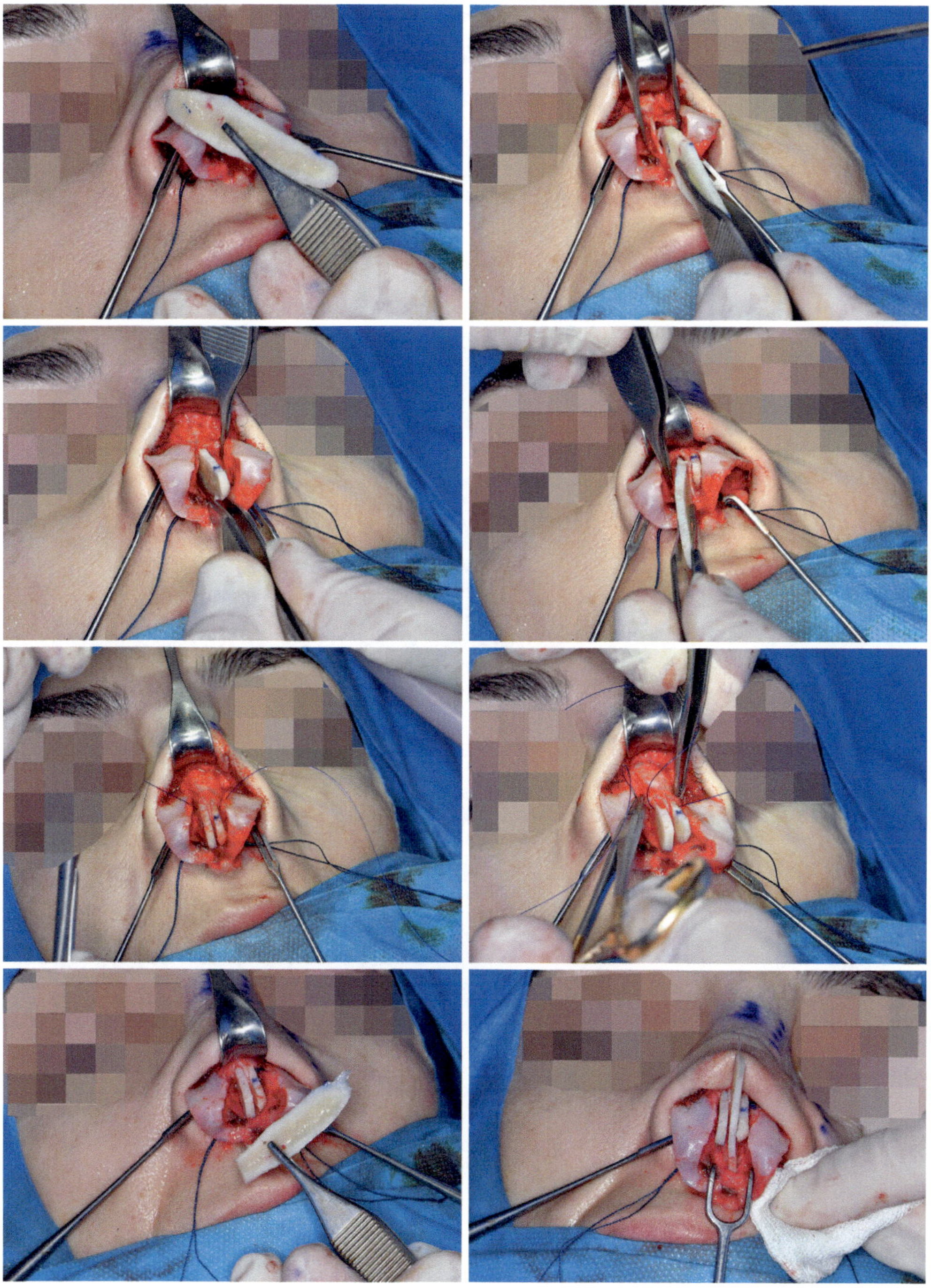

Fig. 10.24 (continued)

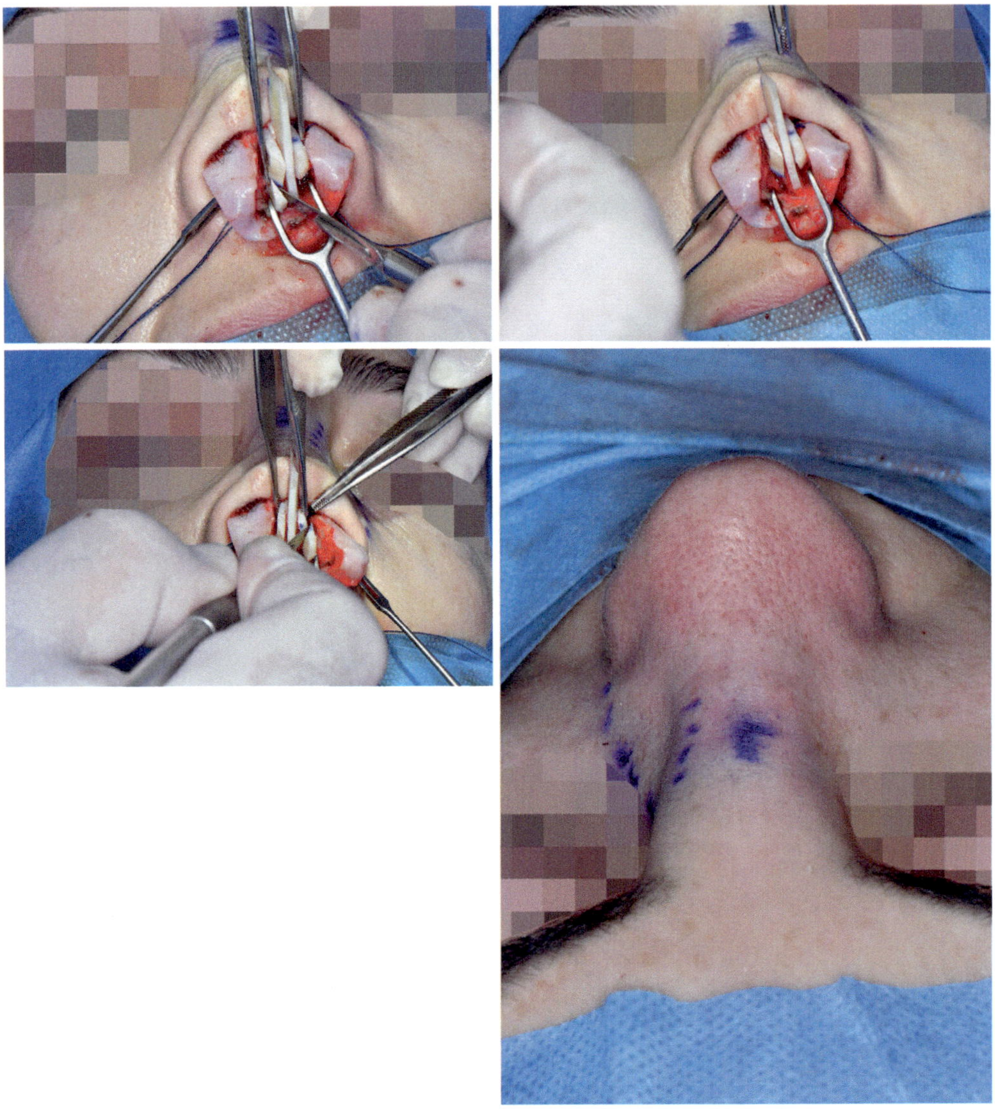

Fig. 10.24 (continued)

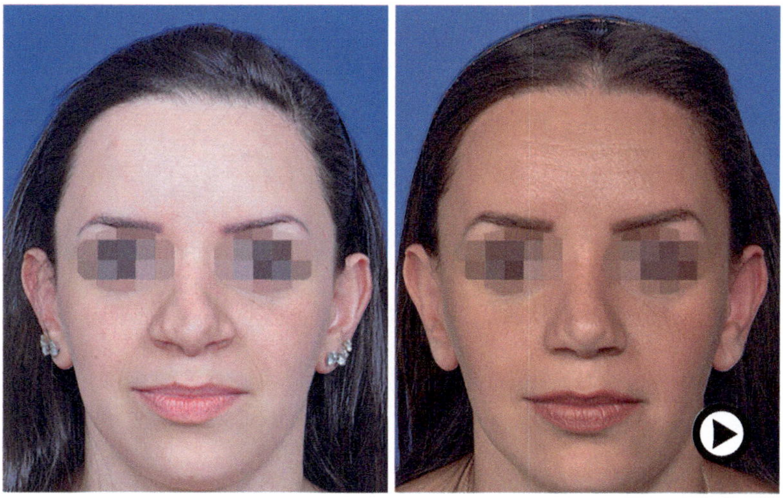

Fig. 10.25 Costal cartilage is used to correct crookedness and tip deformity in a revision rhinoplasty (▶ https://doi.org/10.1007/000-dz4)

References

1. Beeson WH. The nasal septum. Otolaryngol Clin North Am. 1987;20:743–67.
2. Cottle MH. Nasal roof repair and hump removal. AMA Arch Otolaryngol. 1954;60:408–14.
3. Sheen JH. Spreader graft: a method of reconstructing the roof of the middle nasal vault following rhinoplasty. Plast Reconstr Surg. 1984;73:230–9.
4. Rohrich RJ, Hollier LH. Use of spreader grafts in the external approach to rhinoplasty. Clin Plast Surg. 1996;23:255–62.
5. Apaydin F. Segmental reconstruction for nasal septal deviation. Facial Plast Surg. 2013;29:455–63.
6. Byrd HS, Salomon J, Flood J. Correction of the crooked nose. Plast Reconstr Surg. 1998;102:2148–57.
7. Cerkes N. The crooked nose: principles of treatment. Aesthet Surg J. 2011;31:241–57.
8. Sazgar AA. The bony cartilaginous unit: the missing graft in septorhinoplasty. Int J Oral Maxillofac Surg. 2016;45:1006–8.
9. Apaydin F. Septal surgery challenges in rhinoplasty. Facial Plast Surg. 2016;32:351–60.
10. Apaydin F. Bone recycling in nasal septal reconstruction. Facial Plast Surg. 2013;29:473–8.
11. Gibson T, Davis WB. The distortion of autogenous cartilage grafts: its cause and prevention. Br J Plast Surg. 1958;10:257–73.
12. Taştan E, Yücel ÖT, Aydin E, Aydoğan F, Beriat K, Ulusoy MG. The oblique split method: a novel technique for carving costal cartilage grafts. JAMA Facial Plast Surg. 2013;15:198–203.
13. Apaydin F. Oblique split technique: a game changer in costal cartilage sculpting. Plast Aesthet Res. 2019;6:9.

11 Dorso-Caudal Deviations of the Septum

11.1 Introduction

Crooked noses can affect the dorsal and/or caudal segments of the L-strut framework. Isolated deviations of the caudal and dorsal segments were addressed in previous chapters. In this chapter, the management of the deviations affecting the dorsal segment, caudal segment, and the junction between these segments will be focused on (Fig. 11.1).

I observed some interesting findings in patients with crooked noses or badly deviated septums within the past 24 years [1]:

1. The main reason for causing a deviation is usually one or more fractures that are usually located more anterior on the nasal septal cartilage. The posterior part of the septal cartilage is usually straight and less affected by these fractures, although they are deviated. Therefore, a good amount of cartilage or a bony-cartilaginous graft can be obtained without touching the deviated L-strut framework (Fig. 11.2).
2. Most crooked noses and badly deviated septums are the result of childhood trauma [2]. Like the theory of use and disuse of Lamarck, the obstructed nasal passage is used less often during breathing, which is why it stays narrower during the child's development [3]. On the contralateral side, the nasal airway becomes much wider and in time the inferior turbinate can go for compensatory hypertrophy because of the bigger amount of respiratory air passing through. This situation serves as an advantage regarding the use of an L-strut graft because there is space where this graft can be inserted on the concave side, and it rarely causes nasal obstruction (Fig. 11.3).
3. The caudal segment was found to be thinner and weaker in these patients, most probably because of bearing less pressure during the child's development.

In this kind of deviation, there are three options: (1) splinting, (2) resecting and reconstructing, (3) cutting and overlapping.

Supplementary Information The online version contains supplementary material available at https://doi.org/10.1007/978-3-031-74734-2_11. The videos can be accessed individually by clicking the DOI link in the accompanying figure caption or by scanning this link with the SN More Media App.

© The Author(s), under exclusive license to Springer Nature Switzerland AG 2025

F. Apaydın, *Septal Surgery Challenges in Rhinoplasty*,
https://doi.org/10.1007/978-3-031-74734-2_11

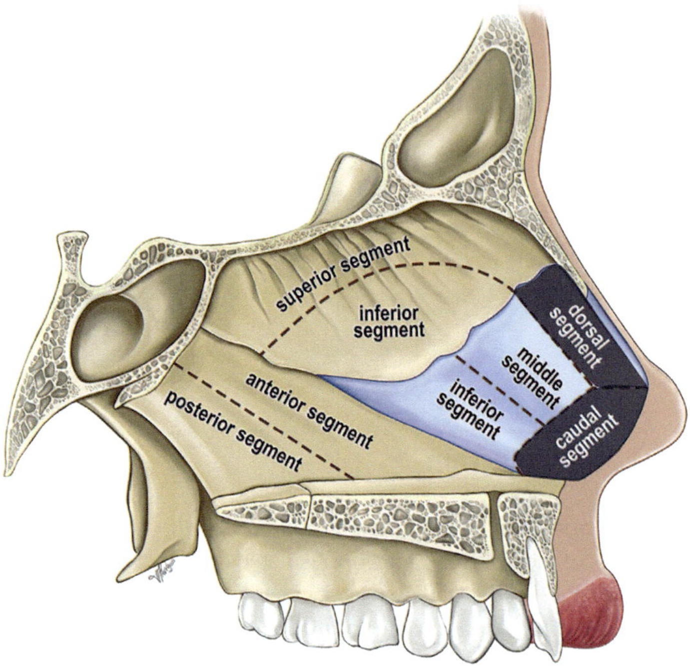

Fig. 11.1 The L-strut framework is composed of the dorsal and caudal segments. Deviations of this framework create a challenge for the surgeon

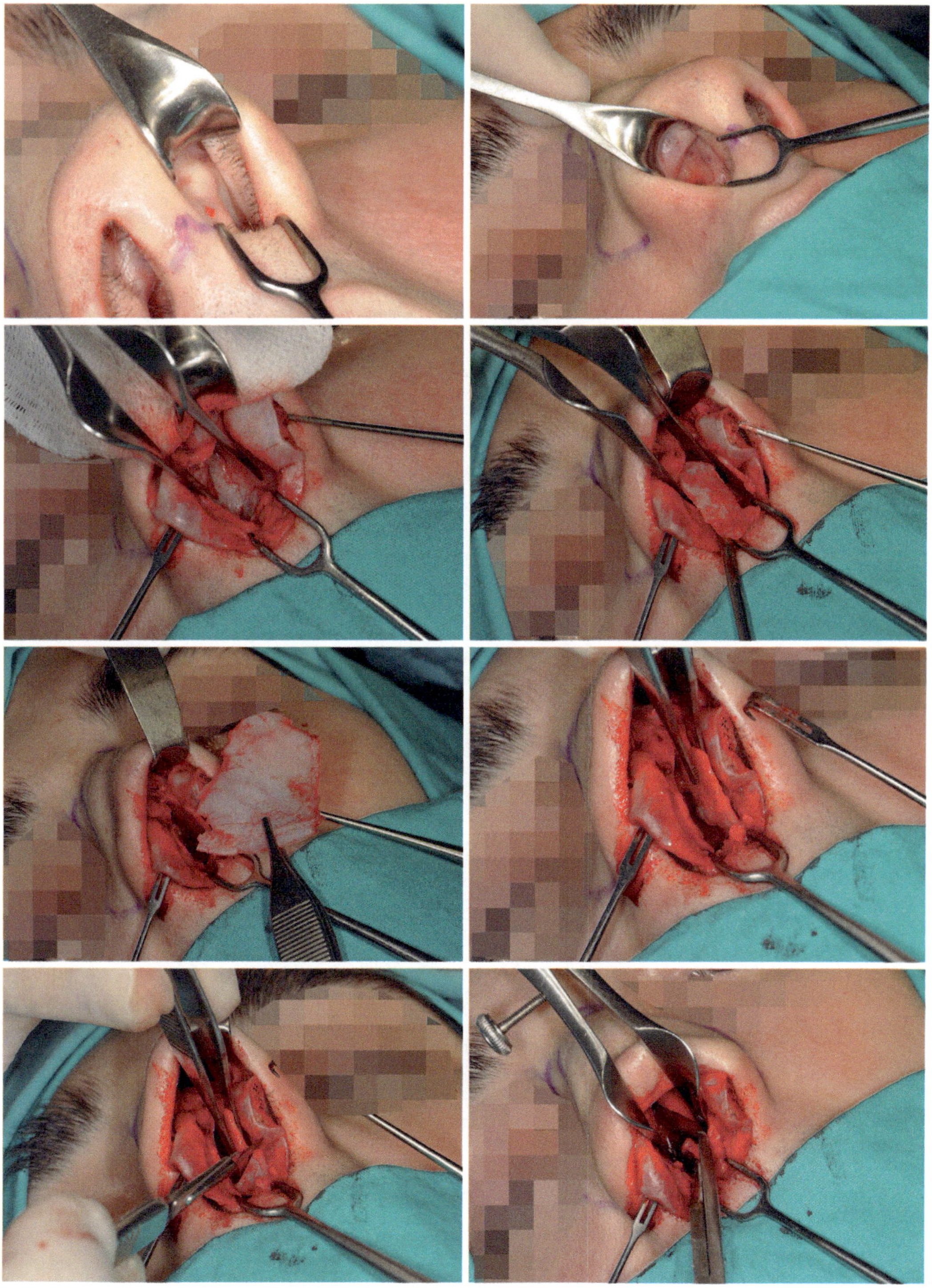

Fig. 11.2 A 21-year-old young man with a crooked nose. During the external approach, three fracture lines were seen, and the fractured segments of cartilage were removed by following the fracture lines. The posterior part of the septal cartilage was not affected by these fractures, and it was straight. A caudal septal replacement graft was sculpted from the harvested cartilage. It was sutured to the anterior nasal spine and to the dorsal segment, which was later supported by a spreader graft. A columellar strut was sutured to the spreader graft and to the caudal septal replacement graft

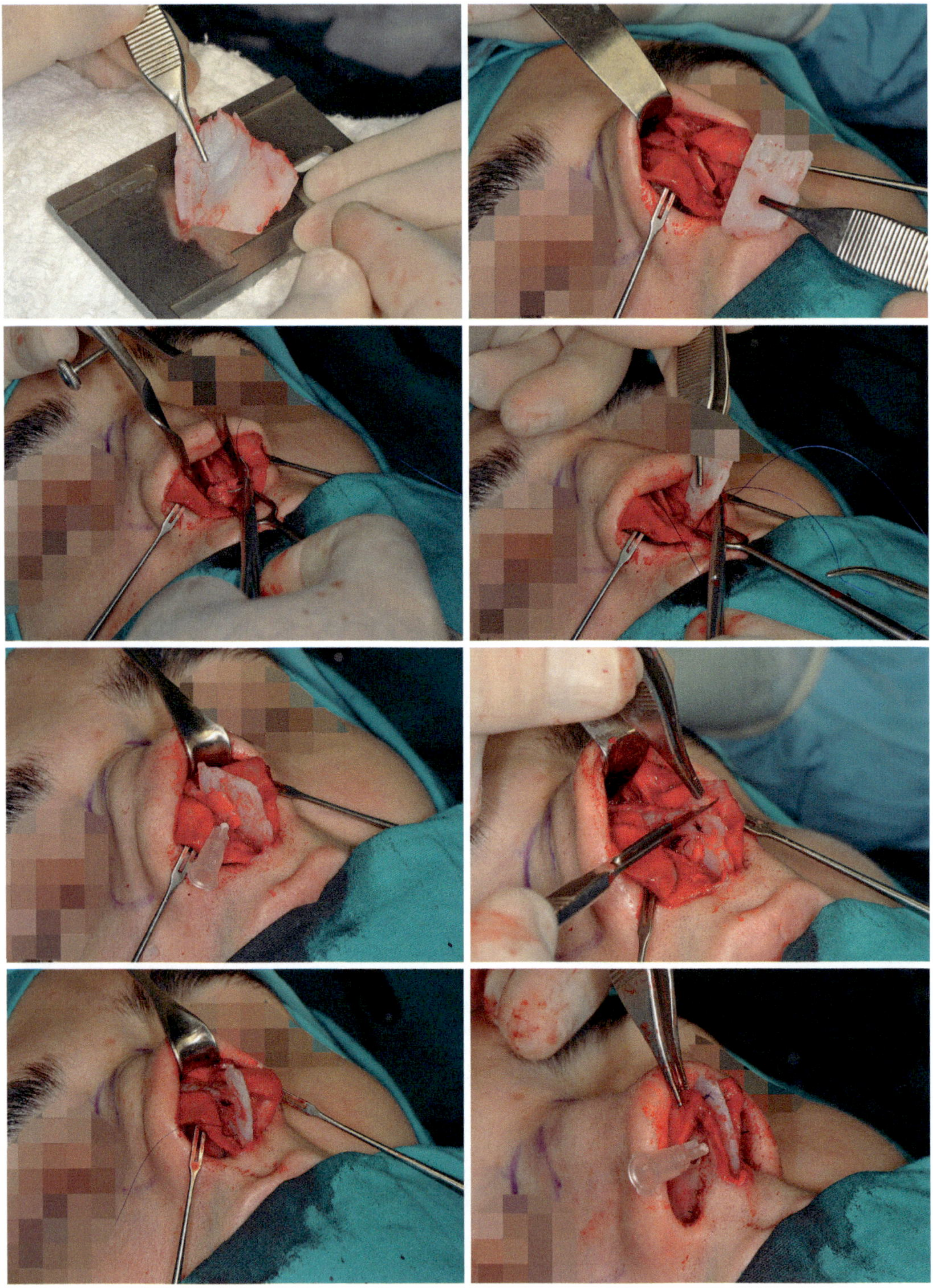

Fig. 11.2 (continued)

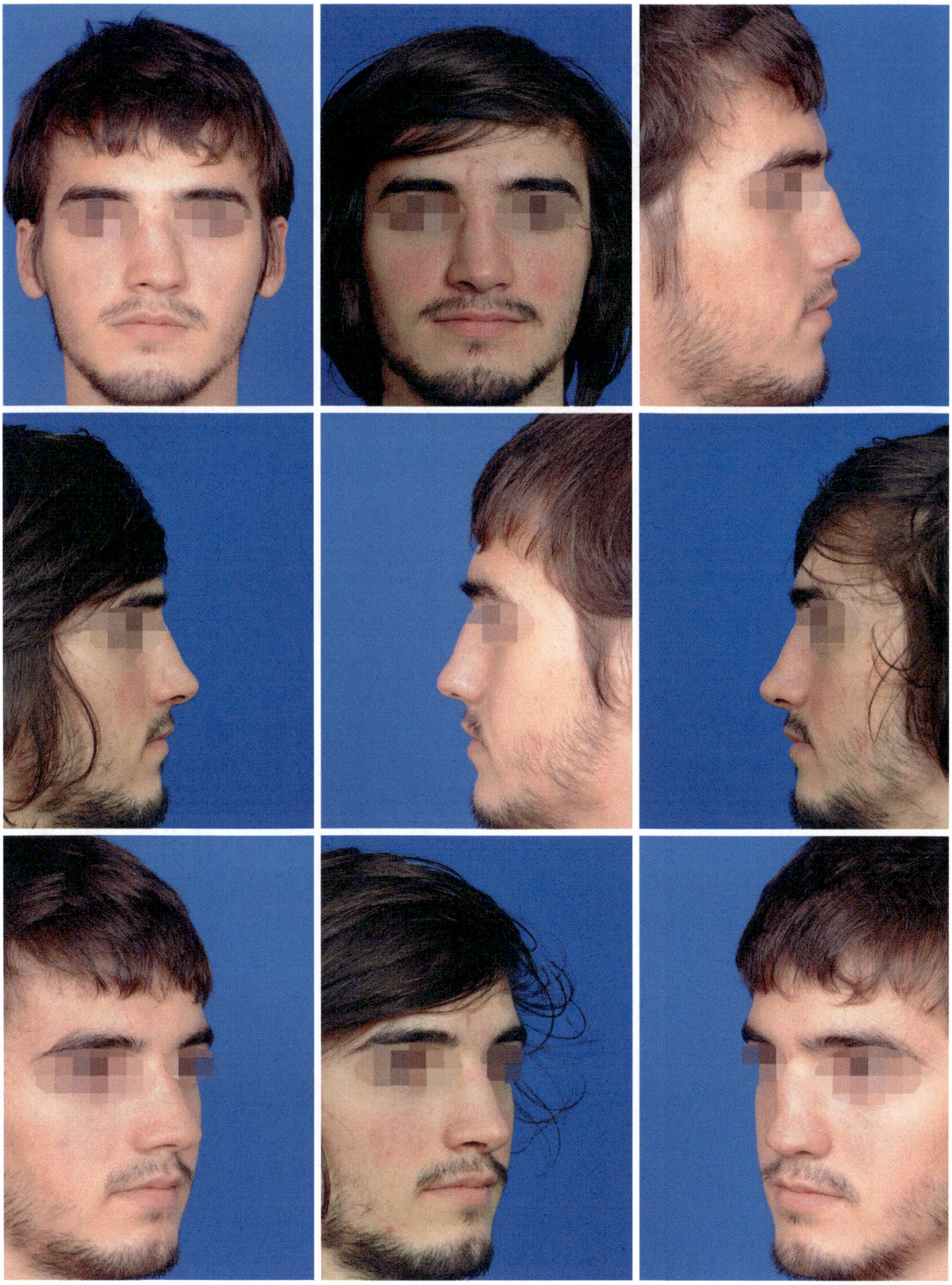

Fig. 11.2 (continued)

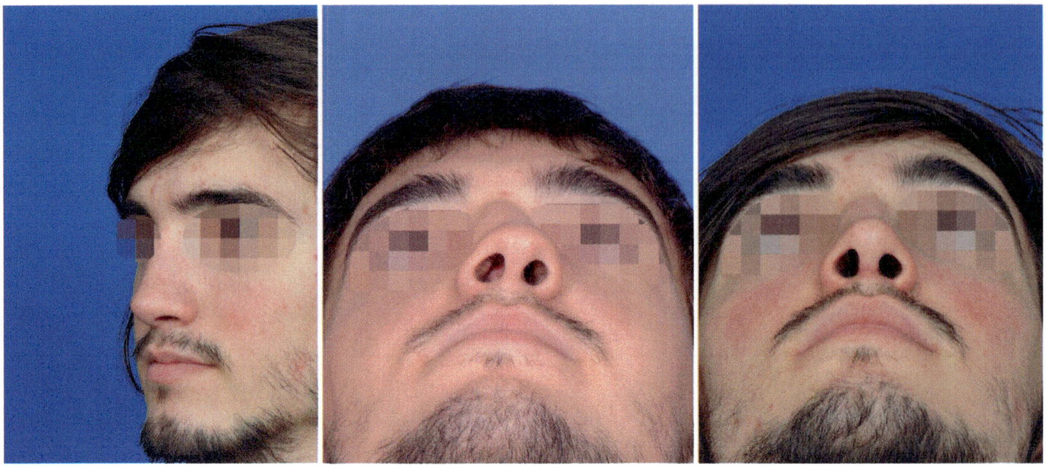

Fig. 11.2 (continued)

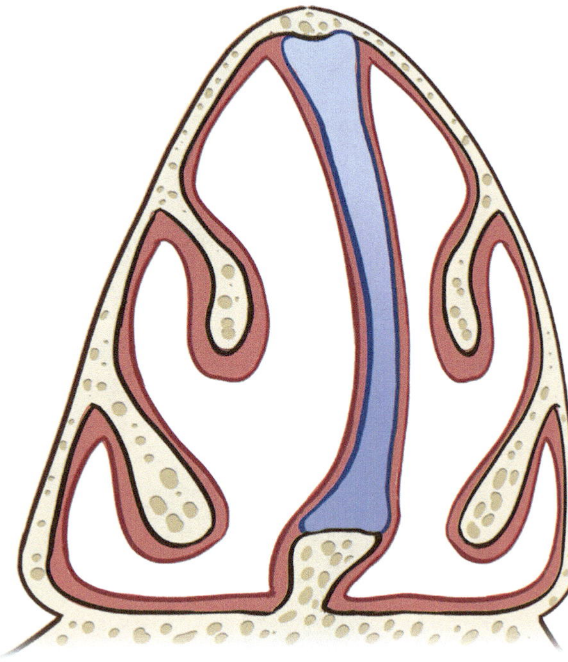

Fig. 11.3 One of the main reasons for crooked noses is childhood trauma. In these kinds of cases, I observed that one nasal passage was always smaller than the other. I think it is due to the theory of use and disuse of Lamarck. The obstructed nasal passage is used less often during breathing, and it stays narrower during the child's development. On the contralateral side, the nasal airway becomes wider

11.2 Splinting Methods

Splinting of the L-strut framework without resection offers many advantages. First, it is easier to decide on profile, rotation, and projection because the original nasal septum is preserved. Second, because the central main support is preserved, it is much easier to add splinting grafts around it. However, it should also be kept in mind that recurrence is more often seen with these methods.

11.2.1 Spreader Grafts

They are described in detail in Chap. 11. Therefore, spreader grafts alone can sometimes be the solution to this kind of problem. However, the spreader grafts should be slightly bigger, especially in height, splinting a bigger surface of the L-strut framework (Fig. 11.4). In addition, when there is an angle of deflection due to a fracture line and if this line is resected, this type of modified spreader graft is very effective for coupling the dorsal and caudal segments together (Fig. 11.5). The deviated caudal segment can be corrected simply by trimming the caudal portion adjacent to the anterior nasal spine or by cross-hatching and splinting (Figs. 11.6, 11.7, and 11.8).

11.2.2 Caudal Septal Extension Grafts and Batten Grafts

Both grafts are very useful in correcting deviations in the caudal segment. If they are put as a bigger graft, they can also be helpful in correcting the deviations at the junction (Fig. 11.9). They can be used together with splinting spreader grafts to correct such deviations (Figs. 11.10 and 11.11). However, these two kinds of grafts are not always successful in correcting the deviations at the junction.

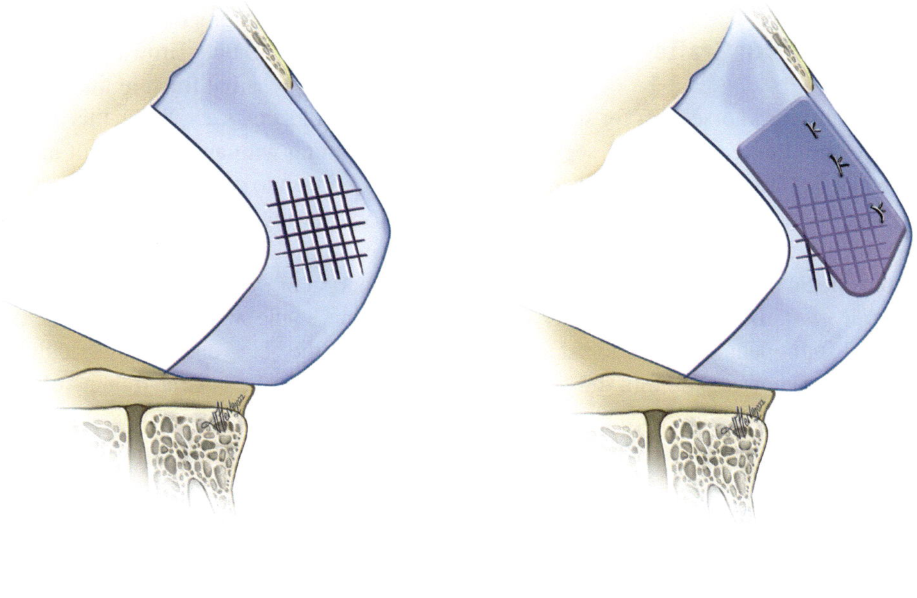

Fig. 11.4 Spreader grafts can be sculpted into a bigger and stronger graft to splint the deviations of the L-strut framework

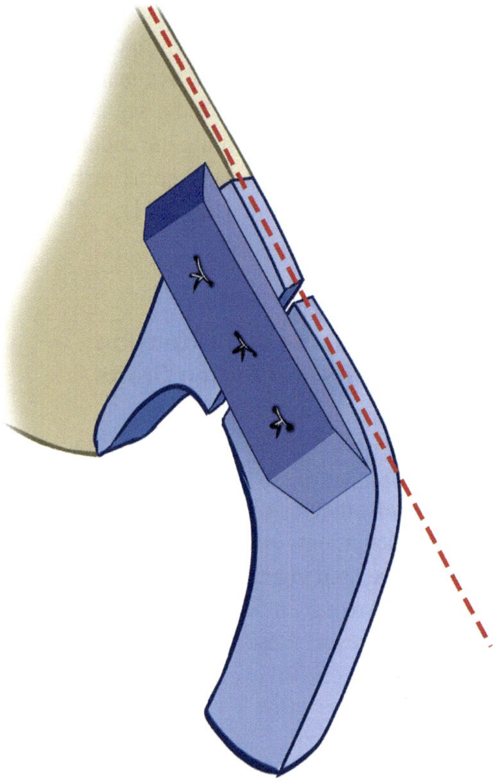

Fig. 11.5 If there is an angle of deflection due to a fracture line, this line can be resected, and a bigger spreader graft is very useful in keeping the dorsal and caudal segments together

11.2.3 L-Strut Grafts

This is my workhorse graft for specific situations where the dorsal and caudal segments and the junction between them are crooked (Fig. 11.12). In fact, I found out that this was the situation in a lot of cases. Cartilage and/or bone harvest is the most critical part to obtain a big piece to use as an L-strut graft. Before I harvest any cartilage or bone, I start opening the subdorsal tunnels with a Freer elevator as 3–5 mm tunnels in height, reaching the upper third of the nose. Then I open the tunnels below by leaving a 3–5 mm of mucoperichondrium attached to the septal cartilage on one side or both sides. It is aimed to leave 12–15 mm of dorsal and cartilage height on the L-strut framework in place when possible. In some instances, a narrower strip has been left while maintaining the integrity of the L-strut framework and supported by the L-strut graft [4, 5]. I used to crosshatch the L-strut framework to break the memory causing the deviation and splint it with the L-strut graft [6]. I almost always use a spreader graft on the contralateral side to counterbalance the midline septal cartilage, fixate the L-strut graft much better, and keep it in the midline (Figs. 11.13, 11.14, and 11.15). It worked well during the last 20 years, during which I observed only a few recurrences of deviation.

Many goals can be reached by using the L-strut graft [1]:

1. Splint the deviated dorsal segment
2. Splint the deviated caudal septum
3. Splint the junction of the dorsal and caudal septum
4. Support the nasal tip as a caudal extension graft
5. The remaining L-shaped framework is used as a scaffold to help keep the original integrity and shape of the nose

I have changed my approach to the L-strut framework in recent years. When I operate on a case with a crooked nose and septum, I try to identify the deflection site by putting the dorsal and caudal segments in a straight position with the help of two Brown-Adson forceps unless there is a visible fracture line. It is usually in the form of a dog's ear. When this dog ear is resected, splinting with an L-strut graft and spreader graft is enough to correct the deviation since the memory causing the deflection is eliminated. However, in some cases, the deflection reaches the outer margin of the L-strut framework, and a full cut is done at the angle of deflection. It is surprising that the cut ends get straight immediately. However, the L-strut framework is destabilized. The L-strut framework is stabilized again using the L-strut graft and spreader graft. I use a small trick in this step. After I identify the deflection site and plan the cut line, I place the L-strut graft or spreader graft on the concave side, and the graft is sutured to the dorsal segment or caudal segment on both sides of the resection. After the L-strut framework is secured by either of these

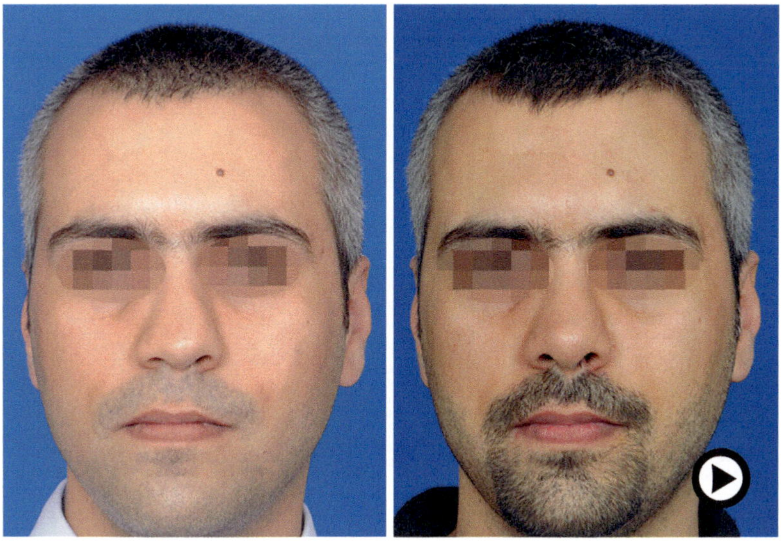

Fig. 11.6 Ethmoid bone and bilateral spreader grafts are used to splint the L-strut framework (▶ https://doi.org/10.1007/000-dzb)

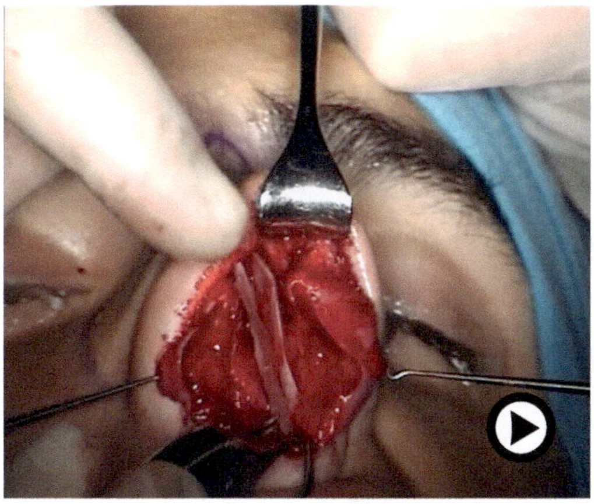

Fig. 11.7 Ethmoid bone and bilateral spreader grafts are used to splint the L-strut framework in a crooked nose (▶ https://doi.org/10.1007/000-dz6)

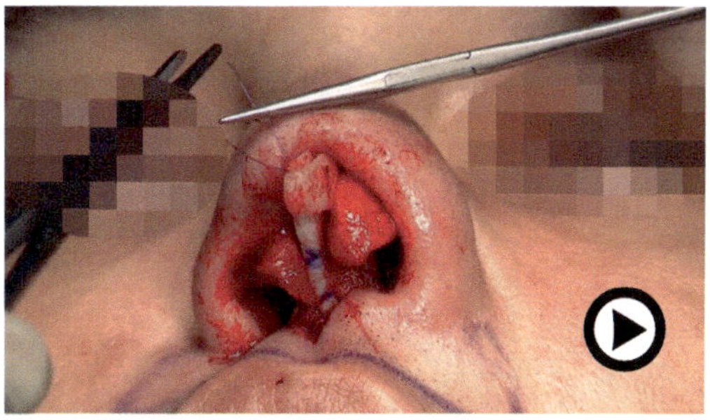

Fig. 11.8 Costal cartilage is used for a total septal reconstruction for a Binder's syndrome patient (▶ https://doi.org/10.1007/000-dz7)

two grafts, the full cut is performed. After the cut, a spreader graft is sutured so that the dorsal segment of the nasal septum is supported from both sides, which keeps the dorsal segment straight.

We published the use of the L-strut graft in 119 patients with very badly deviated septums from 2000 to 2019. The most common type of material for the L-strut graft was cartilaginous in 100 (84.03%), bony-cartilaginous in 11 (9.24%), and bony in 8 (6.72%) patients [1] (Fig. 11.16). As can be seen, the main source of this graft is septal cartilage. Since 2019, I have been using this graft more often in patients with crooked noses (Fig. 11.17).

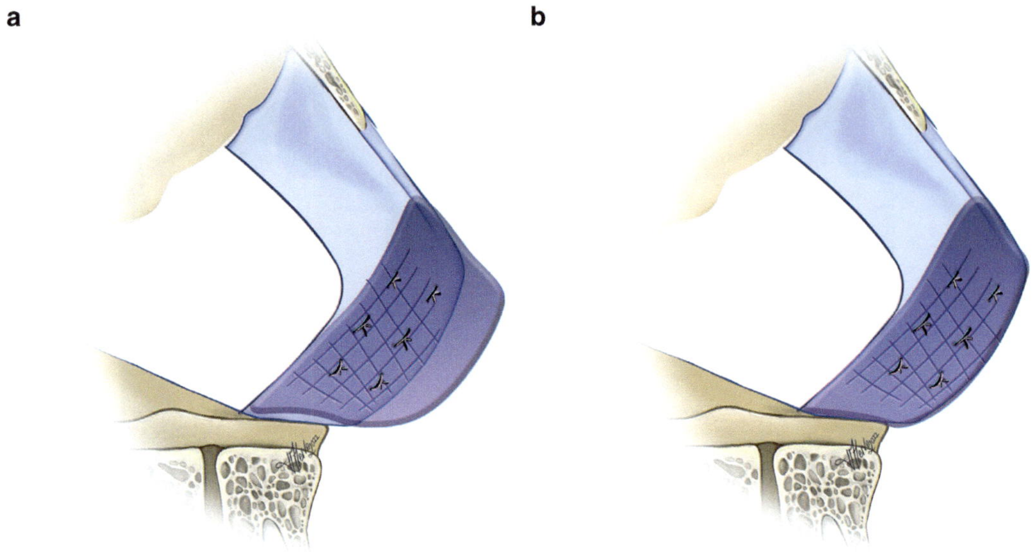

Fig. 11.9 Caudal septal extension grafts and batten grafts are very effective in splinting and correcting the deviations of the caudal septum (**a**, **b**)

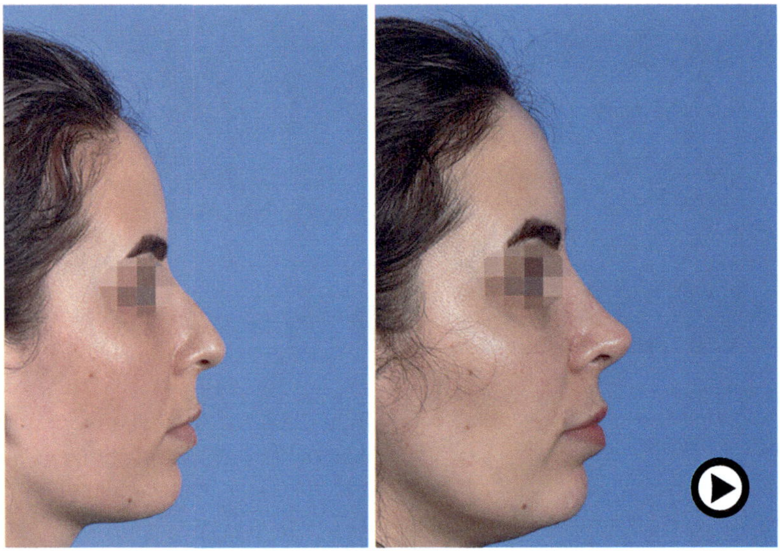

Fig. 11.10 Caudal septal extension graft and an unilateral spreader graft are sutured in opposing sides of the septum (▶ https://doi.org/10.1007/000-dz8)

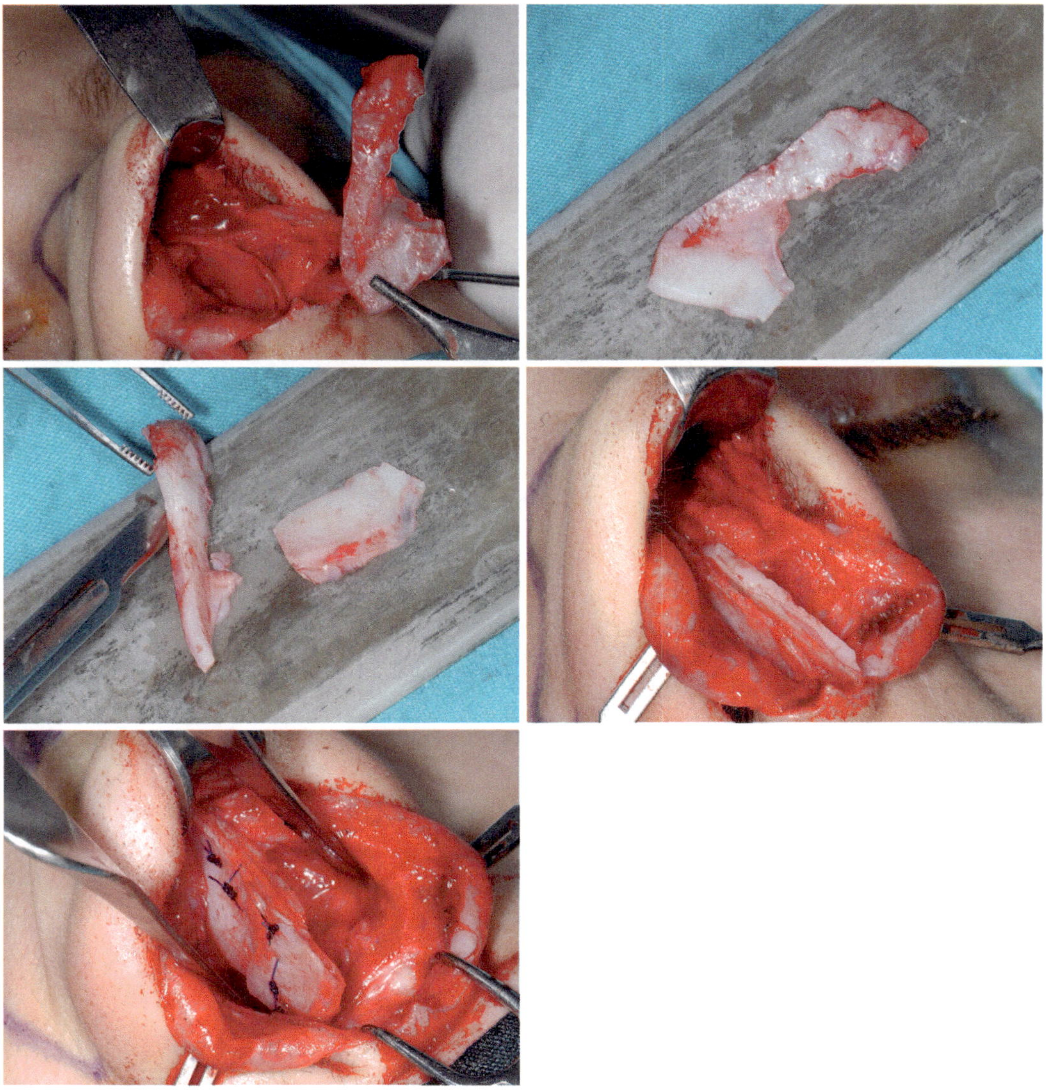

Fig. 11.11 Caudal septal extension grafts and batten grafts are sometimes used with splinting spreader grafts

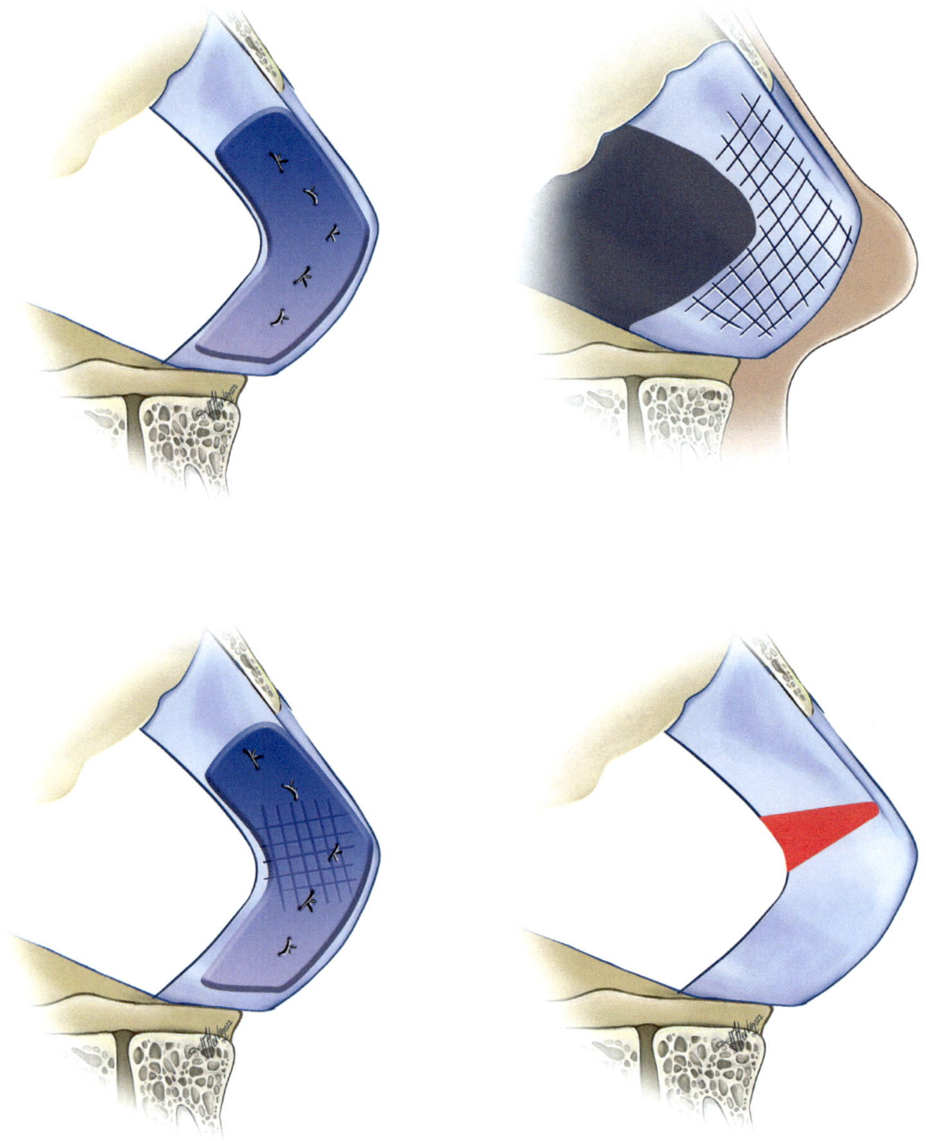

Fig. 11.12 L-strut grafts are the best option for me to splint and correct the deviations affecting the L-strut framework in cases of C-shaped crookedness (1). There are four scenarios in my experience: (1) If the L-strut framework is weak, it can be applied directly on the concave side (2); (2) If the framework is strong, cross-hatching can be used to break the memory, and then the L-strut framework and splinting with the L-strut graft work well (3, 4). If there is a prominent angle of deflection or fracture line, it can be partially (5, 6) or totally resected and then splinted (7, 8)

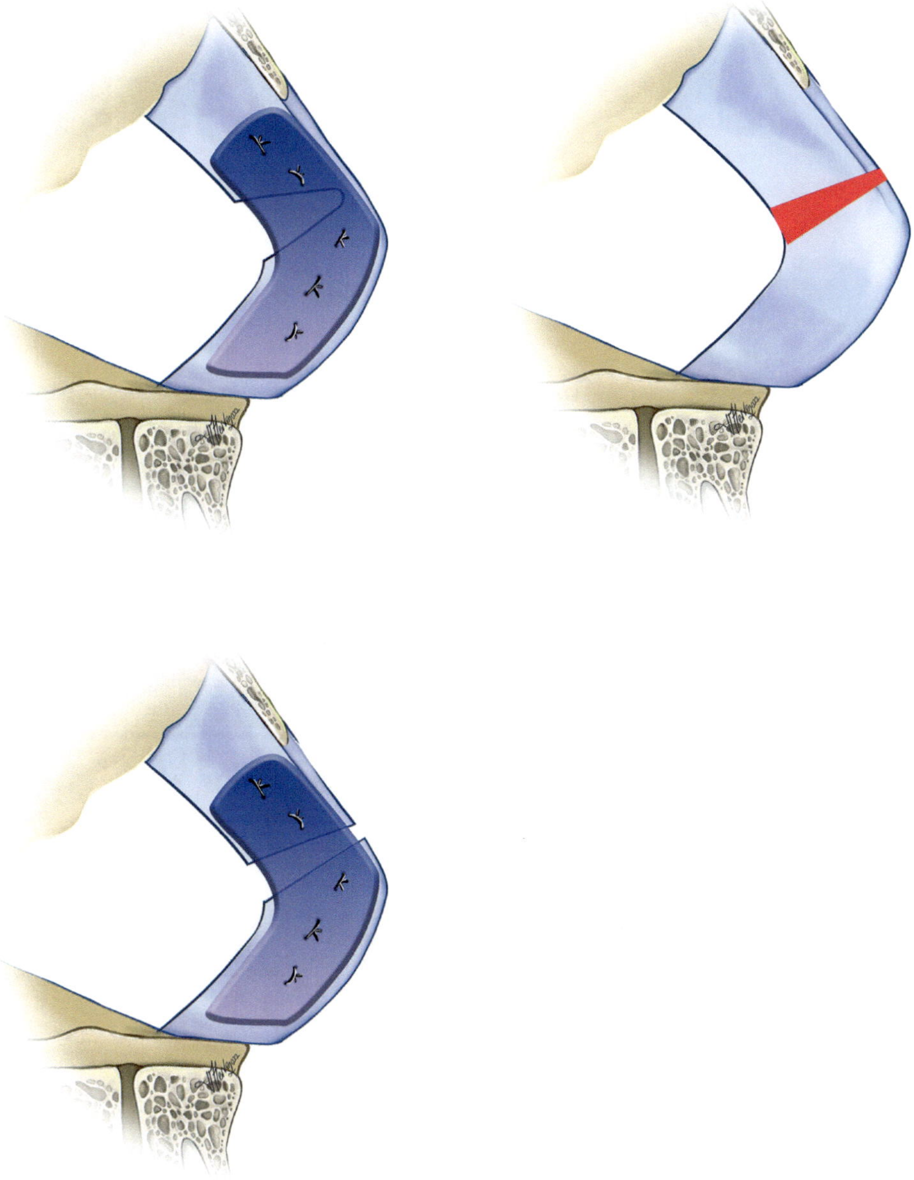

Fig. 11.12 (continued)

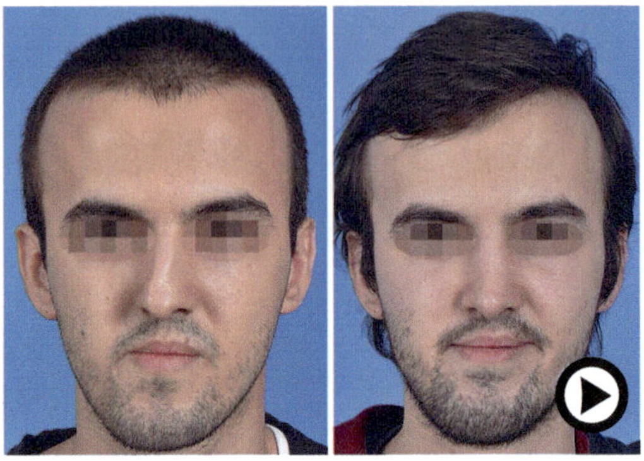

Fig. 11.13 L-strut graft and bilateral spreader grafts are used to reconstruct the septum in a crooked nose patient (▶ https://doi.org/10.1007/000-dz9)

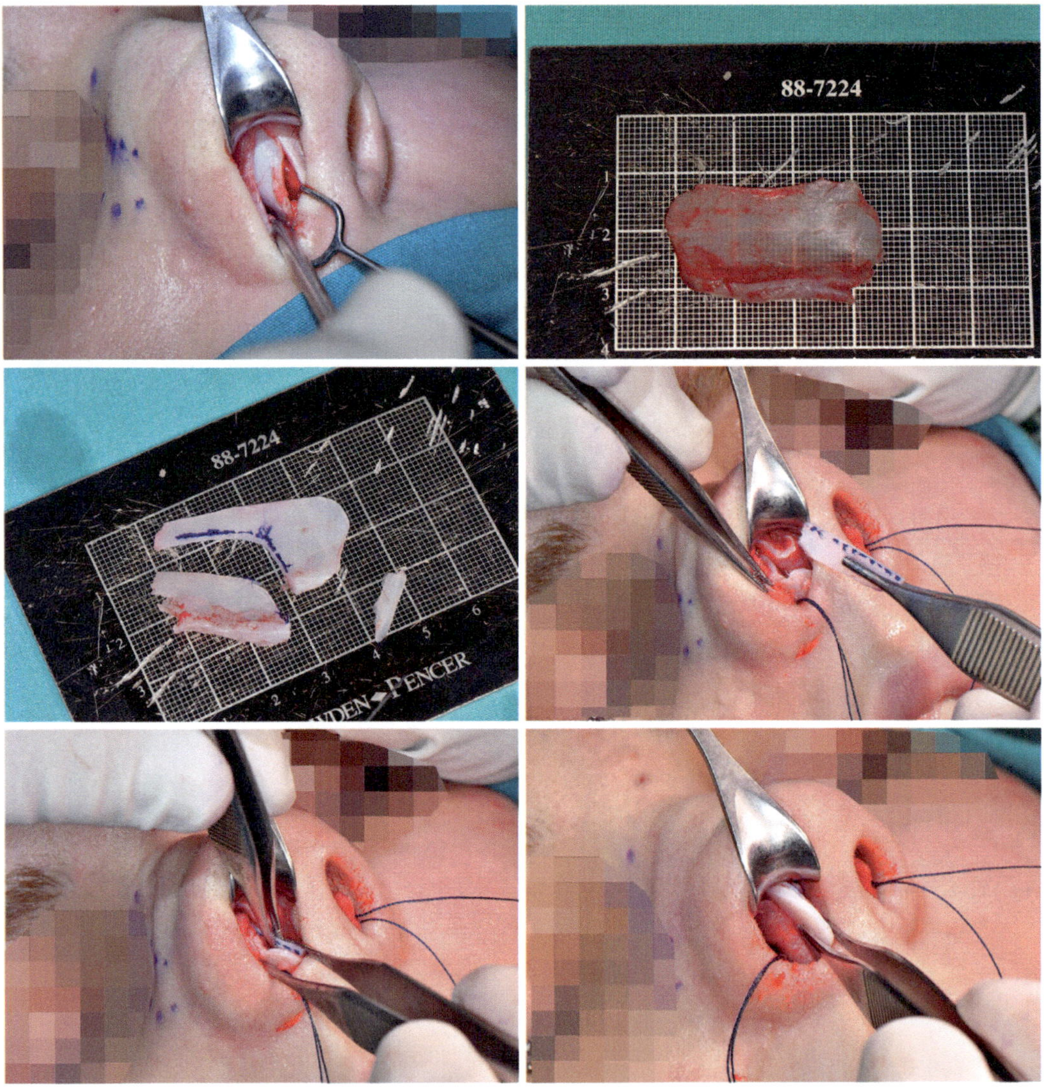

Fig. 11.14 L-strut grafts can be used together with spreader grafts endonasally in crooked noses

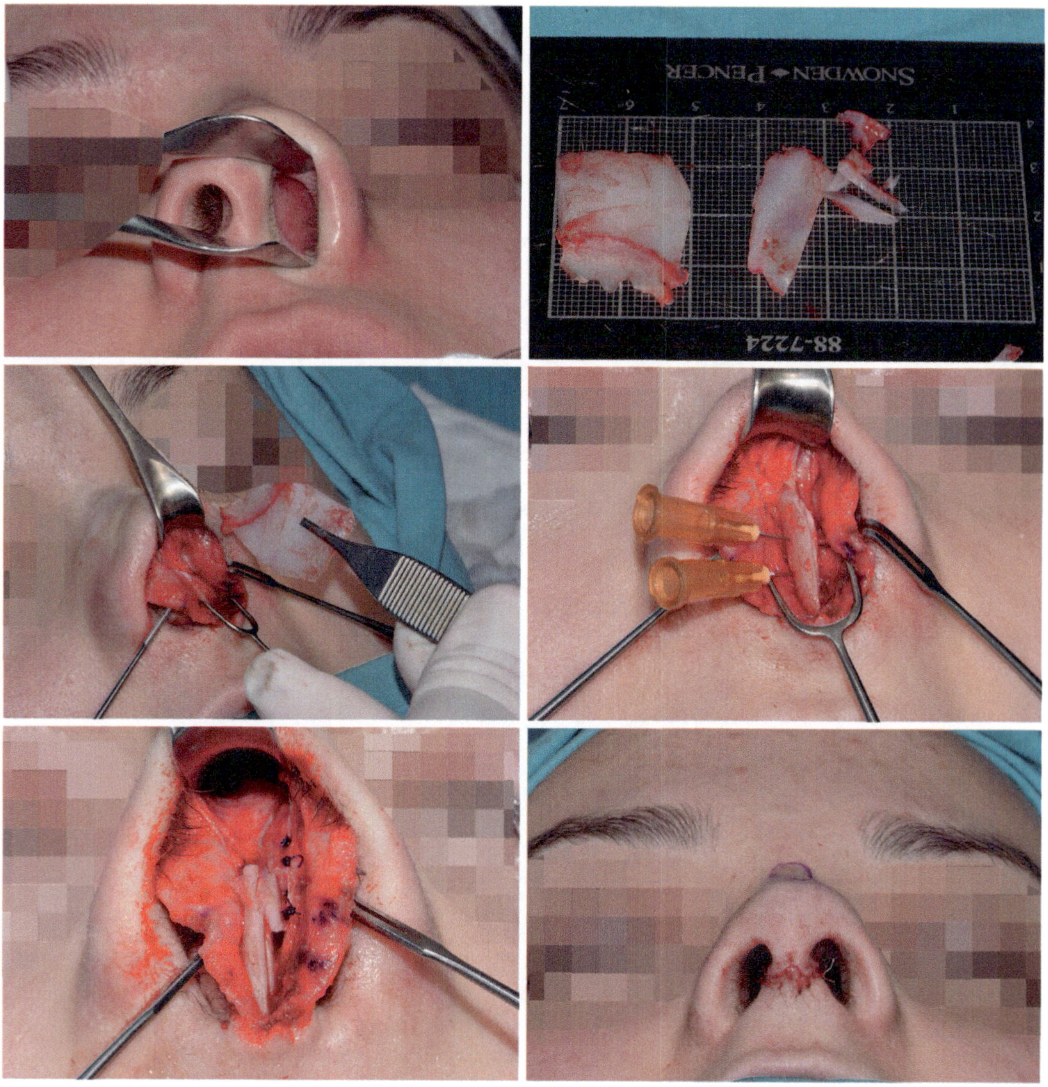

Fig. 11.15 L-strut grafts can be cartilaginous, bony, and bony-cartilaginous

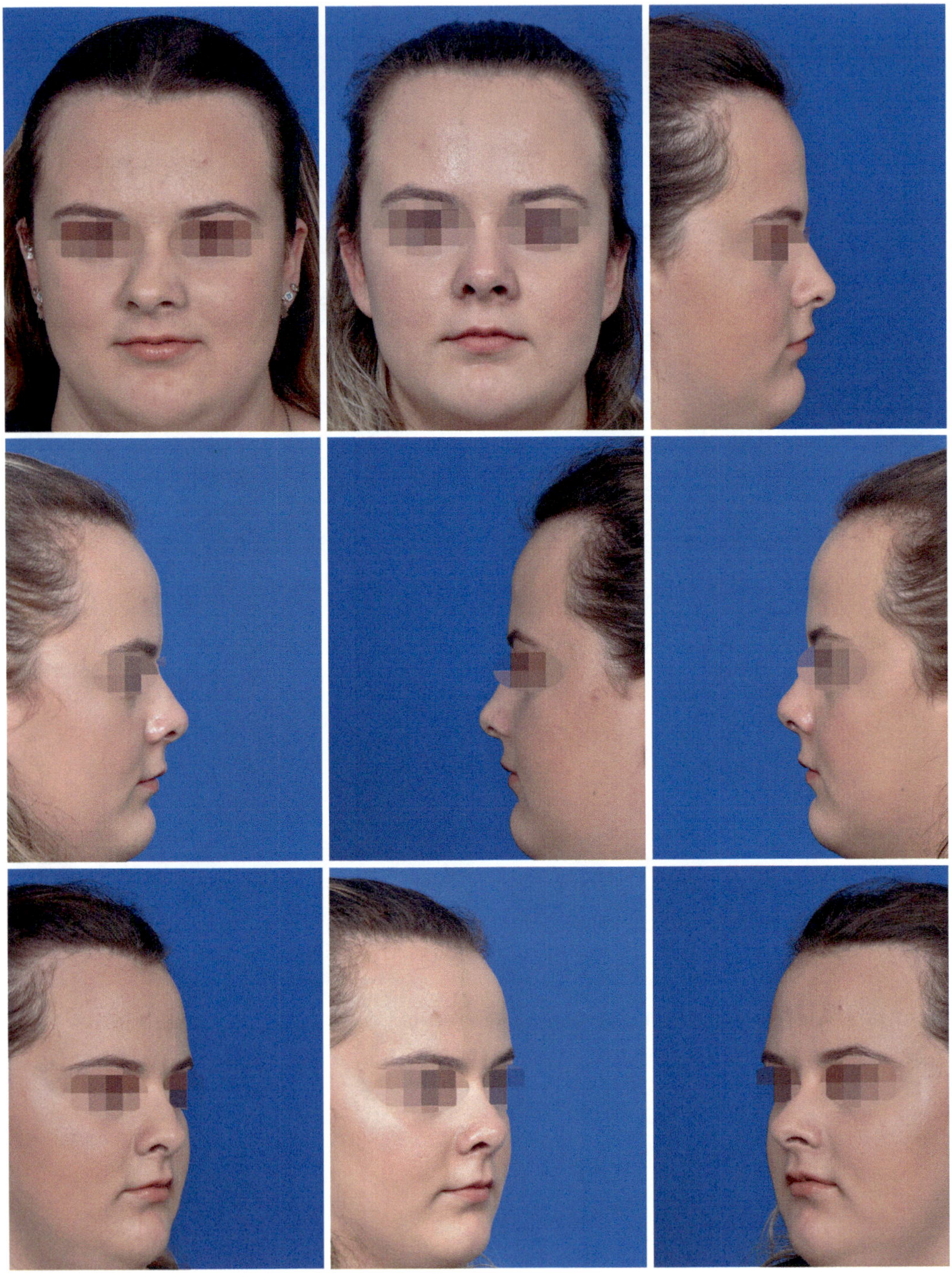

Fig. 11.15 (continued)

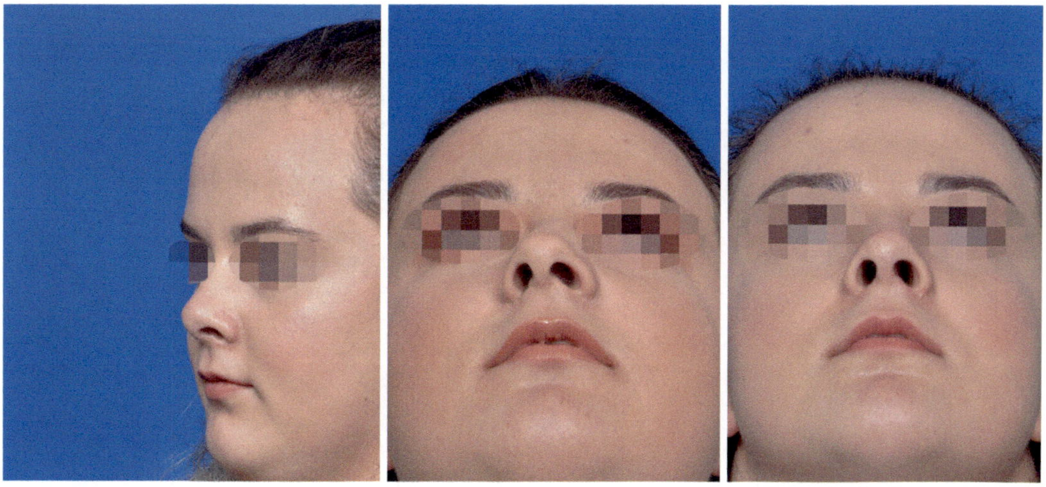

Fig. 11.15 (continued)

Fig. 11.16 Preoperative and second-year postoperative pictures of a 23-year-old patient. Her left nasal passage was totally obstructed. A bony-cartilaginous L-strut graft was inserted on the right side and a spreader graft on the left side

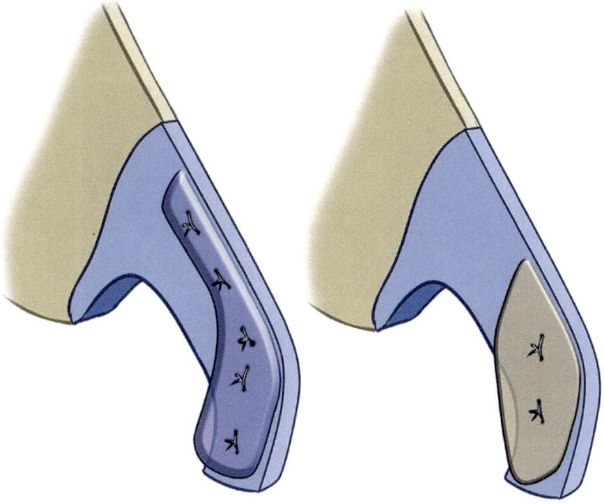

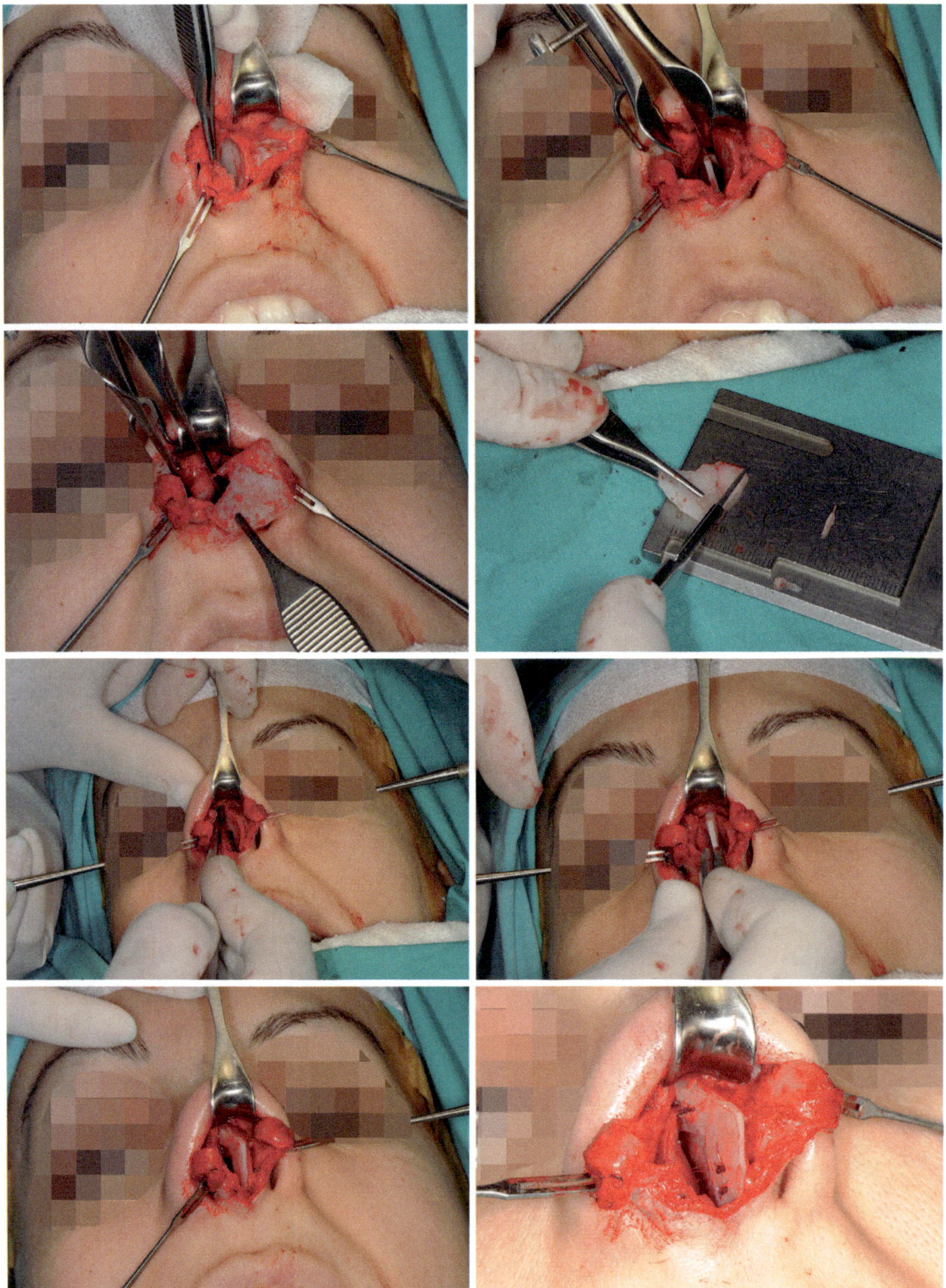

Fig. 11.17 In a revision rhinoplasty case with crookedness, an L-strut graft could be carved from the septal cartilage. Ear cartilage was harvested for the lateral crural strut graft and columellar strut. Postoperative pictures were taken 1 year after surgery

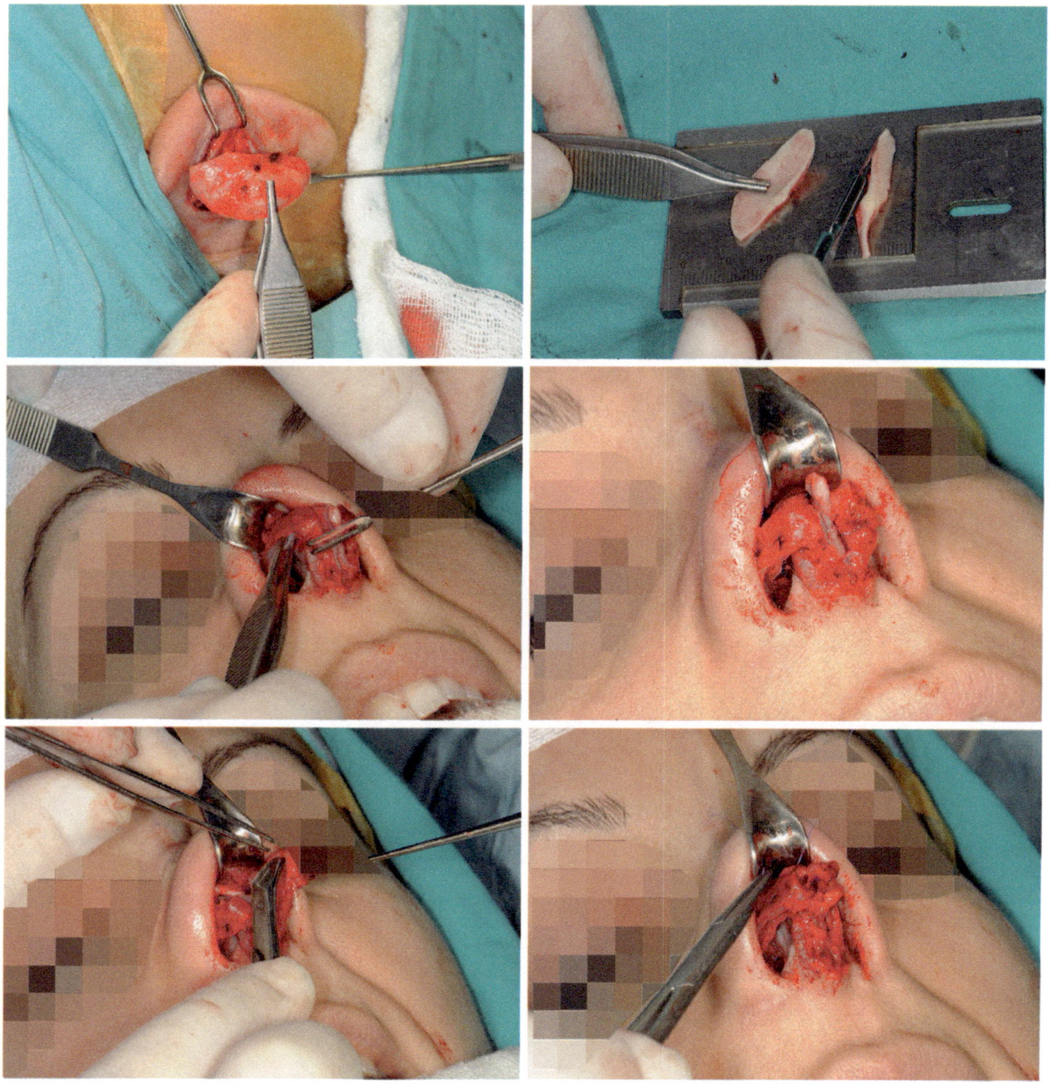

Fig. 11.17 (continued)

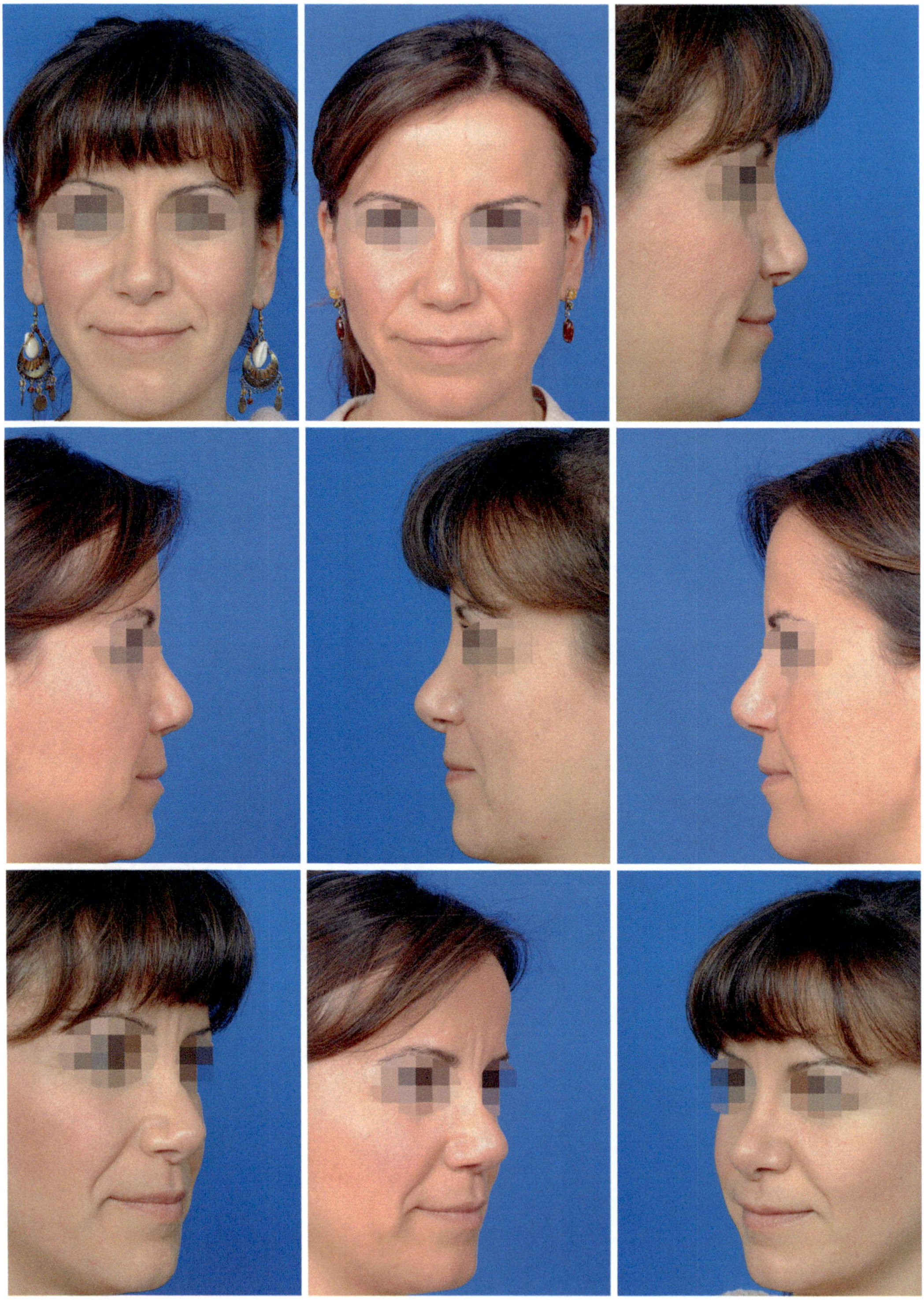

Fig. 11.17 (continued)

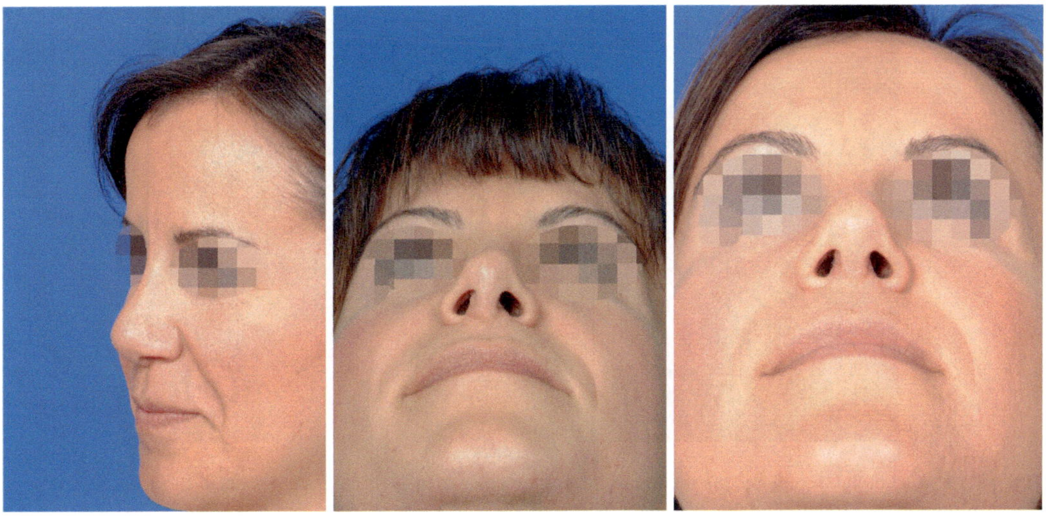

Fig. 11.17 (continued)

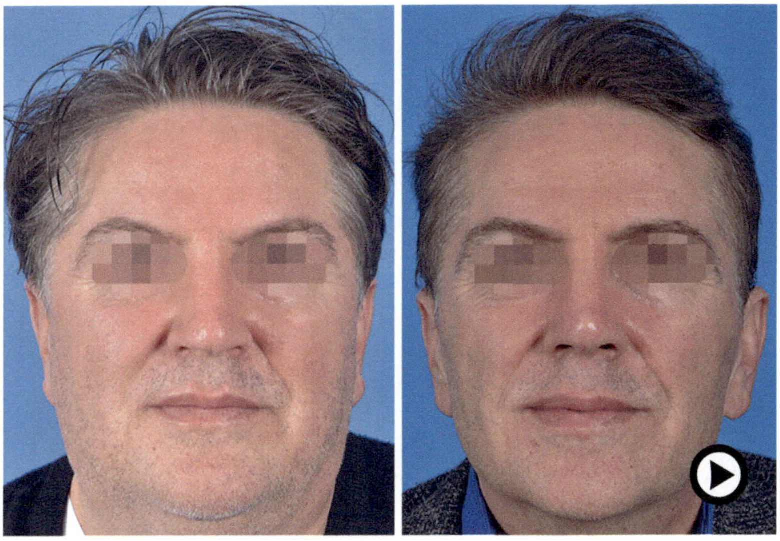

Fig. 11.18 A caudal septal replacement graft was performed to correct a caudal septal deviation using costal cartilage (▶ https://doi.org/10.1007/000-dza)

11.3 Resecting and Reconstructing Methods

11.3.1 Subtotal Septal Reconstruction

In severely crooked noses, sometimes the surgeon meets fracture lines identified in the dorsal and caudal segments, and there is no other way than removing these fractured pieces of cartilage. In most cases, a large piece of cartilage at the keystone area can be preserved. The harvested cartilage can then be sutured to the remaining cartilaginous septum either as spreader grafts or as a new L-strut [7, 8] (Figs. 11.18, 11.19, 11.20, 11.21, 11.22, and 11.23). I do like this method in selected cases (Figs. 11.24, 11.25, 11.26, 11.27, and 11.28).

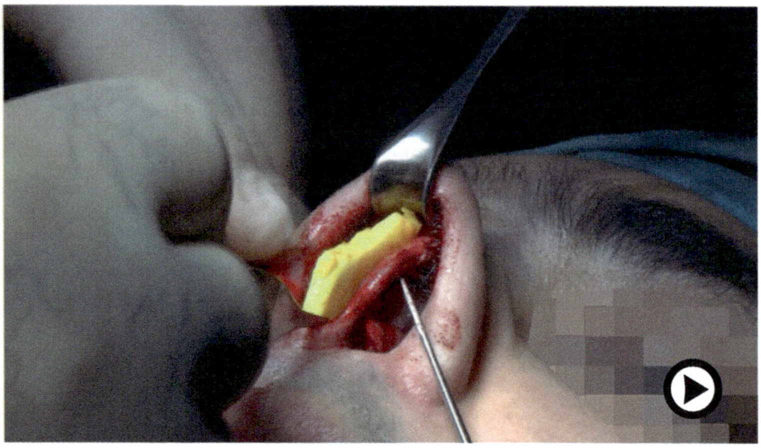

Fig. 11.19 A subtotal septal reconstruction is performed using an L-strut graft designed from costal cartilage (▶ https://doi.org/10.1007/000-dz5)

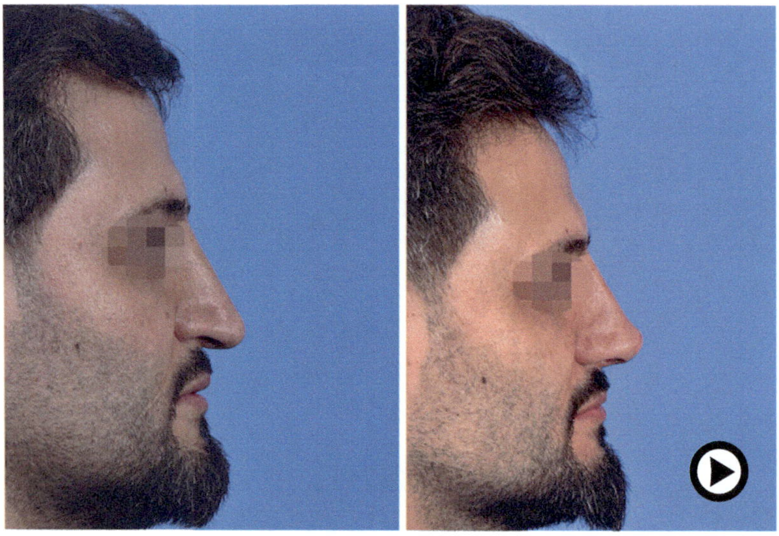

Fig. 11.20 A revision rhinoplasty using costal cartilage was performed in a crooked nose patient (▶ https://doi.org/10.1007/000-dzc)

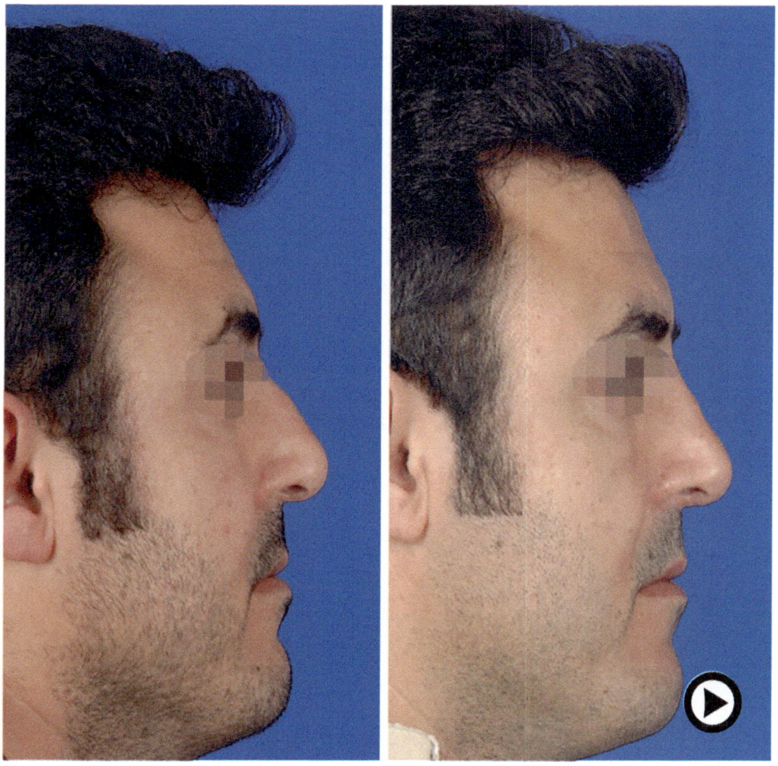

Fig. 11.21 Subtotal septal reconstruction is performed in a traumatic nose using a caudal septal replacement graft from septal cartilage (▶ https://doi.org/10.1007/000-dzd)

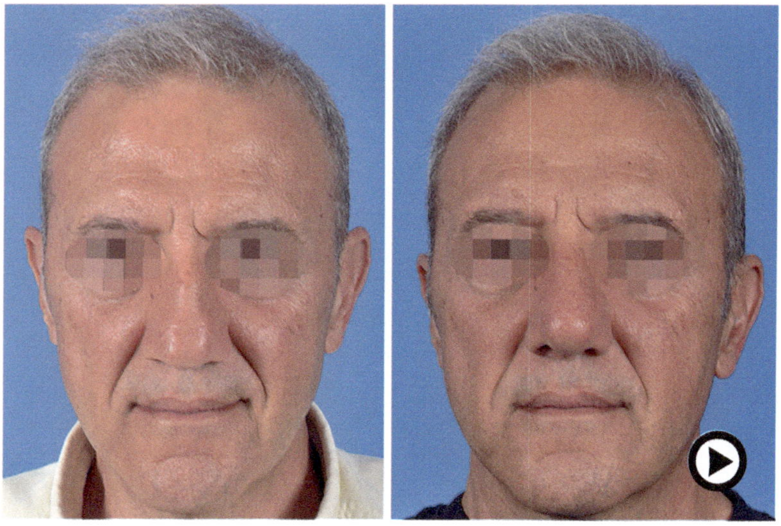

Fig. 11.22 A subtotal septal reconstruction was performed using costal cartilage in a patient with two previous septoplasties (▶ https://doi.org/10.1007/000-dze)

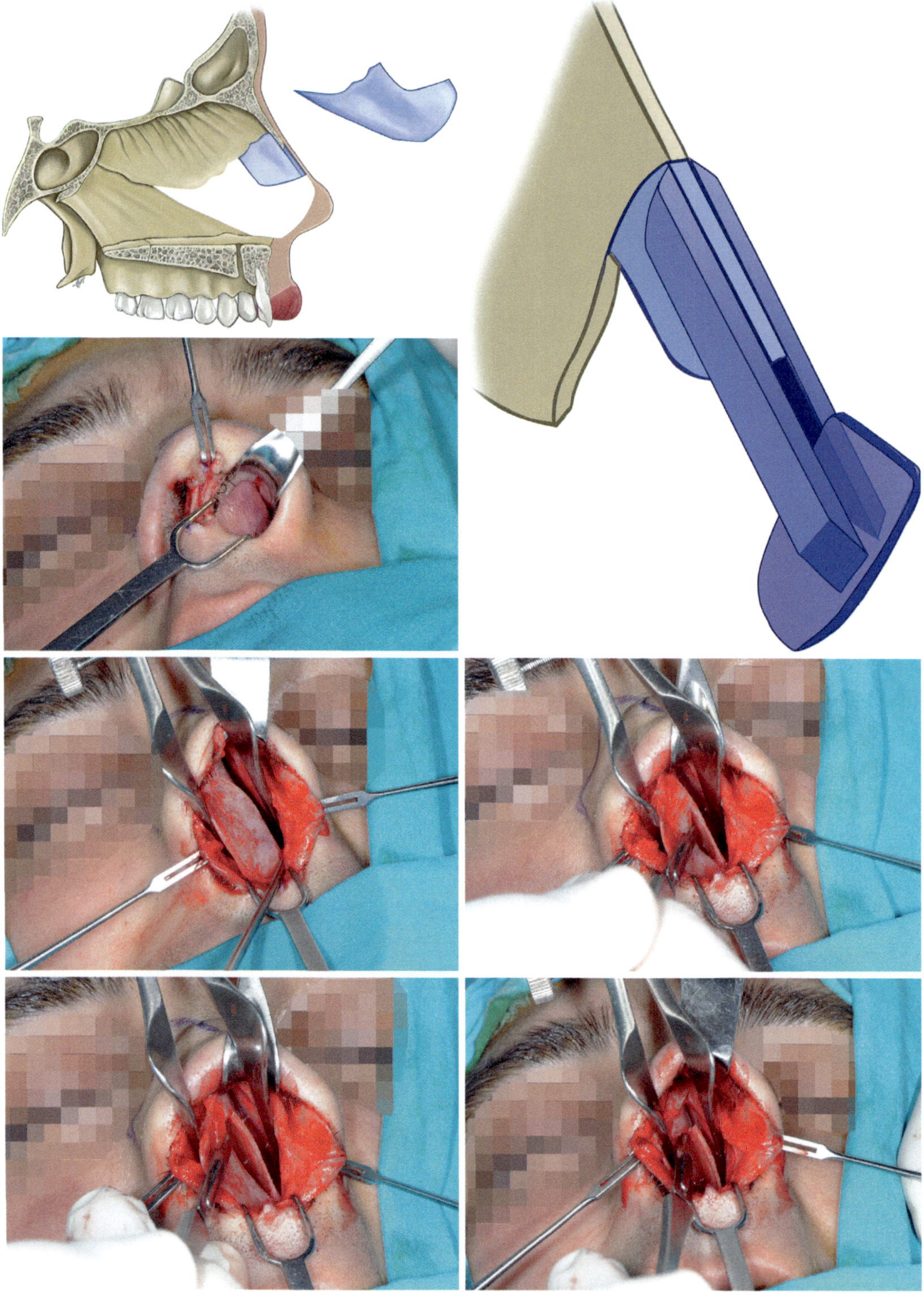

Fig. 11.23 Subtotal septal reconstruction is a powerful but difficult technique in reconstructing severely deviated noses. In more than 90% of cases, the cephalic half of the dorsal segment can be preserved, and this cartilage serves as a strong fixation segment for spreader grafts and/or L-strut grafts

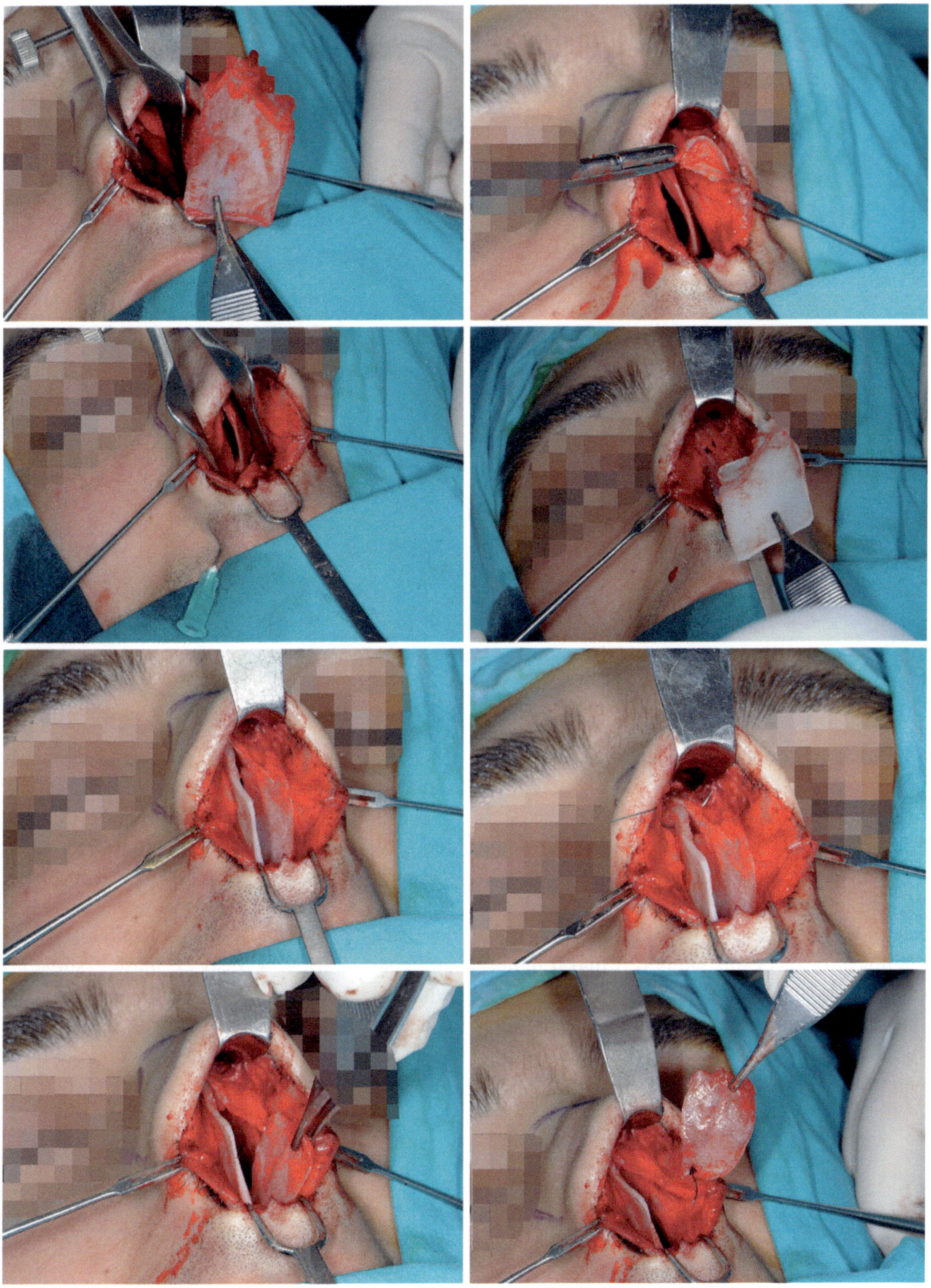

Fig. 11.23 (continued)

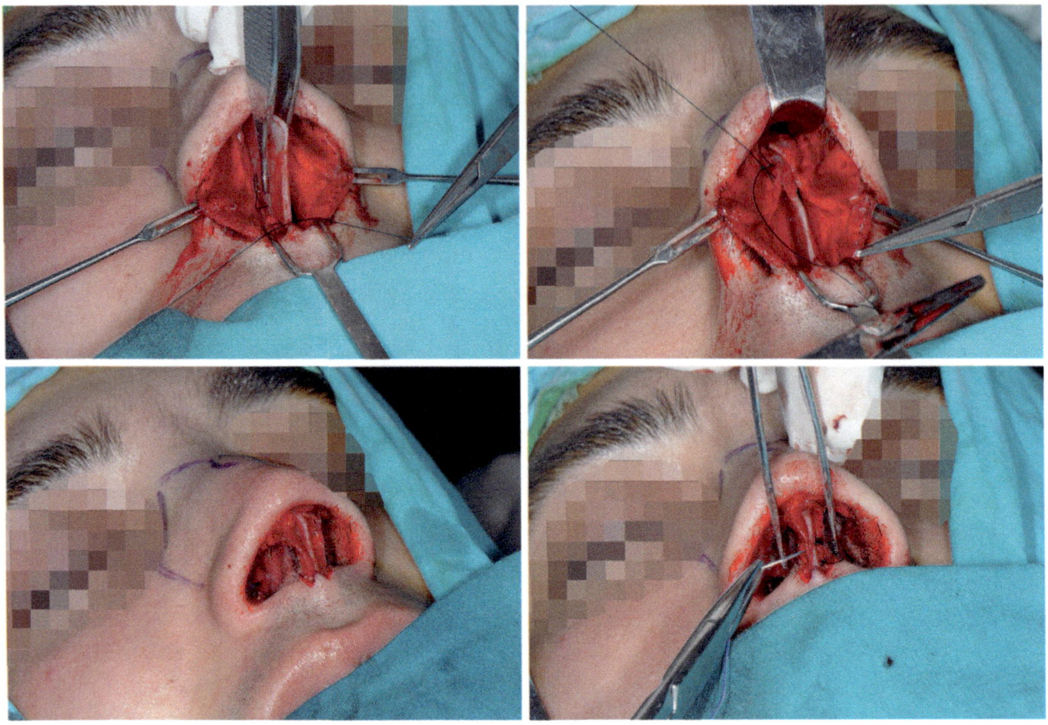

Fig. 11.23 (continued)

11.3.2 Extracorporeal Septoplasty

In severely crooked noses, sometimes the deviation site can be at the joint between the septal cartilage and ethmoid lamina. In these cases, the entire nasal septum can be resected and rebuilt (Figs. 11.29, 11.30, 11.31, and 11.32). I am not in favor of this method. I find it unnecessary and aggressive. Besides, I always do imaging before rhinoplasty, and we agree on a certain shape with the patient. It means that certain profile, projection, and rotation are planned for each individual patient. The nasal septum is always at the center of this new construction, and it is the most important structure to reach the goals of profile, rotation, and projection. If the surgeon removes the whole septal cartilage, it is not easy to replicate the same nasal septum in all cases, especially in the hands of novice surgeons. Surely, I respect master surgeons who have been using this technique for years successfully [9], but I do think that it does not seem like a predictable and reproducible technique for many surgeons.

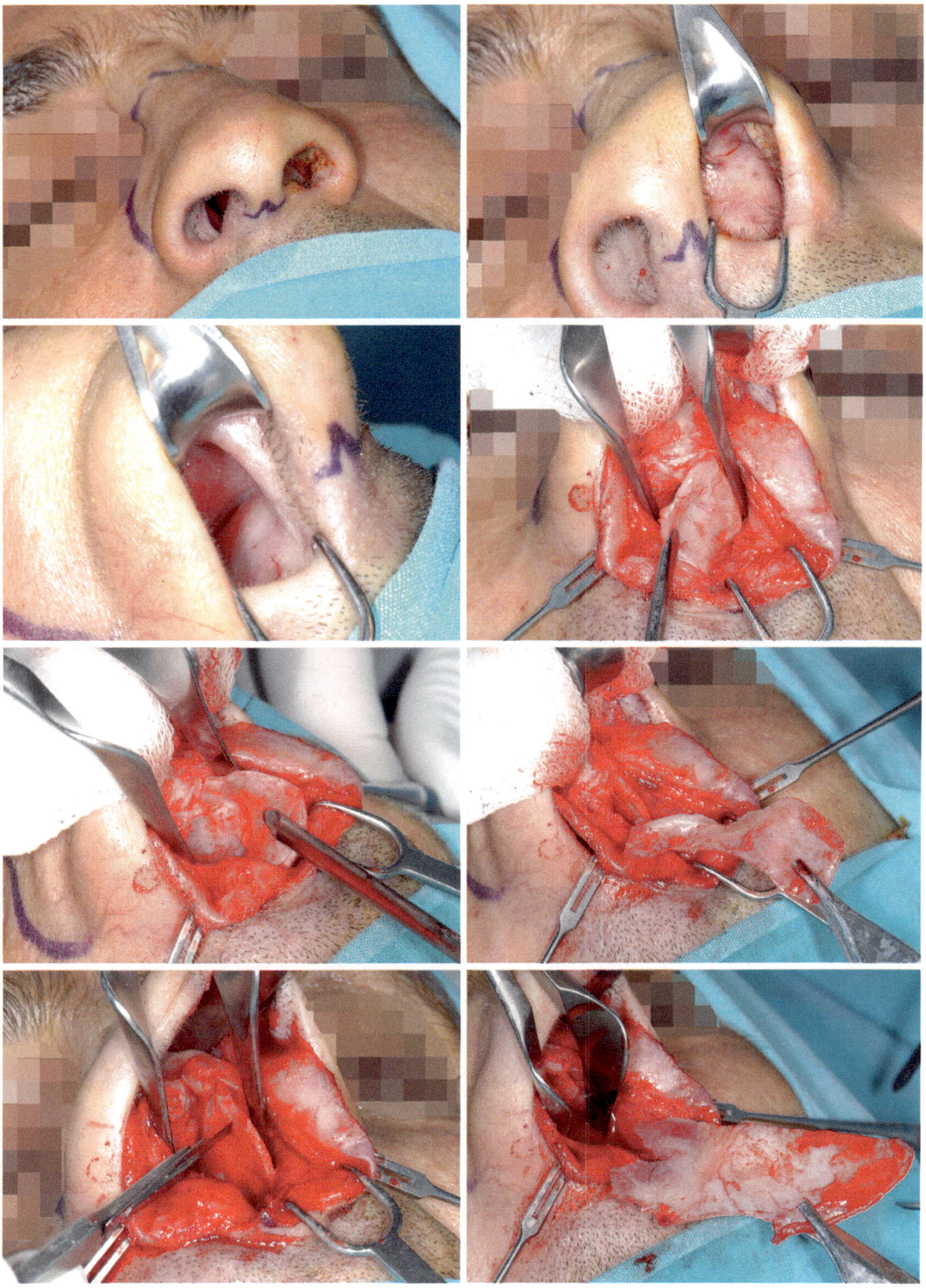

Fig. 11.24 In this case, subtotal septal reconstruction was performed by using a big spreader graft and a caudal septal replacement graft. This is a very strong but difficult technique because the surgeon must use her/his esthetic eye to decide on the projection and rotation

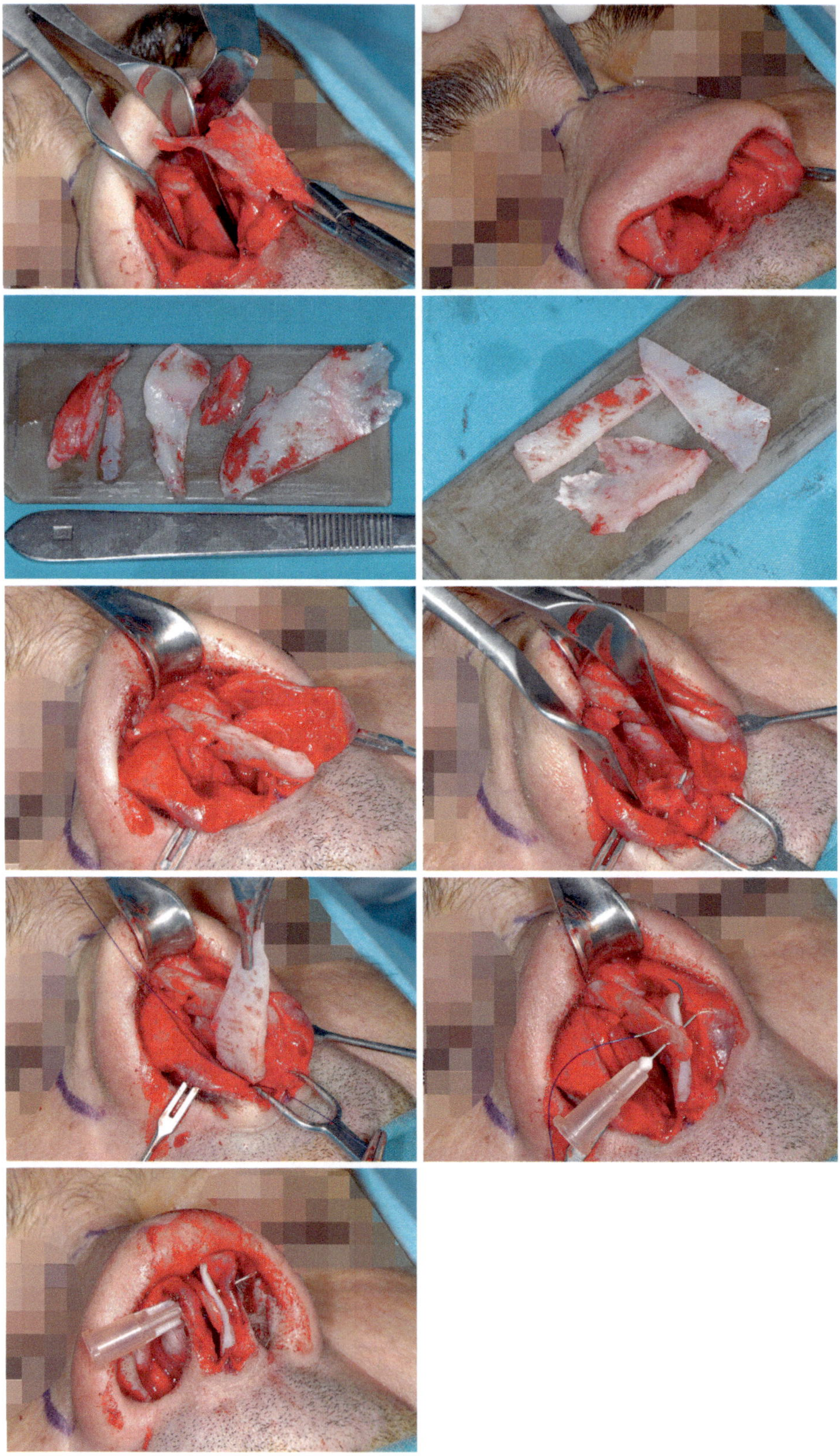

Fig. 11.24 (continued)

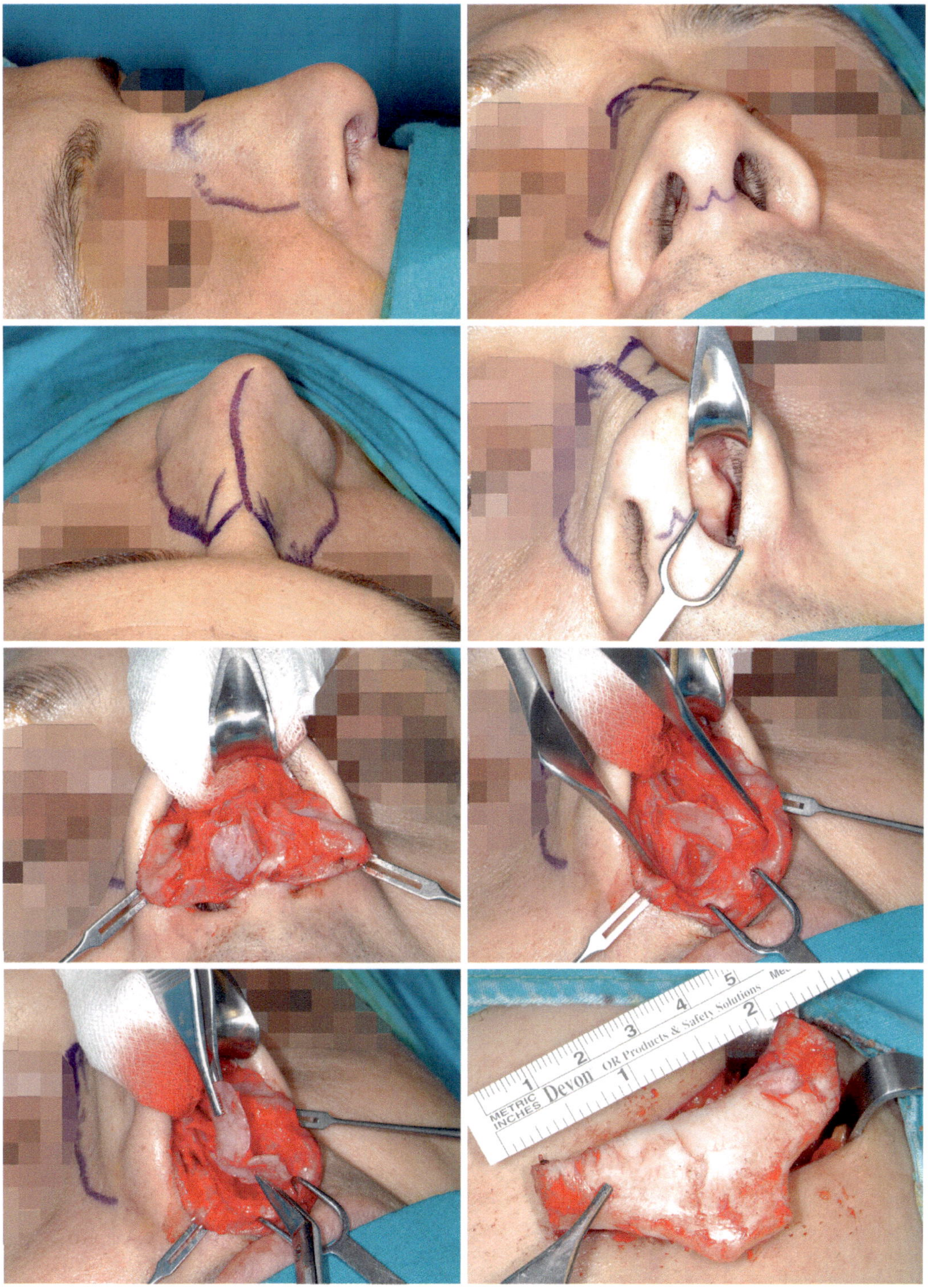

Fig. 11.25 The sixth rib was used as a one-piece L-strut graft in this case. It was sutured to the remaining cartilage at the keystone area and to the anterior nasal spine. I do not use this technique very often because the nose becomes very rigid, and it is not easy to obtain additional grafts for different purposes

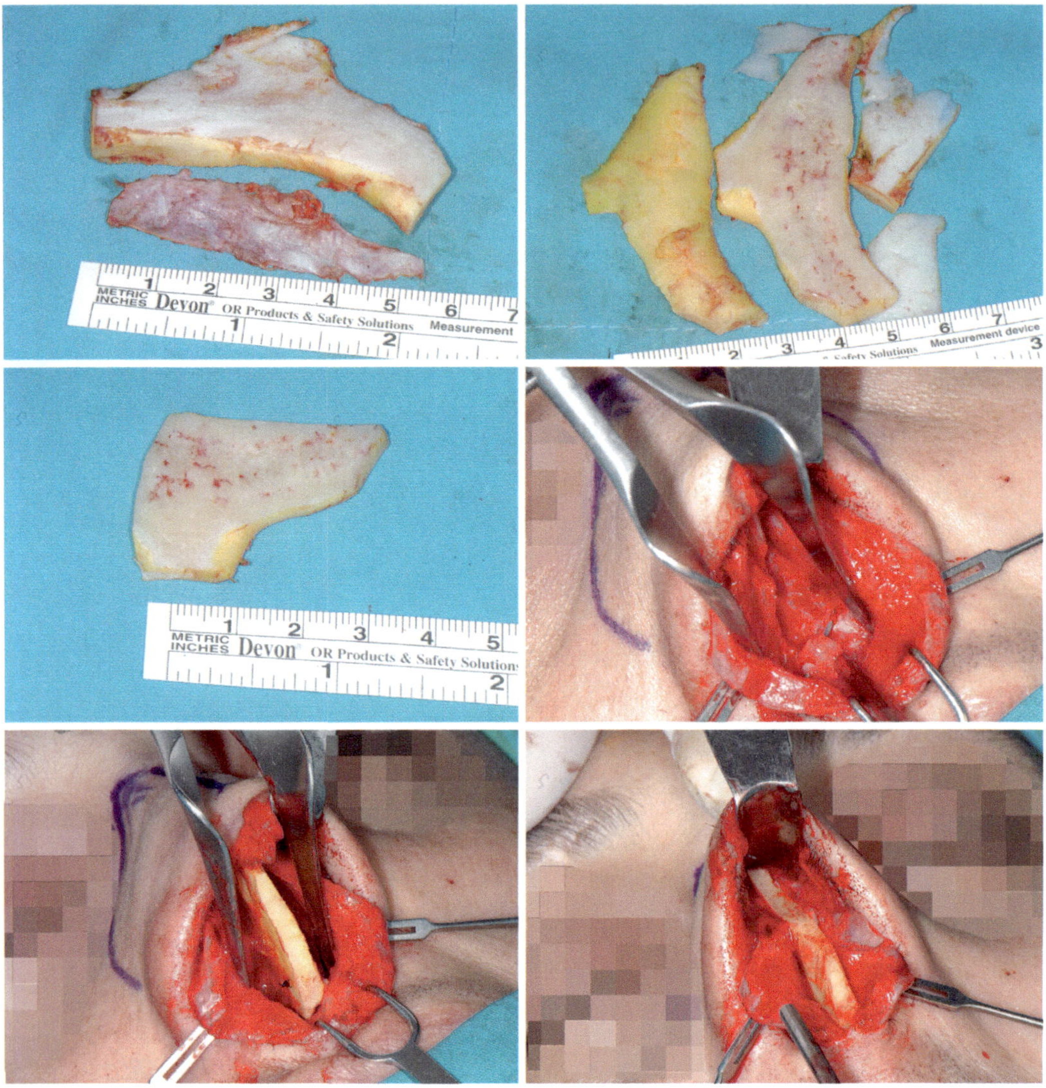

Fig. 11.25 (continued)

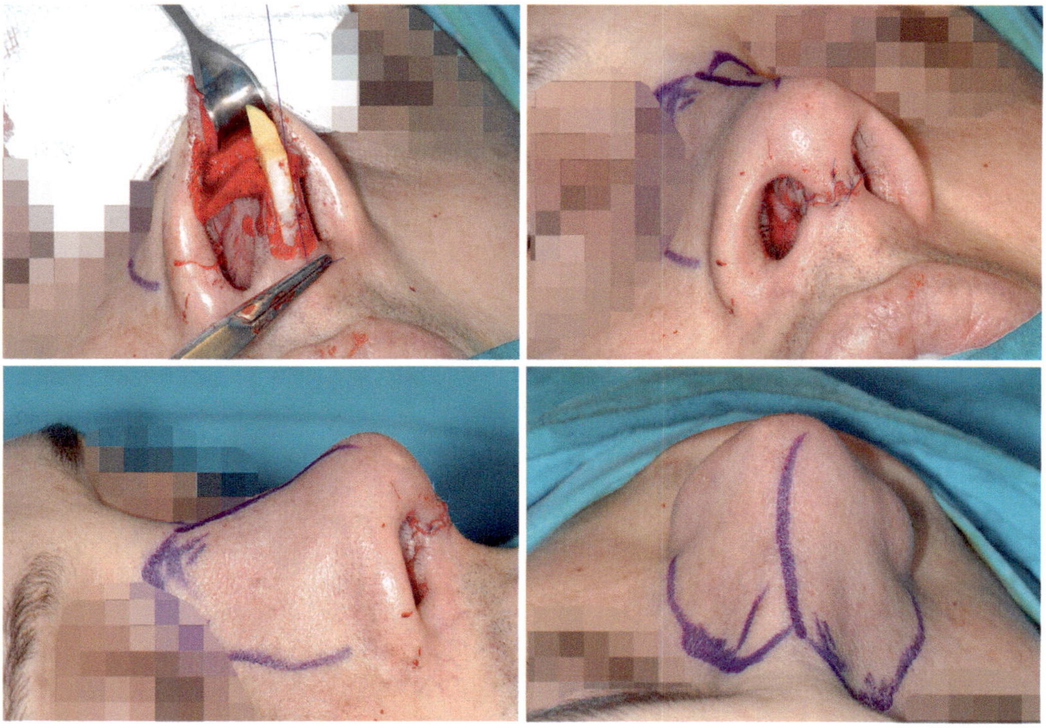

Fig. 11.25 (continued)

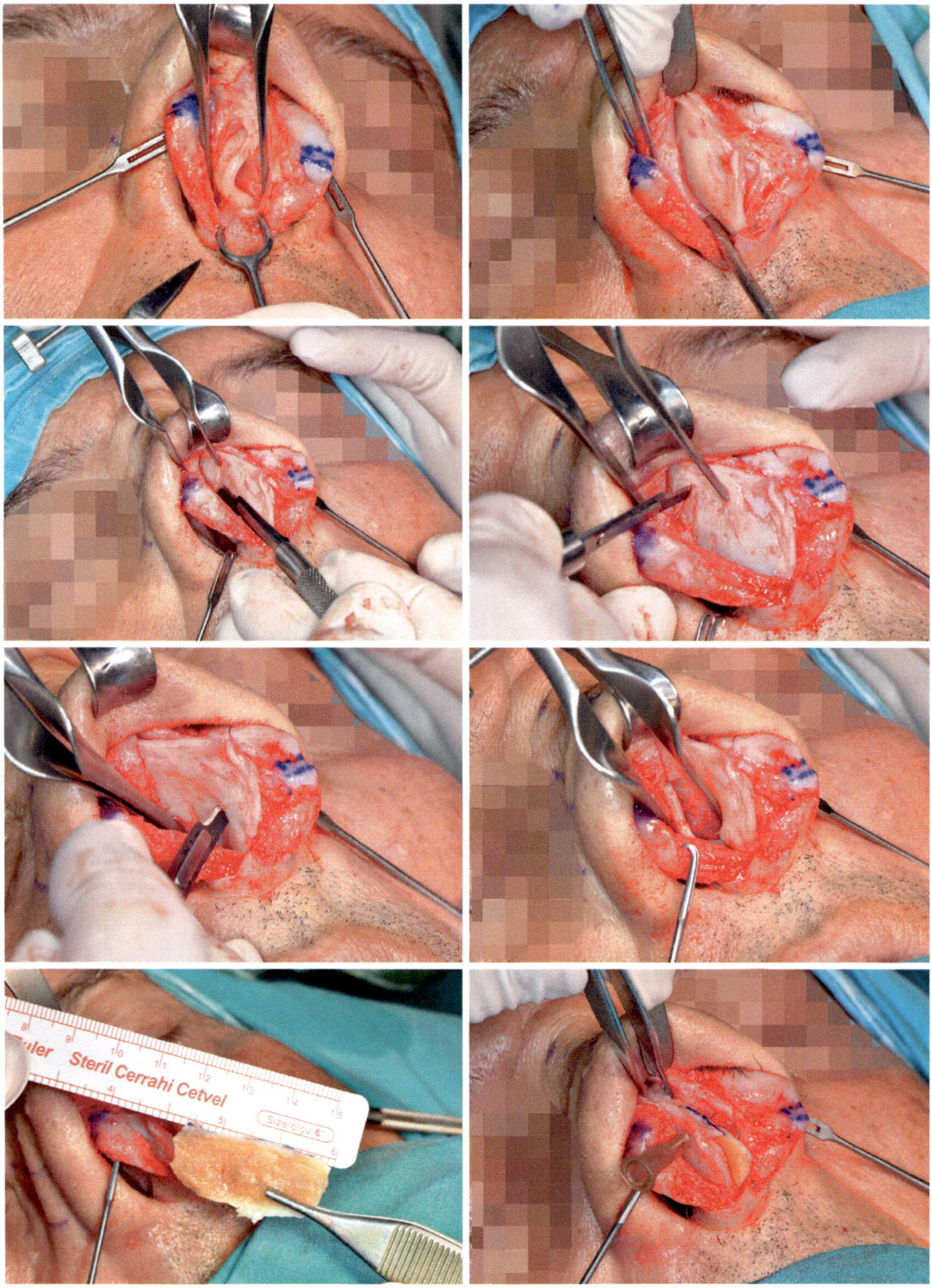

Fig. 11.26 This is a 63-year-old patient who had undergone two previous septoplasties. The oblique split technique helped us to obtain spreader grafts, a caudal septal replacement graft, and a tip graft. The nose is still swollen after 6 months

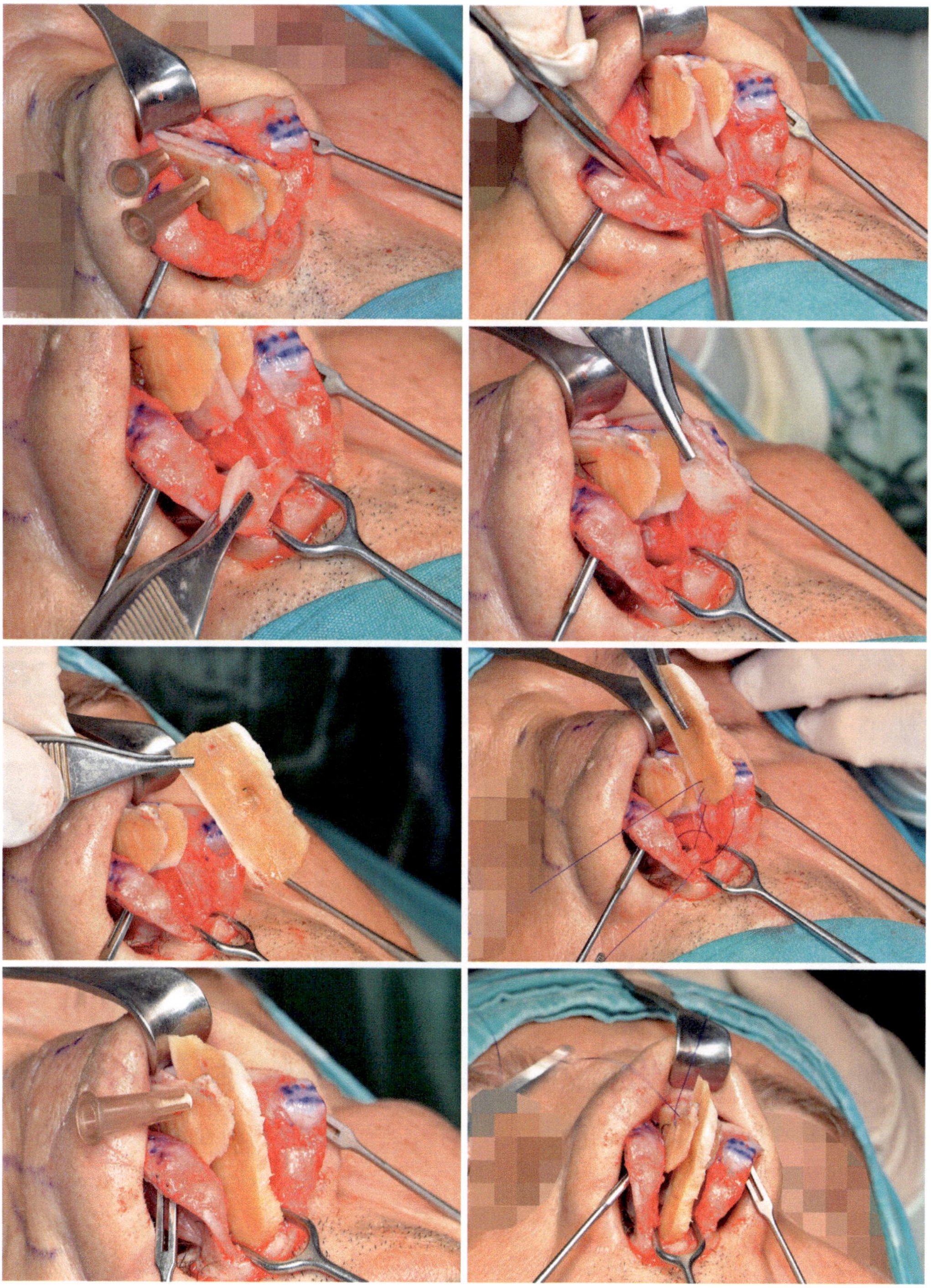

Fig. 11.26 (continued)

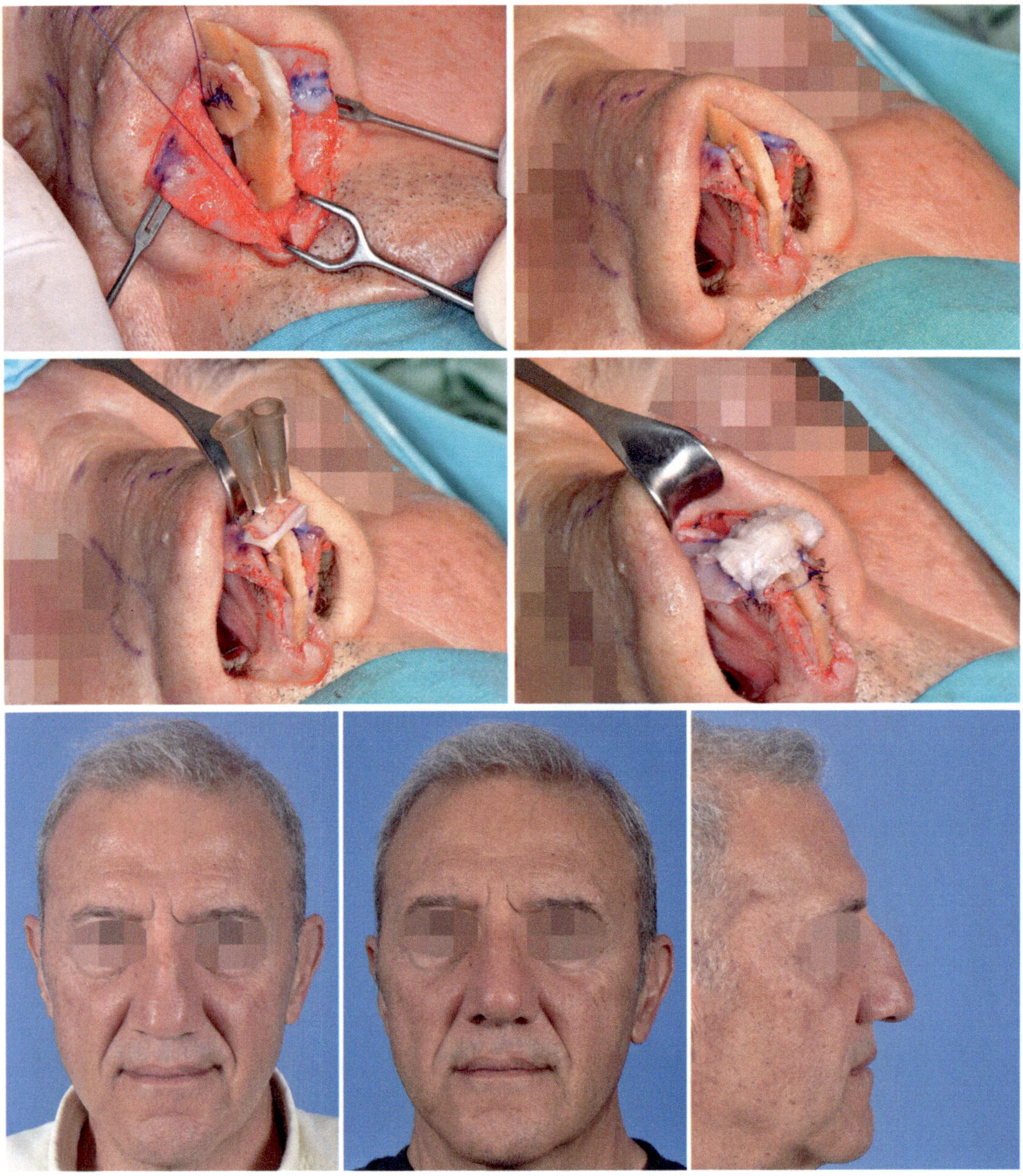

Fig. 11.26 (continued)

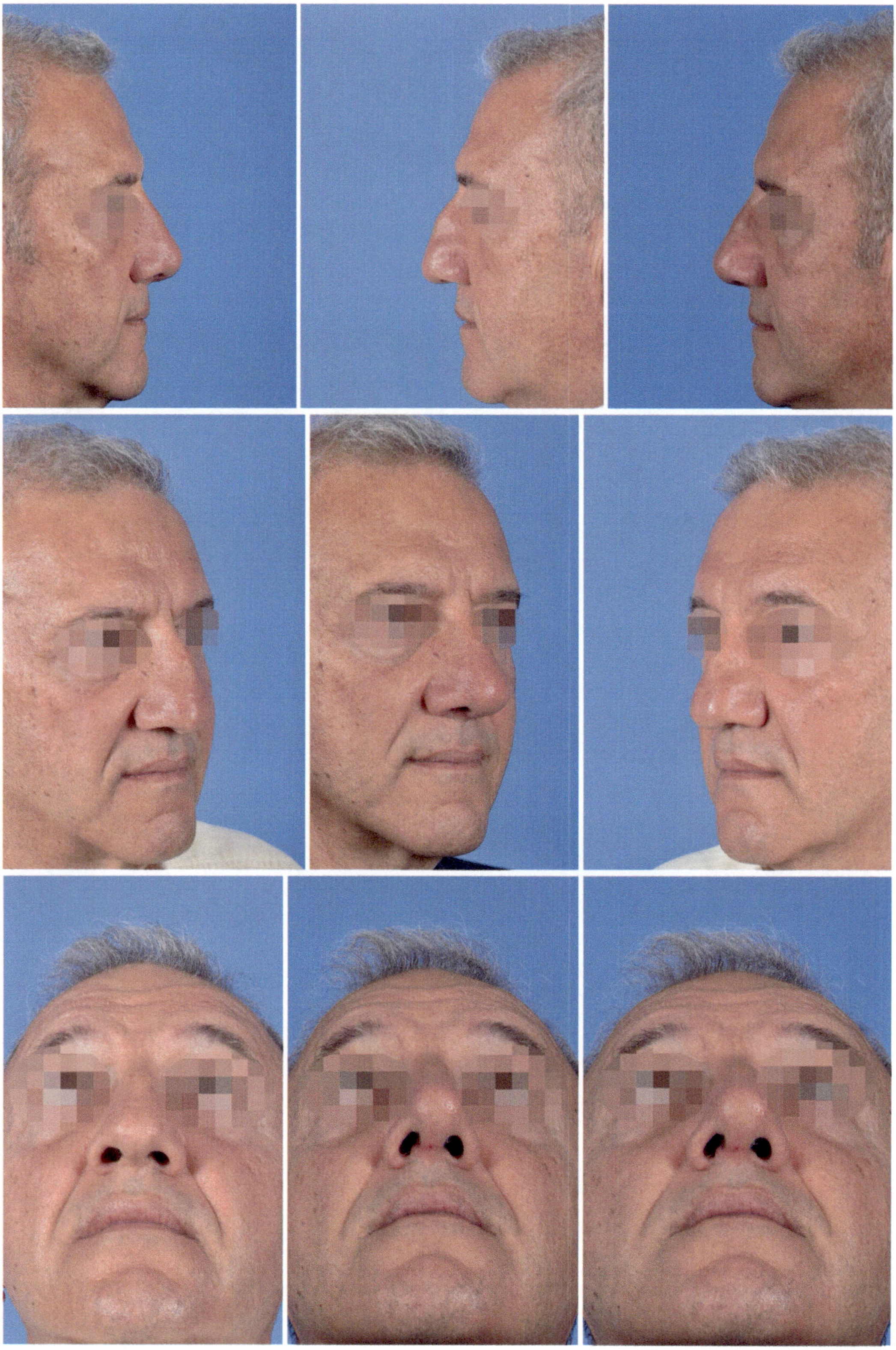

Fig. 11.26 (continued)

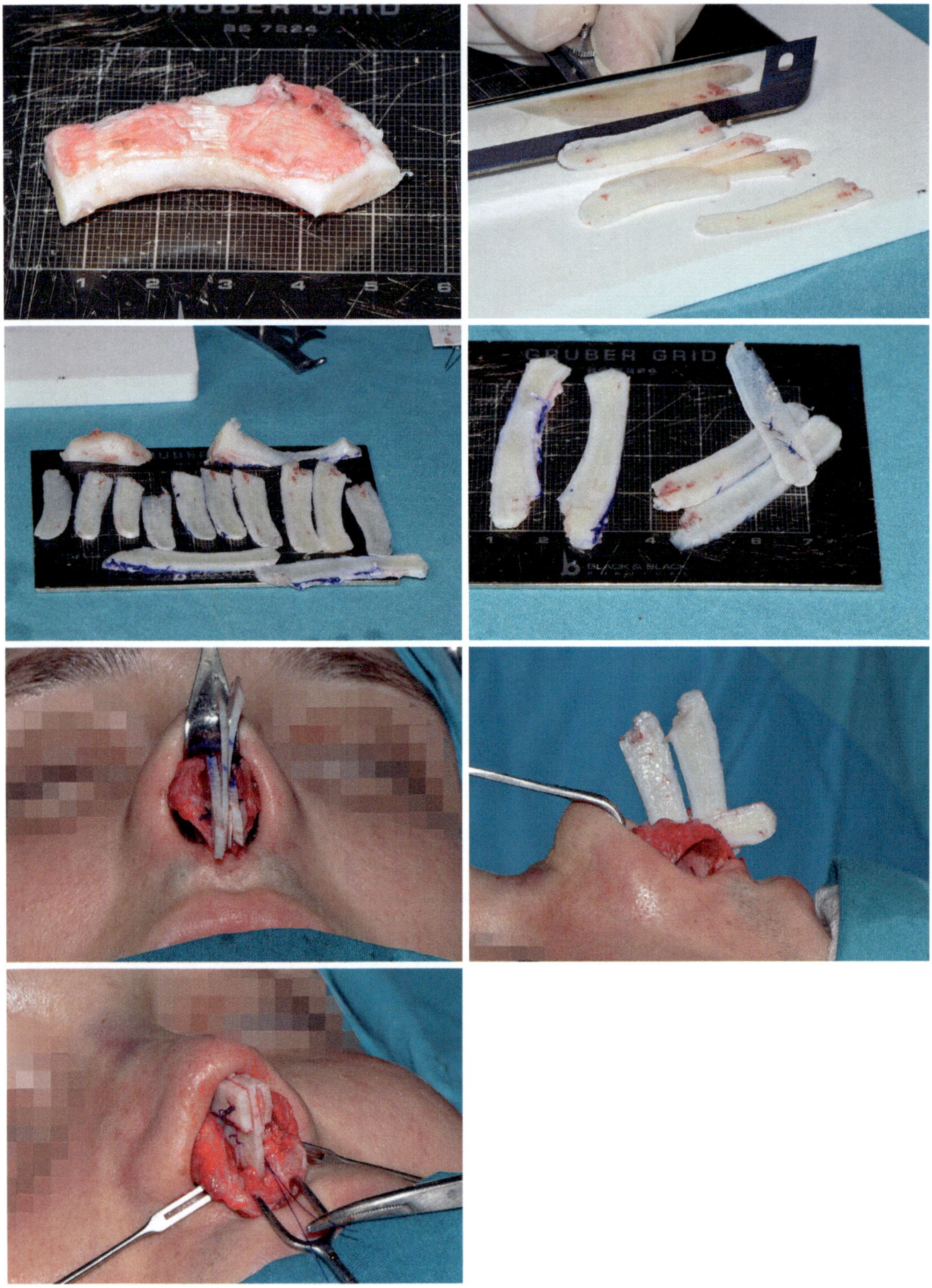

Fig. 11.27 In younger patients, the rib cartilage is softer, and when cut obliquely by using the Chef's knife, the implants obtained are almost like septal cartilage. In a 25-year-old patient, a new septum was created and fixed in place with the help of spreader grafts

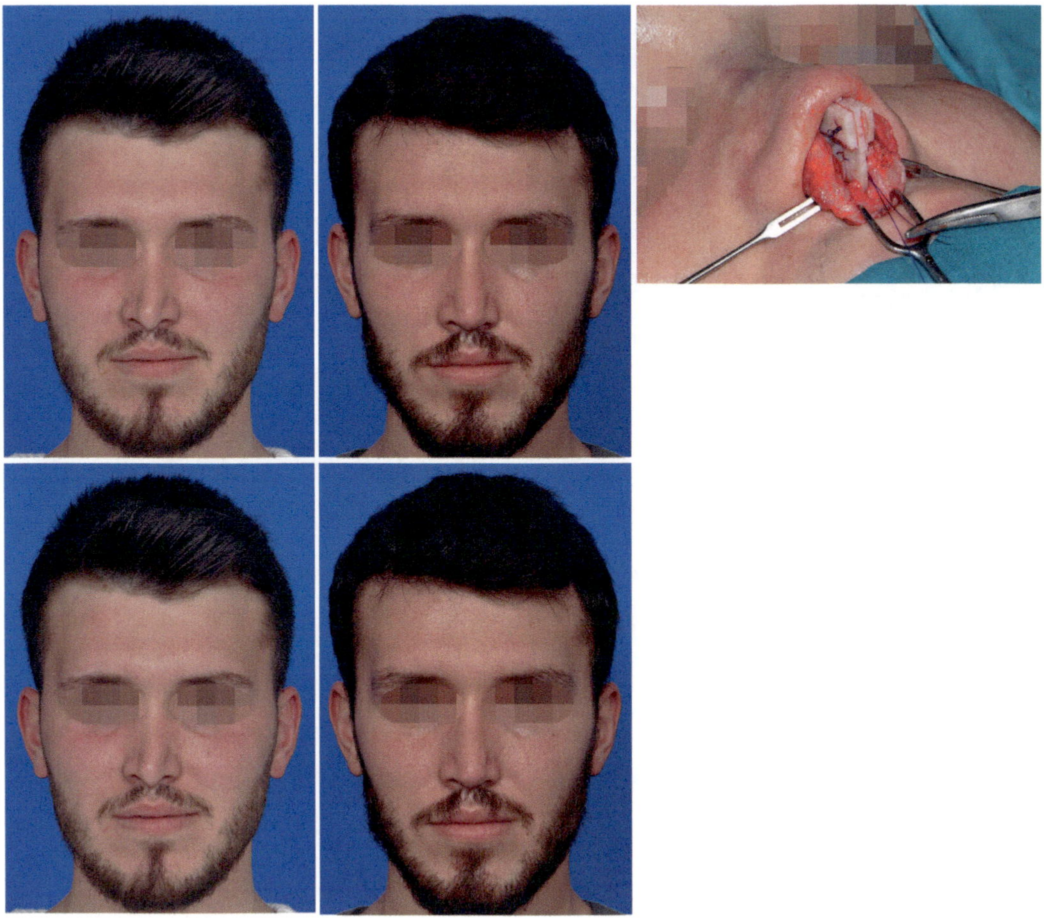

Fig. 11.27 (continued)

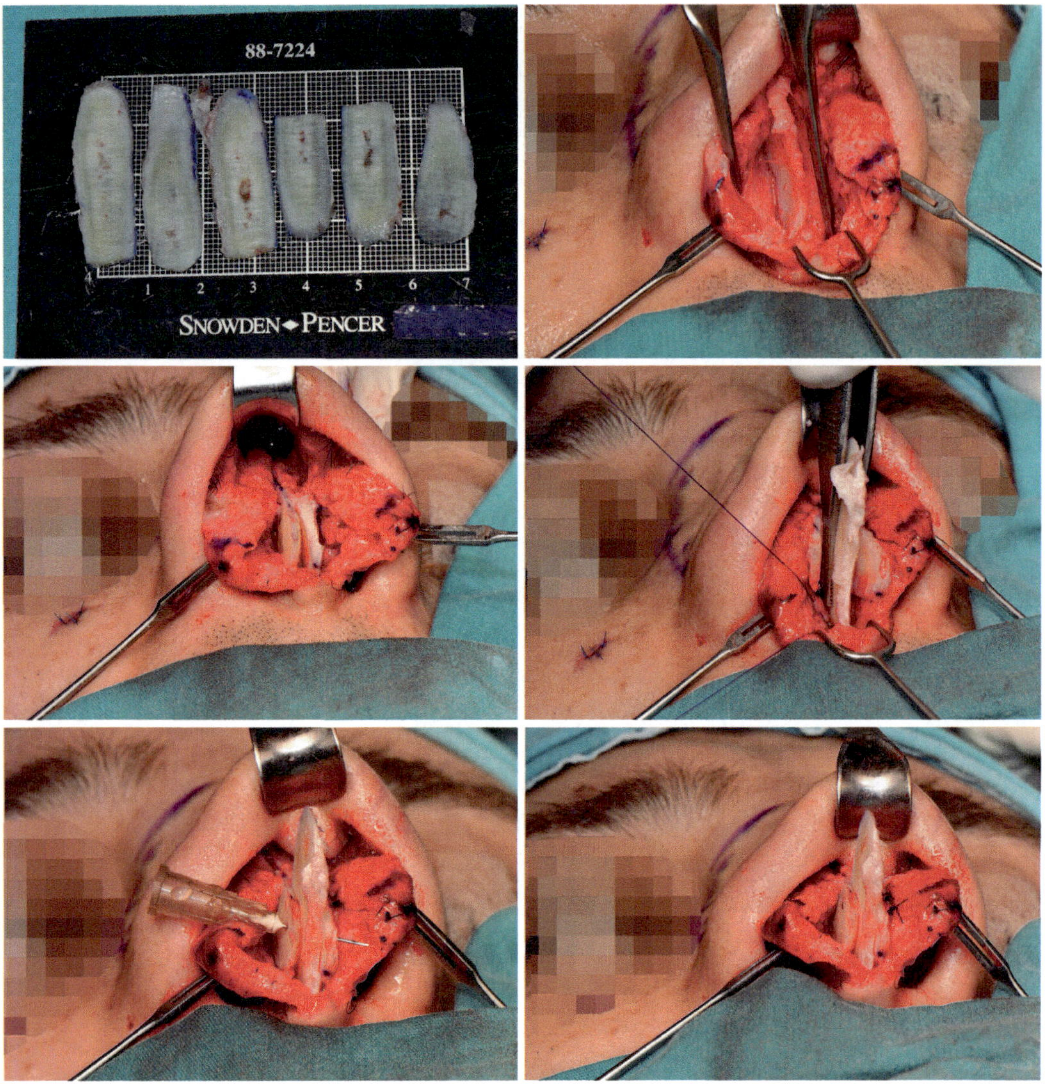

Fig. 11.28 The versatility of the oblique split technique can be better understood in a 38-year-old patient who came in for a revision rhinoplasty. The L-strut framework was reconstructed by splinting spreader grafts and a caudal septal extension graft. A double-layer dorsal onlay graft, covered by fascia, was used for dorsal augmentation. Bilateral wedge excision was performed at the end of surgery. The functional and esthetic results after 1 year were well accepted by the patient

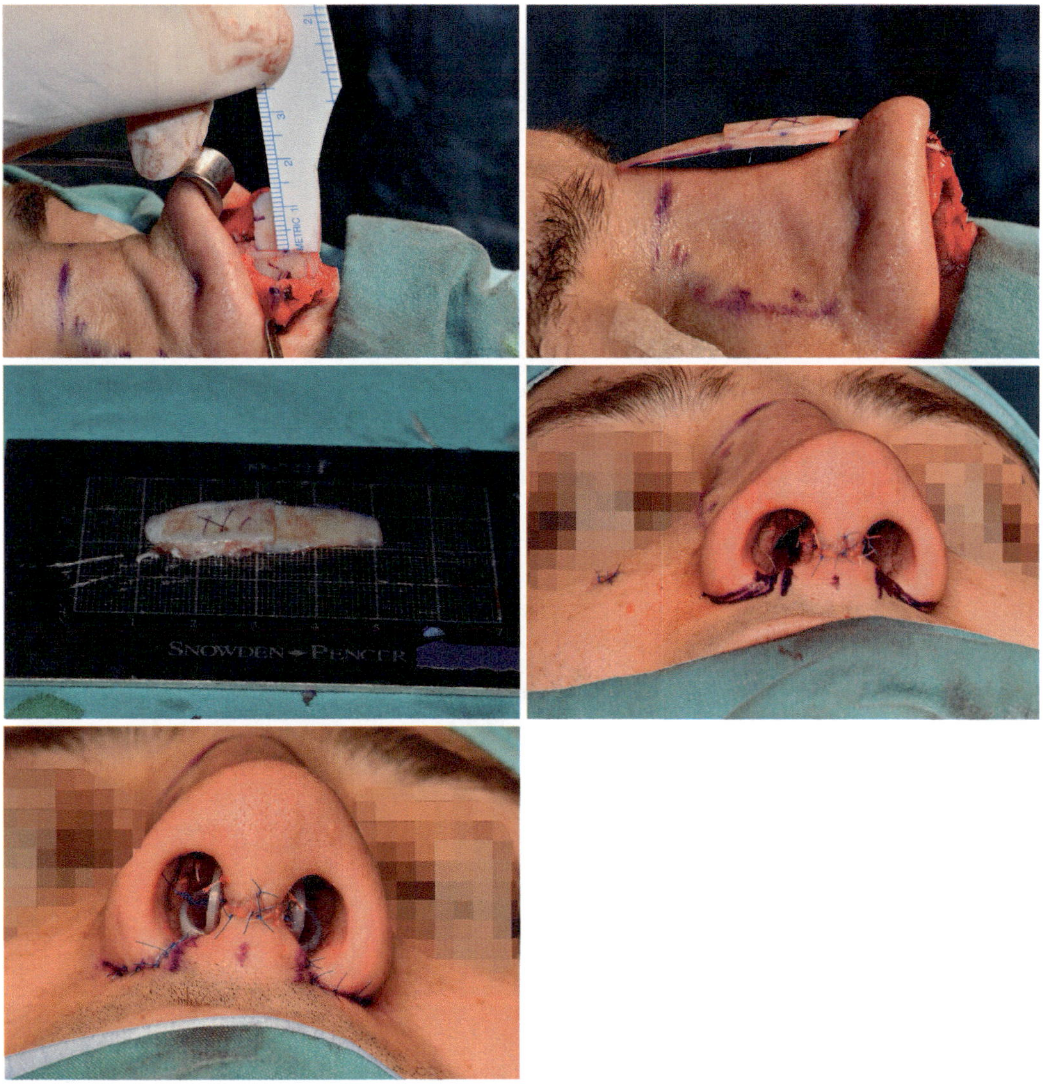

Fig. 11.28 (continued)

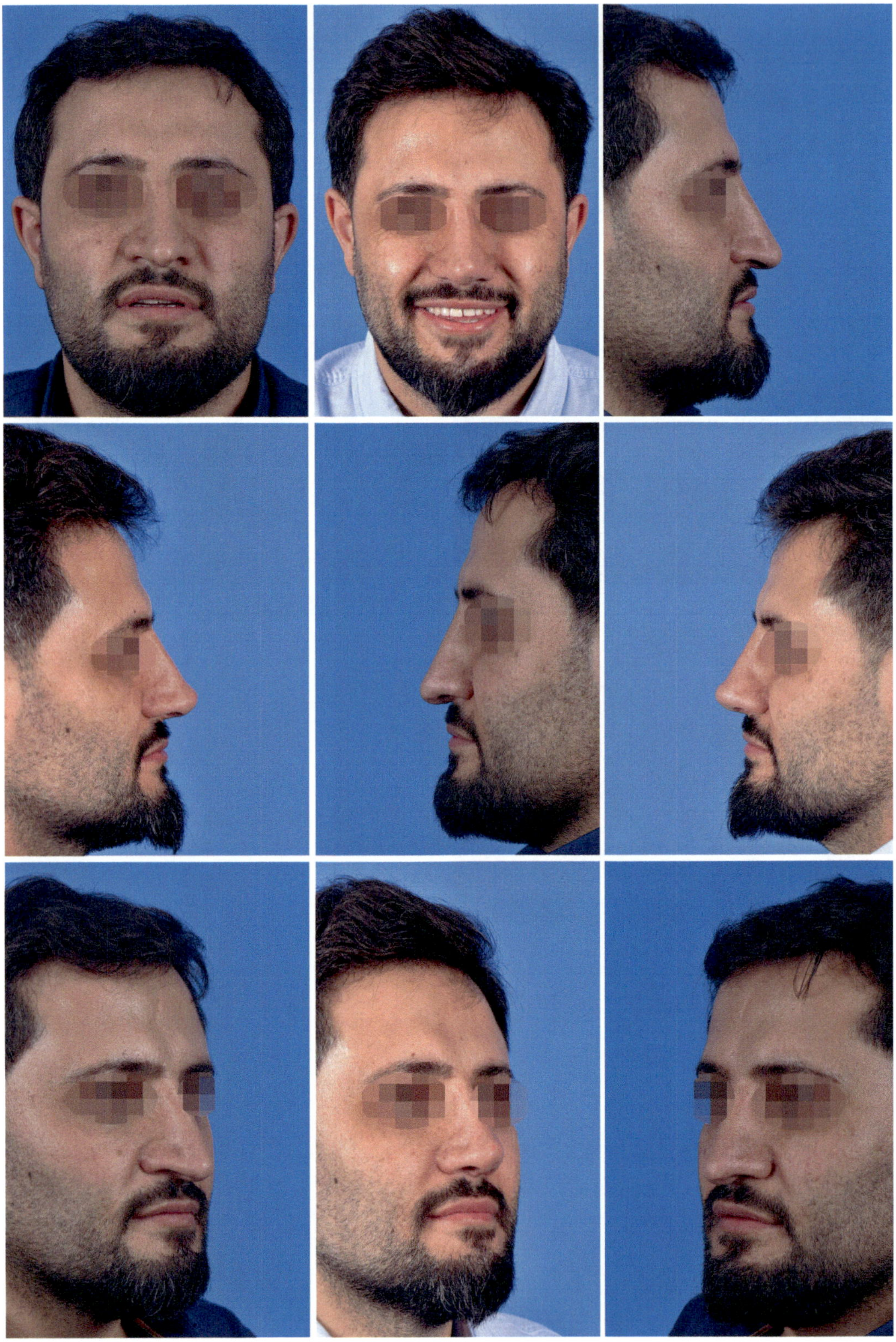

Fig. 11.28 (continued)

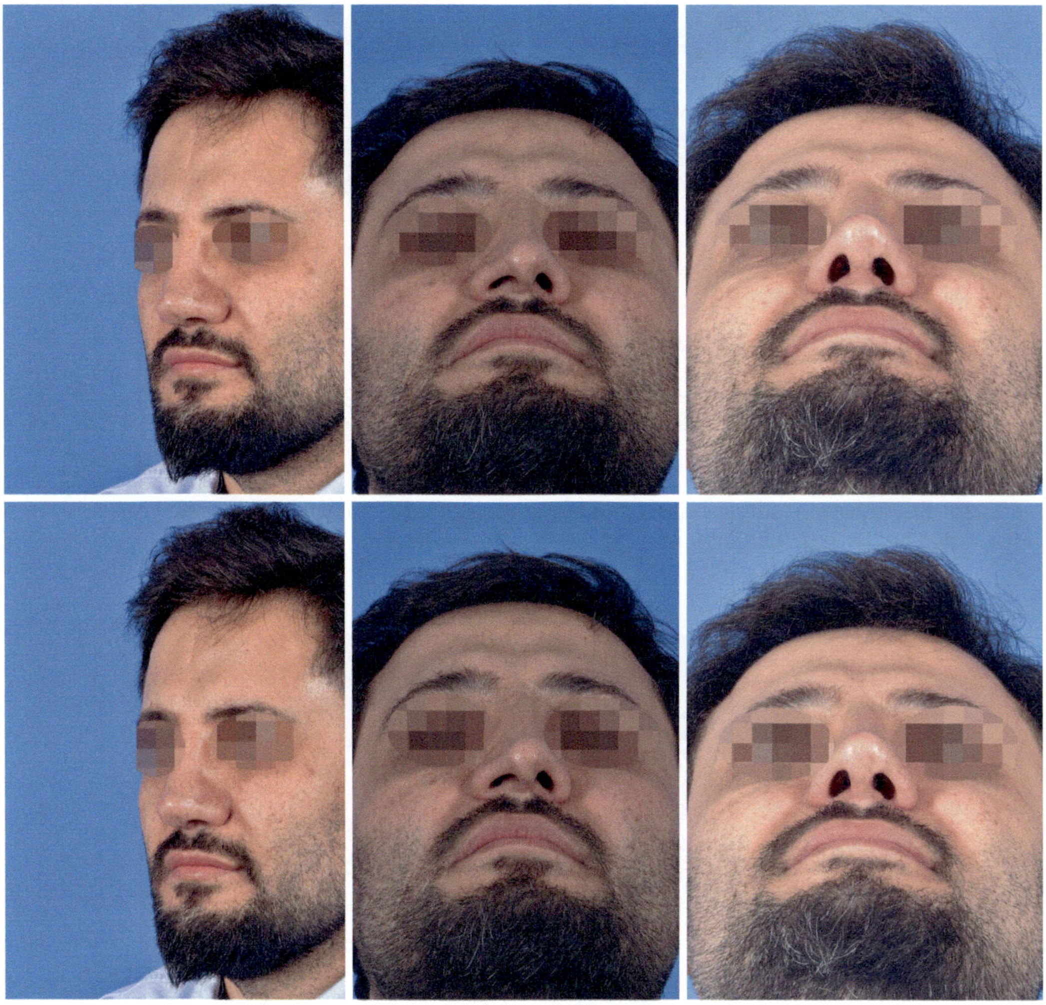

Fig. 11.28 (continued)

Fig. 11.29 Keystone area stabilization suture was performed (▶ https://doi.org/10.1007/000-dzf)

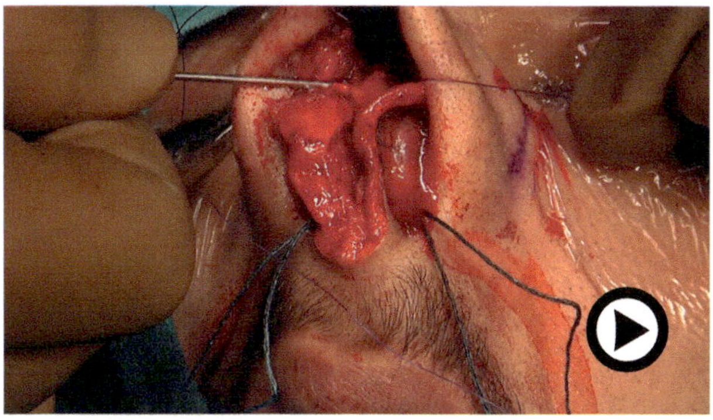

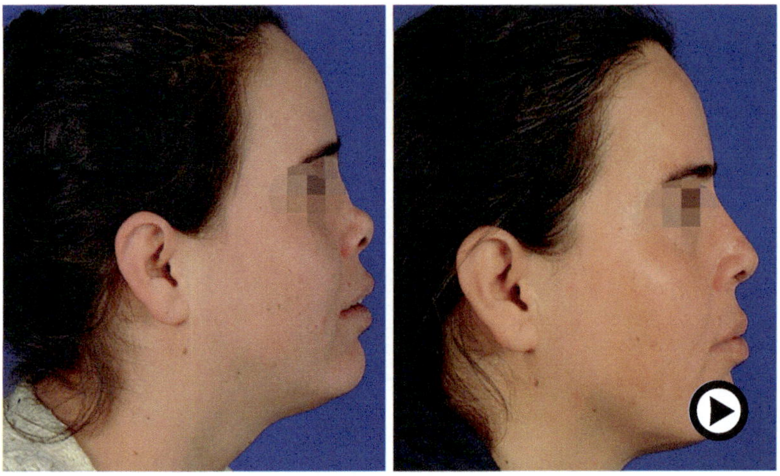

Fig. 11.30 Total septal reconstruction is performed using spreader and caudal septal replacement grafts from costal cartilage (▶ https://doi.org/10.1007/000-dzg)

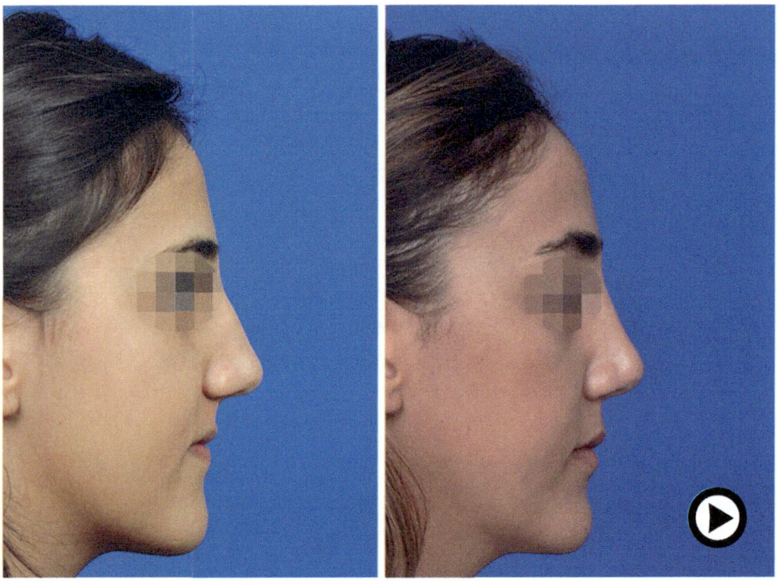

Fig. 11.31 A total septal reconstruction was performed after a total septal removal (▶ https://doi.org/10.1007/000-dzh)

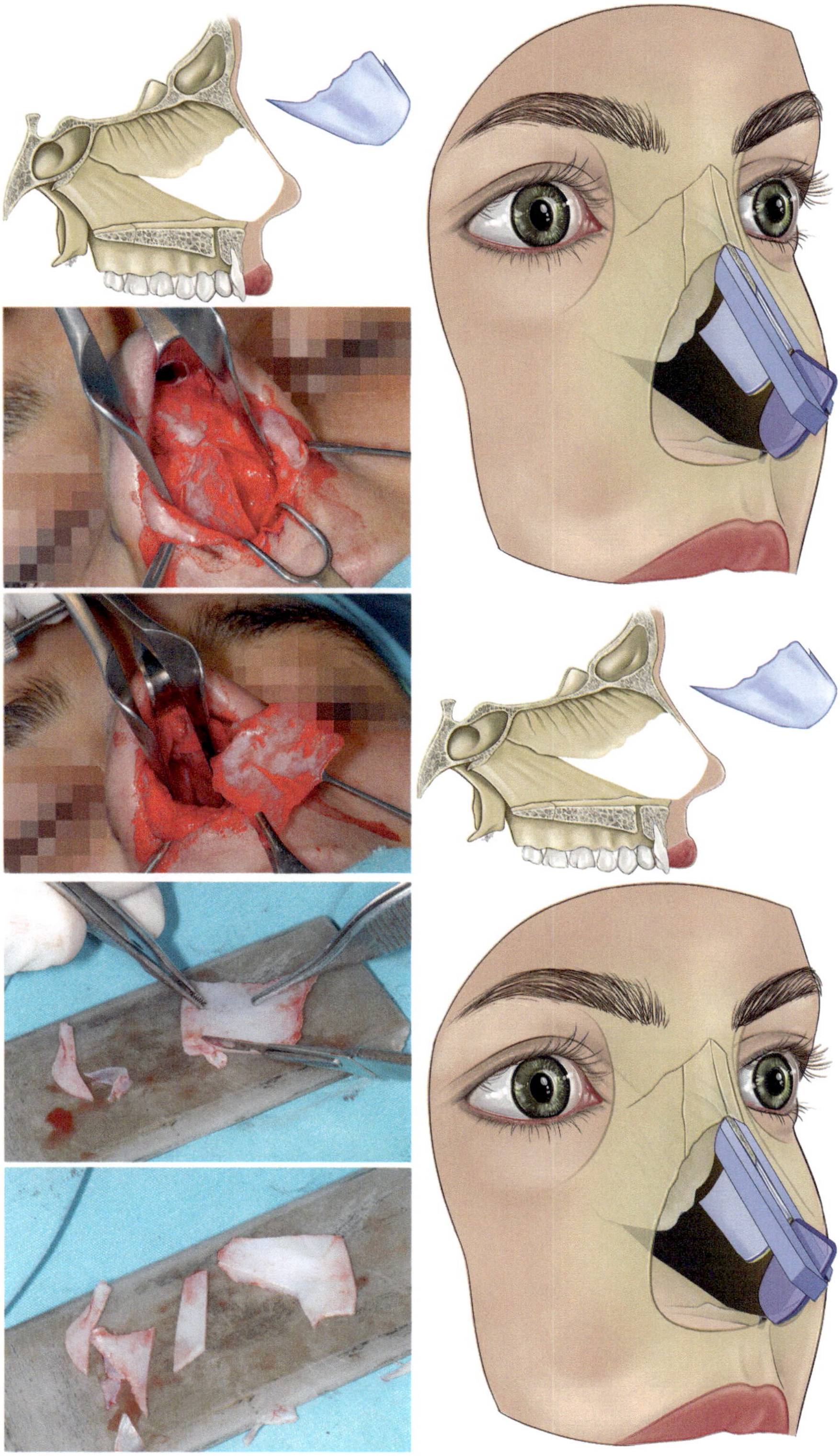

Fig. 11.32 Extracorporeal septoplasty can be done in severely crooked noses where the deviation site affects the joint between the septal cartilage and the ethmoid lamina. The entire nasal septum is resected, sculpted as a new septum on the table, and sutured in place. I did only a few cases with this method, and they were after incidental detachment of the septal cartilage from the ethmoid lamina

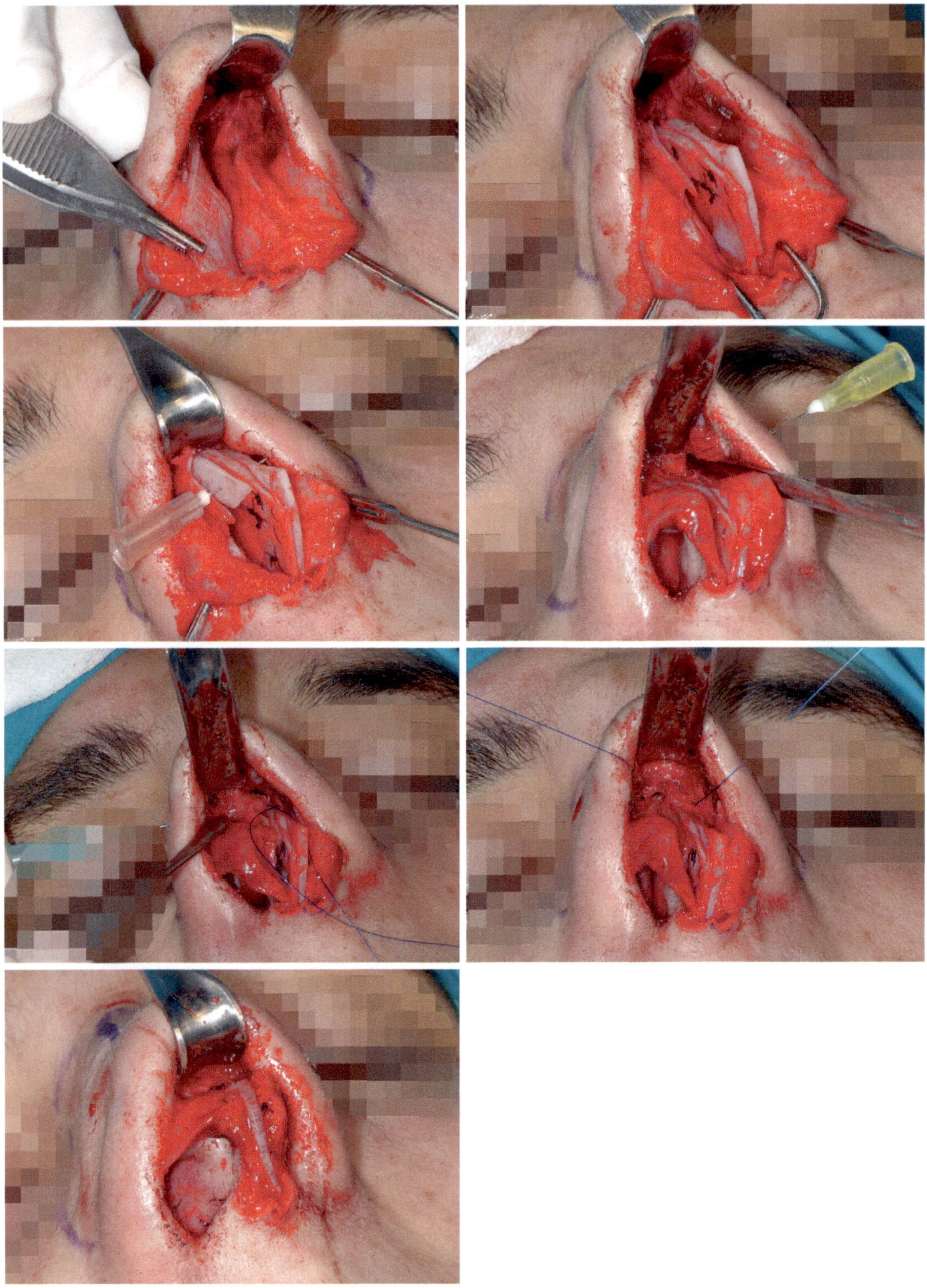

Fig. 11.32 (continued)

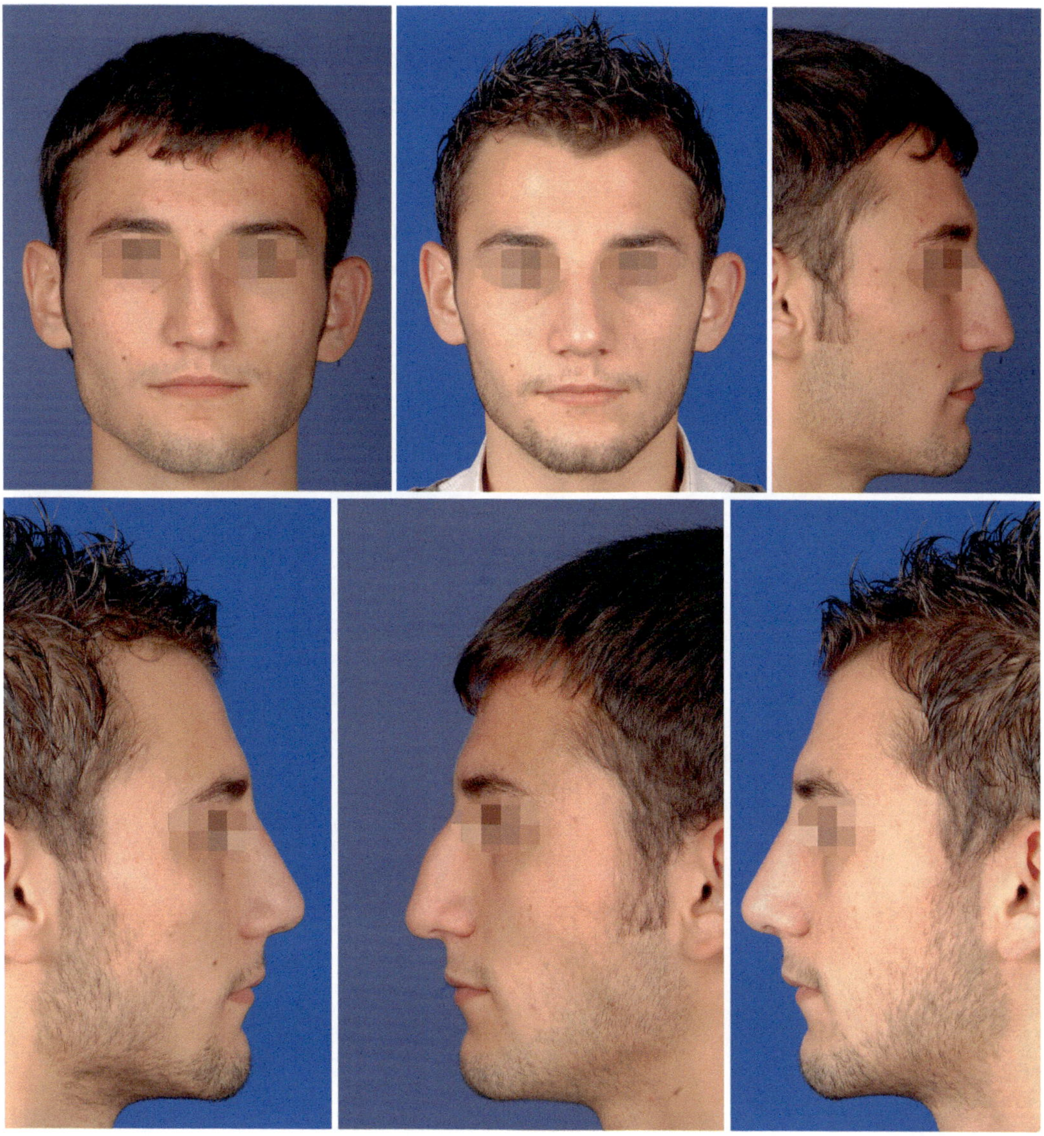

Fig. 11.32 (continued)

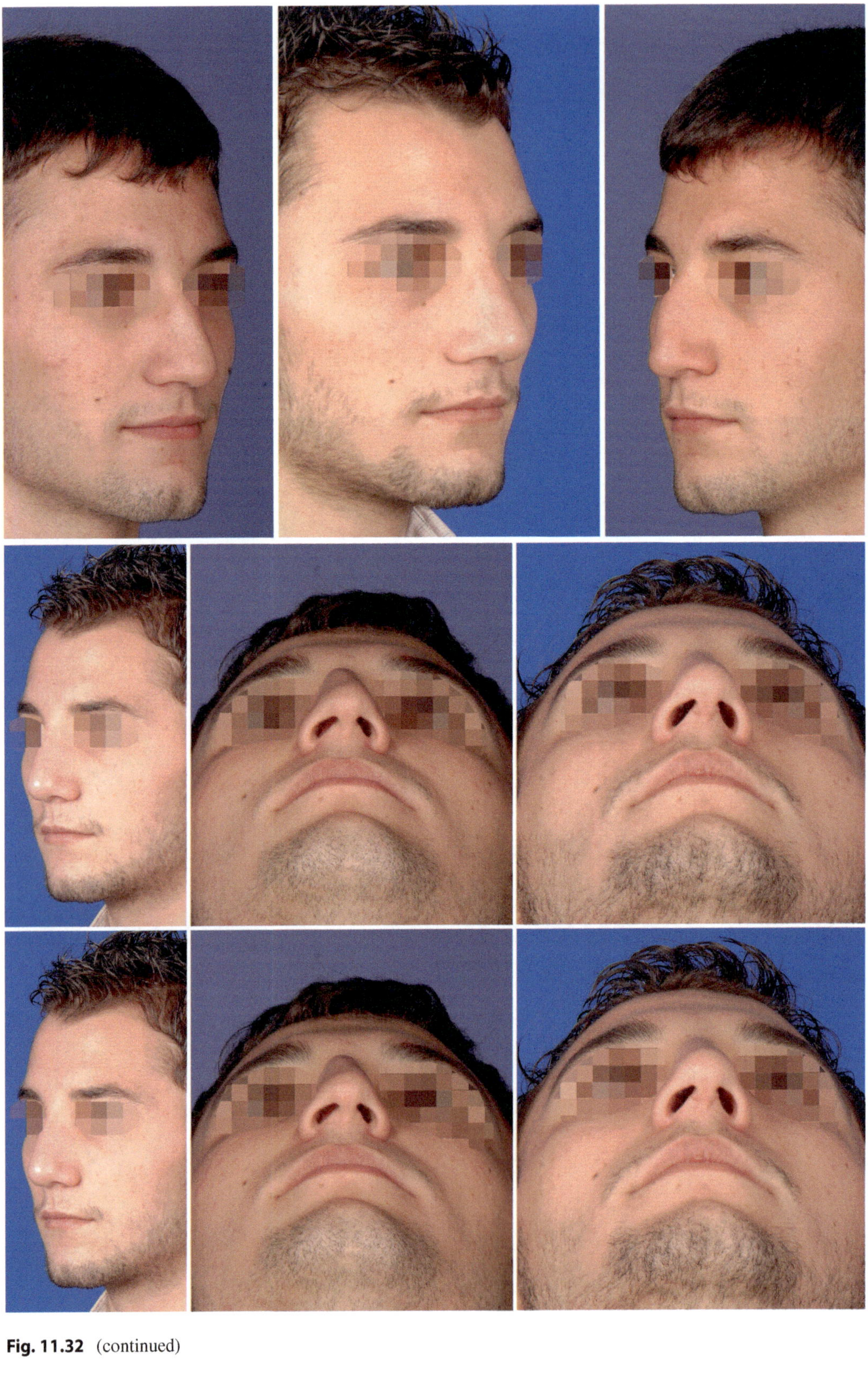

Fig. 11.32 (continued)

11.4 Cutting and Overlapping

The deviated septum is usually larger than the normal nasal septum. Therefore, cutting and overlapping of the septal cartilage, especially at the deflected or mostly deviated portions of the L-strut framework, can be beneficial. In fact, I was never fond of this method. However, in some rare cases, I have found that it can be very useful. I should also point out that, as a structural rhinoplasty surgeon, I always try to add support to this overlap using spreader grafts (Fig. 11.33).

The correction of deformities, including the L-strut framework, is very challenging in rhinoplasty. Therefore, a rhinoplasty surgeon should master all the above-mentioned techniques in order to help patients with crooked noses.

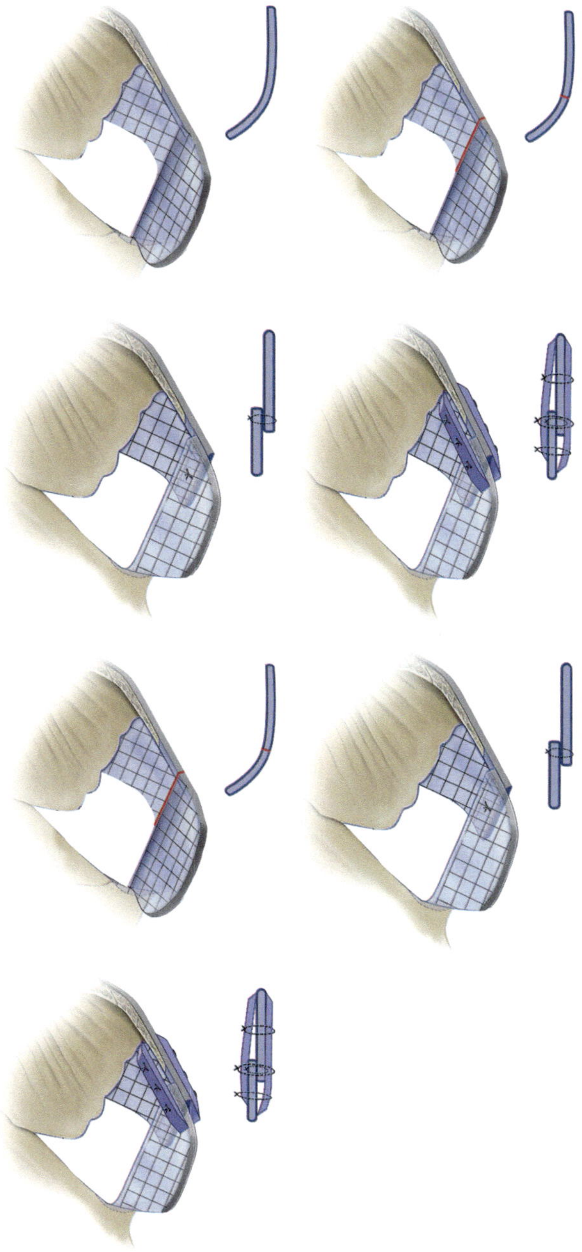

Fig. 11.33 The deviated dorsal segment can be larger than normal, and when a cut is performed at the deflected part, it is possible to overlap the cut edges, suture, and straighten the septum. If additional splinting grafts, such as spreader grafts, are used, the reconstruction becomes much stronger

References

1. Apaydin F, Garcia RFF, Tas V. L-strut graft: a very versatile graft in the management of crooked and traumatic noses. Facial Plast Surg Aesthet Med. 2021;23:110–7.
2. Rohrich RJ, Gunter JP, Deuber MA, Adams WP Jr. The deviated nose: optimizing results using a simplified classification and algorithmic approach. Plast Reconstr Surg. 2002;110(6):1509–23.
3. Evolutionary biology/Jean-Baptiste Lamarck. https://en.wikibooks.org/wiki/Evolutionary_Biology/Jean-Baptiste_Lamarck. Accessed 30 May 2020.
4. Neu BR. Segmental bone and cartilage reconstruction of major nasal dorsal defects. Plast Reconstr Surg. 2000;106(1):160–70.
5. André RF, Vuyk HD. Reconstruction of dorsal and/or caudal nasal septum deformities with septal battens or by septal replacement: an overview and comparison of techniques. Laryngoscope. 2006;116(9):1668–73.
6. Murakami WT, Wong LW, Davidson TM. Applications of the biomechanical behavior of cartilage to nasal septoplastic surgery. Laryngoscope. 1982;92:300–9.
7. Toriumi DM. Subtotal reconstruction of the nasal septum: a preliminary report. Laryngoscope. 1994;104(7):906–13.
8. Apaydin F. Segmental reconstruction for nasal septal deviation. Facial Plast Surg. 2013;29(6):455–63.
9. Gubisch W. Extracorporeal septoplasty for the markedly deviated septum. Arch Facial Plast Surg. 2005;7(4):218–26.

12 Deviations of the Bony Septum

12.1 Introduction

The bony nasal septum comprises the ethmoid lamina, vomer, and maxillary crest. All these structures can show different levels of obstruction when dealing with crooked noses. The process of ossification of the cartilages inside the nose, starting from puberty, can create different anatomic situations for everyone. Besides, in structural rhinoplasty, the main source of grafts is the nasal septal cartilage. However, when it is not sufficient enough, other sources are sought. One of the valuable sources is the bony septum. In this chapter, we will try to address the components of the bony septum in terms of obstruction and as a source of grafts.

12.2 Ethmoid Lamina

The ethmoid lamina is anatomically called as the perpendicular plate of the ethmoid bone. The ethmoid bone is a very special bone in many ways. The ventral surface of this bone forms part of the central part of the anterior skull base. The lower portion forms the roof of the nasal cavity [1]. This sensitive anatomic reality is usually neglected by surgeons, and there is a tendency to think of the ethmoid lamina as an isolated structure. Unfortunately, this is a very big mistake, and the anatomy of the ethmoid bone must always be kept in mind. This is the main reason why this relatively thin plate must be handled with great care by surgeons. In virtual mapping of the ethmoid bone, the upper part must never be touched (Fig. 12.1).

Where do we see deviations in the ethmoid lamina? Usually at the junction with the nasal septum and vomer. The ethmoid is a very thin bone, and it is easy to work on it. My usual routine is to dissect the mucoperiosteum on both sides to reveal the deformities. I like to use Heyman scissors to cut the ethmoid lamina from above and below. This is a relatively easy task because of the thinness of the ethmoid lamina. In most cases, after these two cuts, the ethmoid is usually liberated and easily removed with the help of Blakesley forceps. However, a back cut of the ethmoid is sometimes necessary. I have been using the Joseph elevator to break the ethmoid from the rear portion for years. A long cutting tip of a Piezo machine or a burr is also very useful at this point. If the obtained piece is a straight and big one, it can be used to splint the deviated septal cartilage.

The ethmoid lamina is the preferred splinting material for me and for many surgeons in the management of crooked noses [2–7]. I like using it to splint the dorsal segment, caudal segment, and as an L-strut graft (Figs. 12.2 and 12.3).

Supplementary Information The online version contains supplementary material available at https://doi.org/10.1007/978-3-031-74734-2_12. The videos can be accessed individually by clicking the DOI link in the accompanying figure caption or by scanning this link with the SN More Media App.

© The Author(s), under exclusive license to Springer Nature Switzerland AG 2025

F. Apaydın, *Septal Surgery Challenges in Rhinoplasty*,
https://doi.org/10.1007/978-3-031-74734-2_12

Fig. 12.1 The superior segment of the ethmoid lamina should never be disturbed in order not to have skull base problems

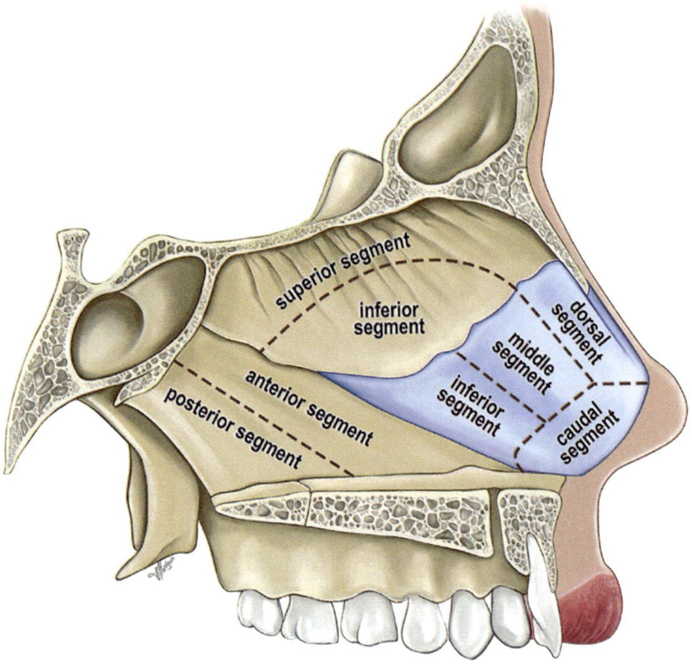

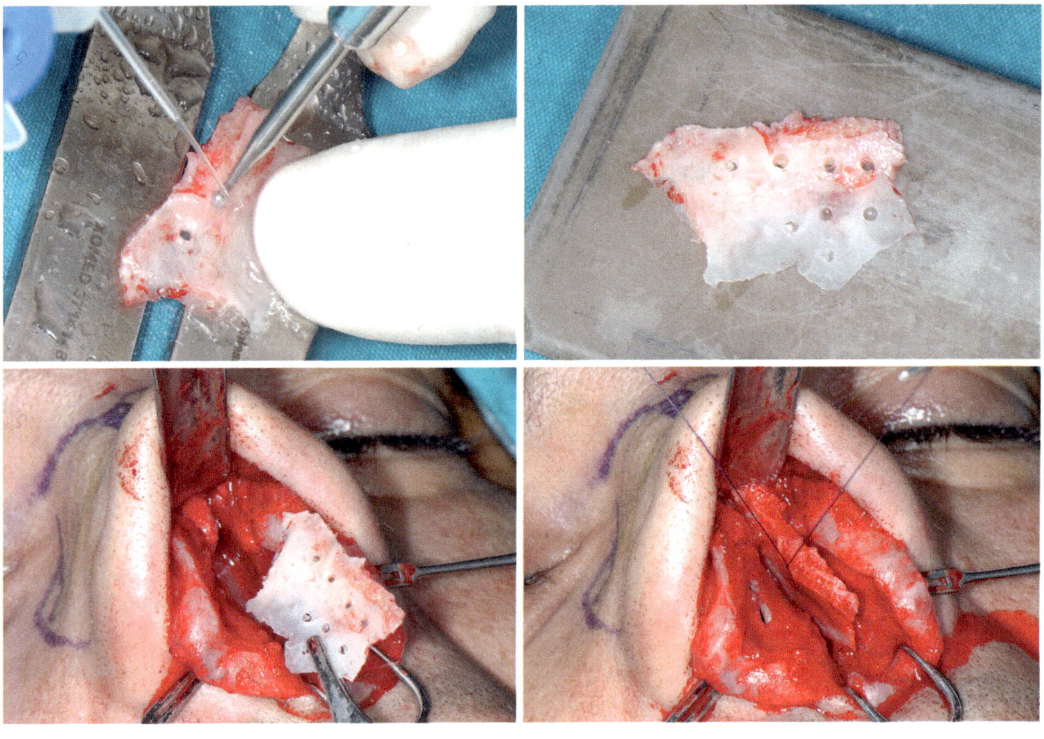

Fig. 12.2 Thin ethmoid bone is a great material for splinting the caudal and/or dorsal segments. Some holes must be opened by using a drill to pass sutures through it

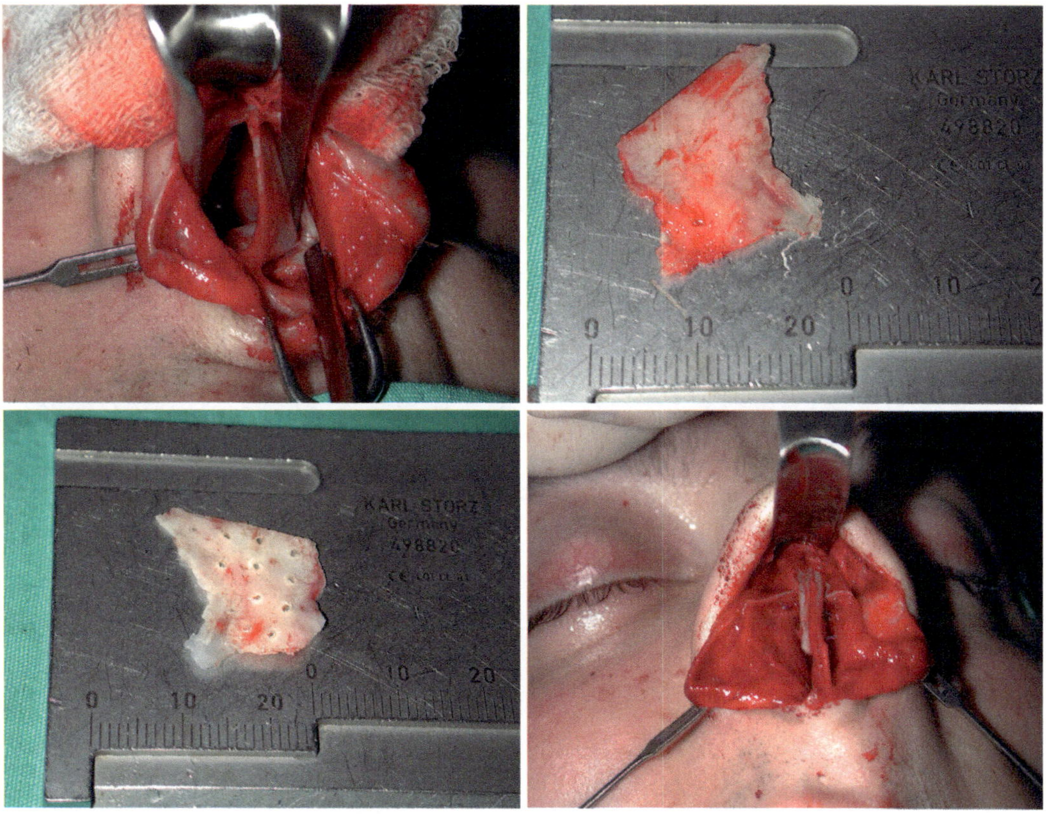

Fig. 12.3 If the ethmoid lamina is bigger, it can be used to splint the L-strut framework

12.3 Ethmoidoseptal Junction

The connection between the septal cartilage and ethmoid lamina is so strong that the septal cartilage and ethmoid plate can be accepted as one anatomical unit. Keeping this fact in mind, the surgeon should plan to harvest septal cartilage and ethmoid lamina together as one piece if there is a need for a bigger graft, such as longer spreader grafts, L-strut grafts, septal extension grafts, or batten grafts (Figs. 12.4, 12.5, and 12.6). I coined the term "hybrid" graft for this kind of bony-cartilaginous graft. Besides, there are times that the septal cartilage is smaller than expected, and in these cases, these hybrid grafts become more important. Having visited and lectured in Latin America and the Far East many times, I witnessed the difficulty that my colleagues are facing every day with this kind of patients where the septal cartilage is so small as a graft material.

In recent years, Sazgar et al. published three papers on this hybrid graft, which they named as "bony-cartilaginous unit." They also reported its use as caudal extension grafts, spreader grafts, lateral crural strut grafts, and for the closure of septal perforations in primary and revision cases [8]. They added that in revision cases, their use as a graft could keep the surgeon away from ear or rib cartilage harvest [9]. They even published an outcome evaluation proving its value in their patients [10]. I also agree with these points that Sazgar et al. brought to our attention after more than 30 years of experience in this kind of graft.

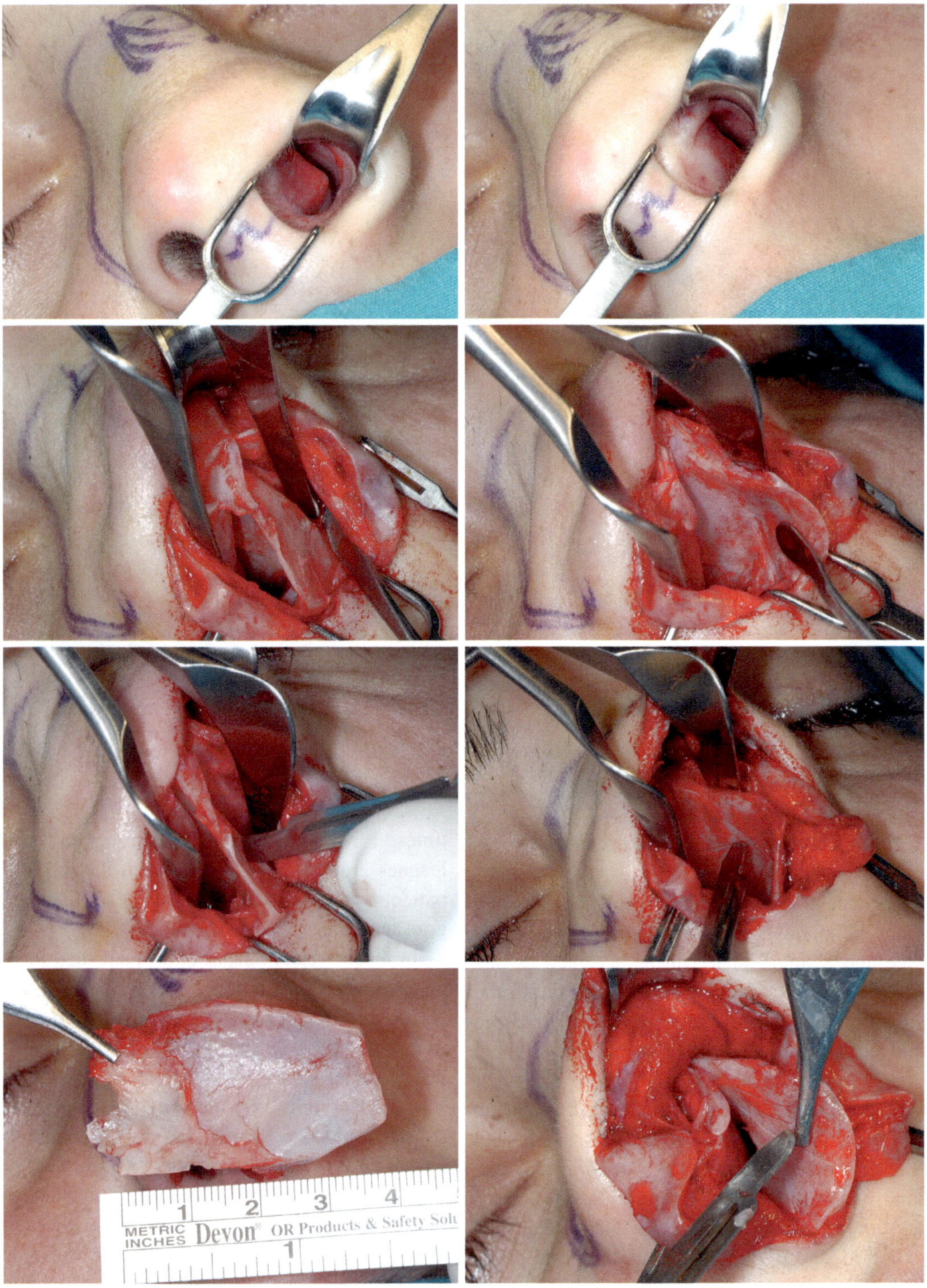

Fig. 12.4 A big bony-cartilaginous (hybrid) graft is used to splint the concave part of a C-shaped deformity after deep cross-hatching

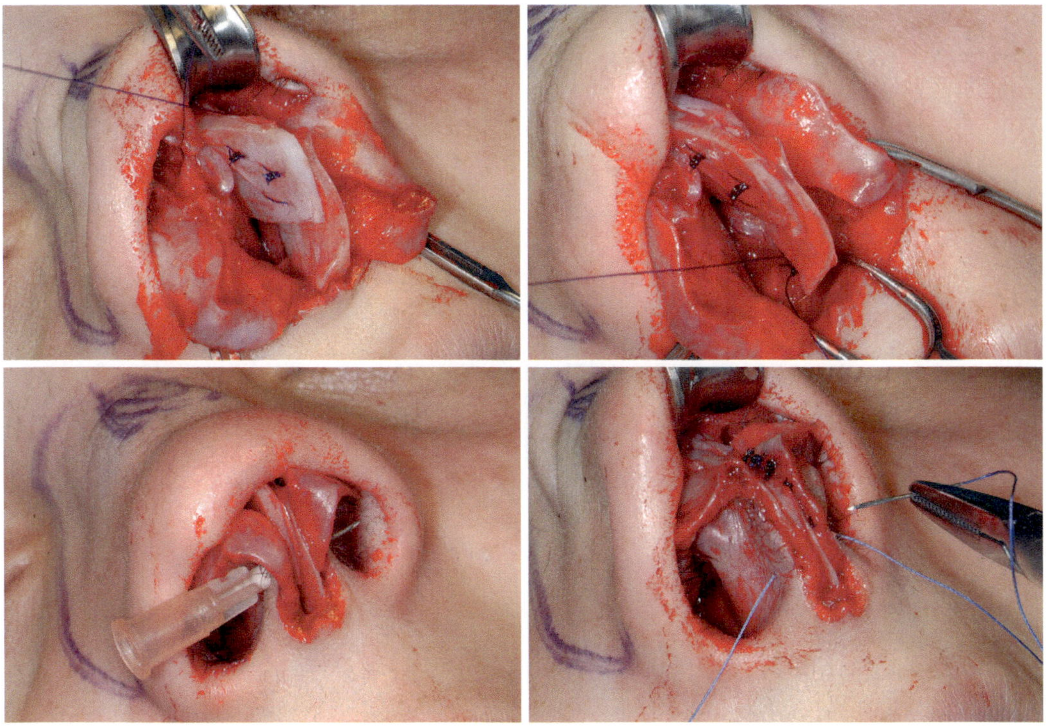

Fig. 12.4 (continued)

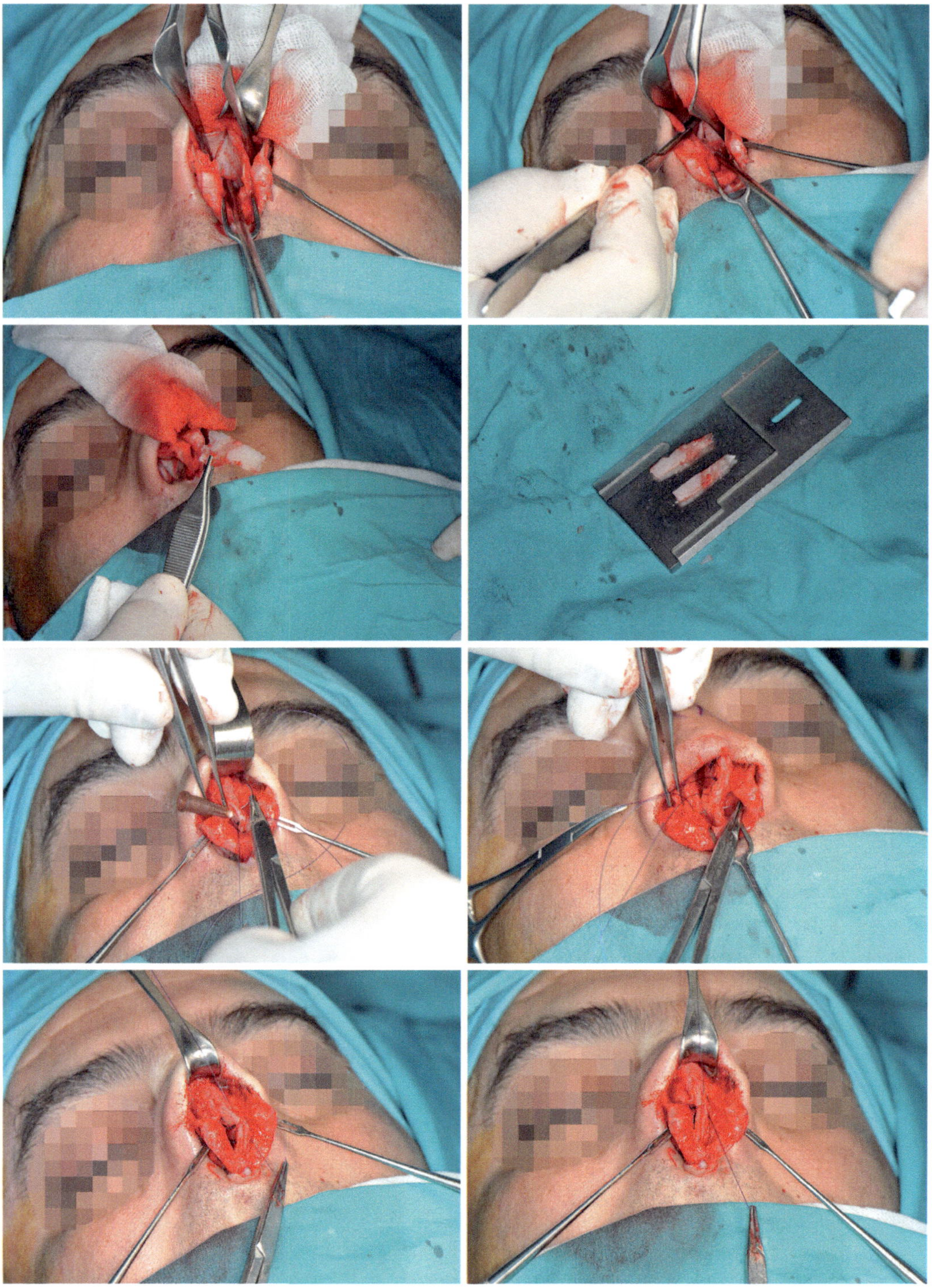

Fig. 12.5 Two splinting bony-cartilaginous grafts were used to splint the dorsal and then the caudal segment. The crookedness was gone, as can be seen in the sixth-month picture

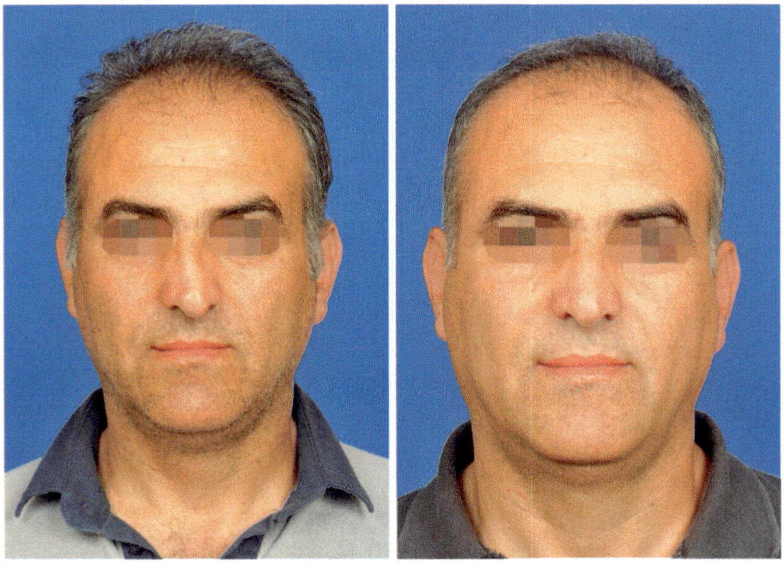

Fig. 12.5 (continued)

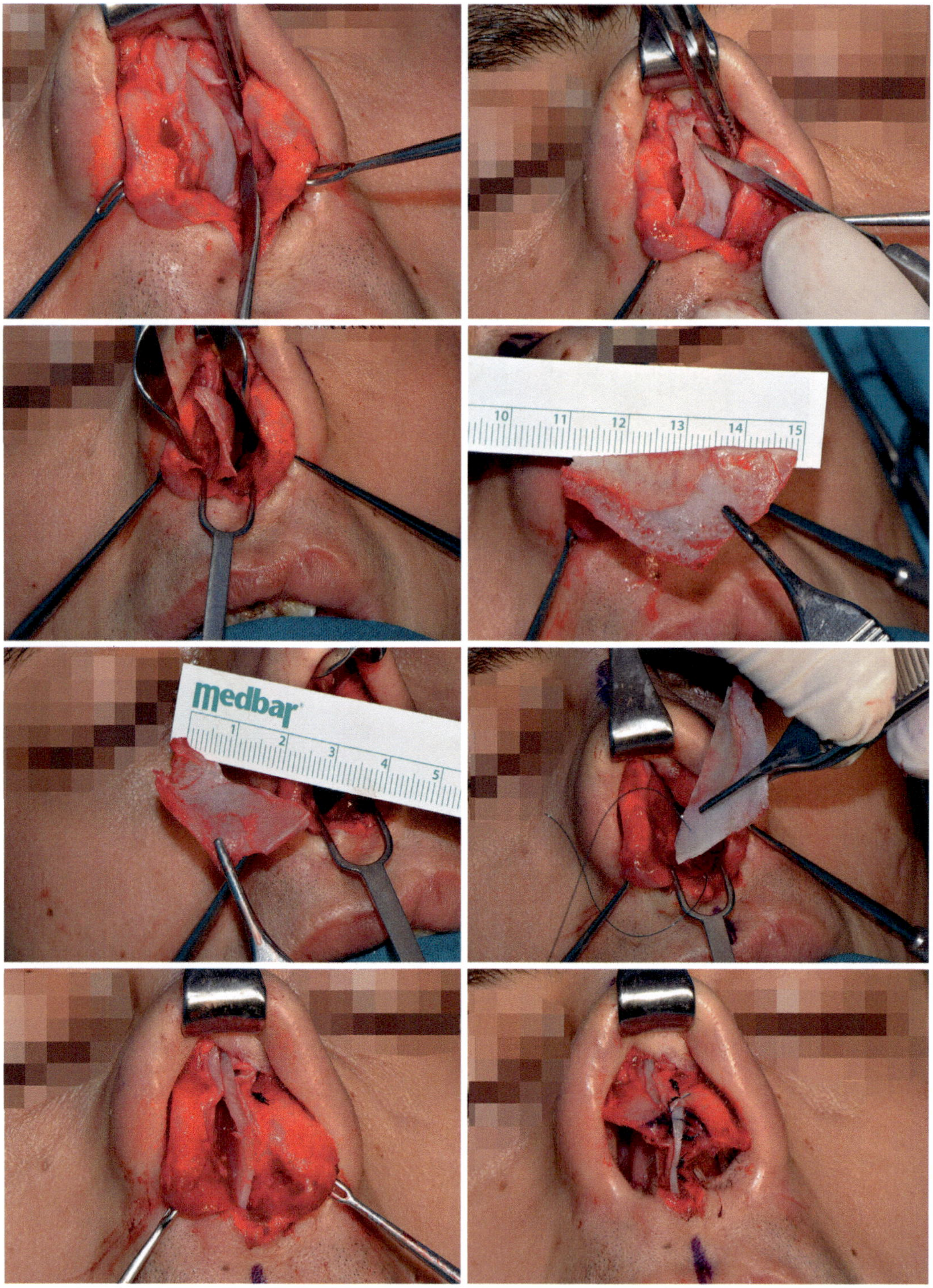

Fig. 12.6 A big bony-cartilaginous graft was used for subtotal septal reconstruction

12.4 Vomer

The vomer is a bilaminar bone that is much thicker than the ethmoid [1]. It is more difficult to cut out than the ethmoid lamina. One lamina usually causes a spur that helps the aerodynamics of the nasal passages. However, if this spur is bigger, it can cause obstruction by itself. Therefore, it must be removed to open the airway. The vomer can be cut horizontally using Heyman scissors or Kaplan-Meyer bone-cutting scissors. The difficulty is in cutting the posterior part of the vomer. After the superior and inferior horizontal cuts, the vomer is forced laterally to break from the posterior part using a strong instrument such as the Joseph elevator. Today, it can be done using the long tips of a Piezo or burrs.

Submucous resection of the septum in the management of septal deviation is still the most popular technique today. In a way, it was popularized even more when structural rhinoplasty techniques became the gold standard during the last two decades. When I was a resident, this was the technique I learned. I used to give all the fragments that I resected from the nose during SMR with great pride to the patient, saying that I had solved all the problems inside the nose. I later learned the Cottle type of septoplasty and reinserting the cartilaginous and bony fragments inside the nose. Still, I was throwing the spur away because it was not suitable to reinsert. Then I remembered that the vomer was a bilaminar bone and decided to shave one lamina causing the spur. I used rongeurs for this purpose, and it worked well to thin the thick vomer to use as a graft. I called this process as "bone recycling" [2] (Fig. 12.7). Like everyone who thinks that they found something new, I was wrong, and it was thought and presented before, in fact, published in 1966 [11].

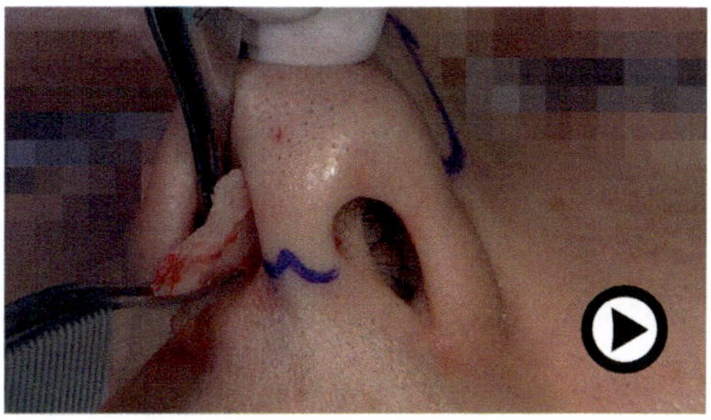

Fig. 12.7 Septoplasty was performed, then the resected bone was reshaped and reinserted into the septal pocket (▶ https://doi.org/10.1007/000-dzk)

Schindylesis is a form of articulation in which a thin plate of bone is received into a cleft or fissure formed by the separation of two laminae in another bone. So, the articulation of the ethmoid lamina with the vomer is a good example of schindylesis [1]. The ethmoid lamina is thin and flat, and its inferior border, which is attached to the septal cartilage, is thicker than the posterior. The vomer is fused with the perpendicular plate and grooved for the inferior margin of the septal cartilage [1] (Figs. 12.8 and 12.9). Therefore, a bigger bony implant can be obtained from the vomer and the ethmoid, preferably under endoscopic guidance (Figs. 12.10 and 12.11).

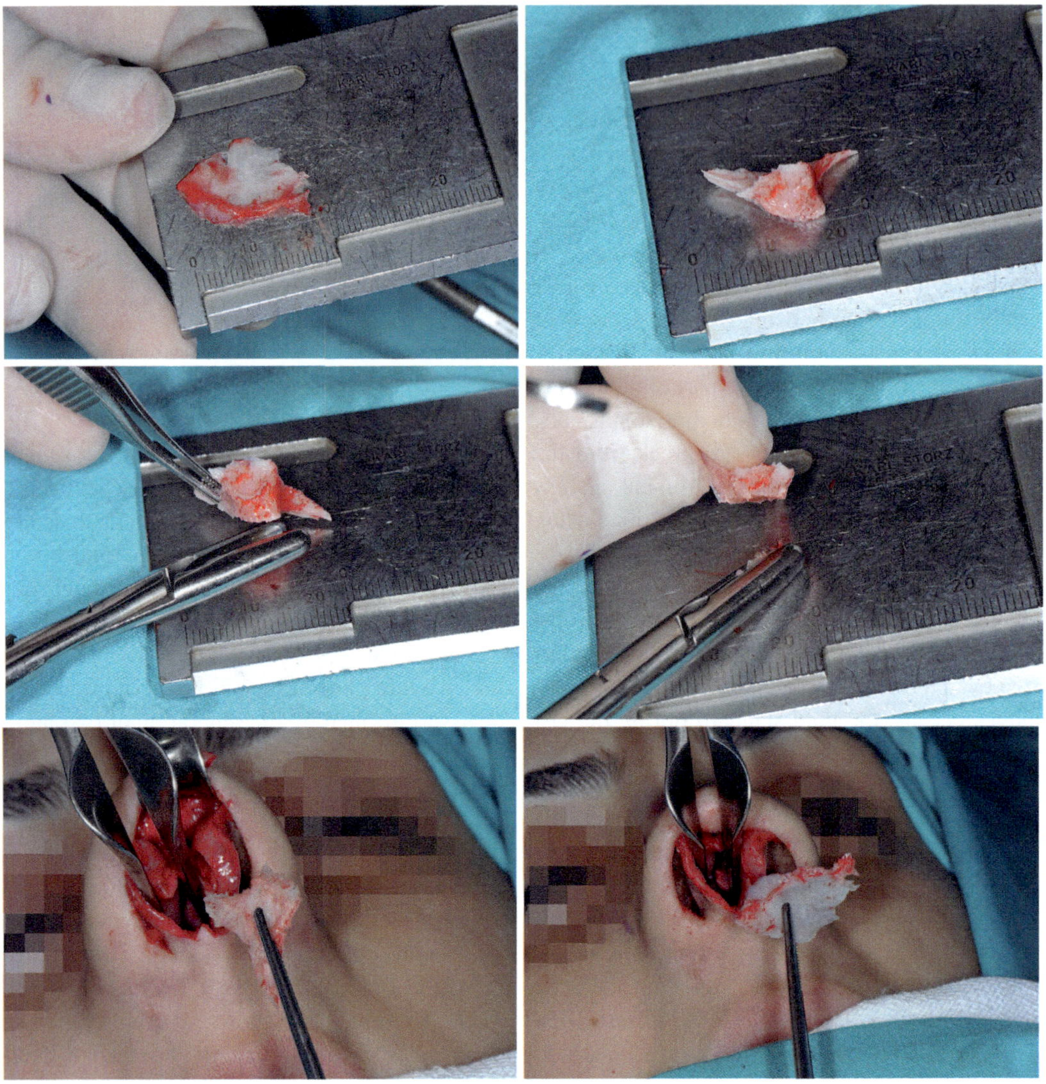

Fig. 12.8 Ethmoid and vomer were removed. The vomer was thinned by rongeur. Both of them were reinserted in the nose

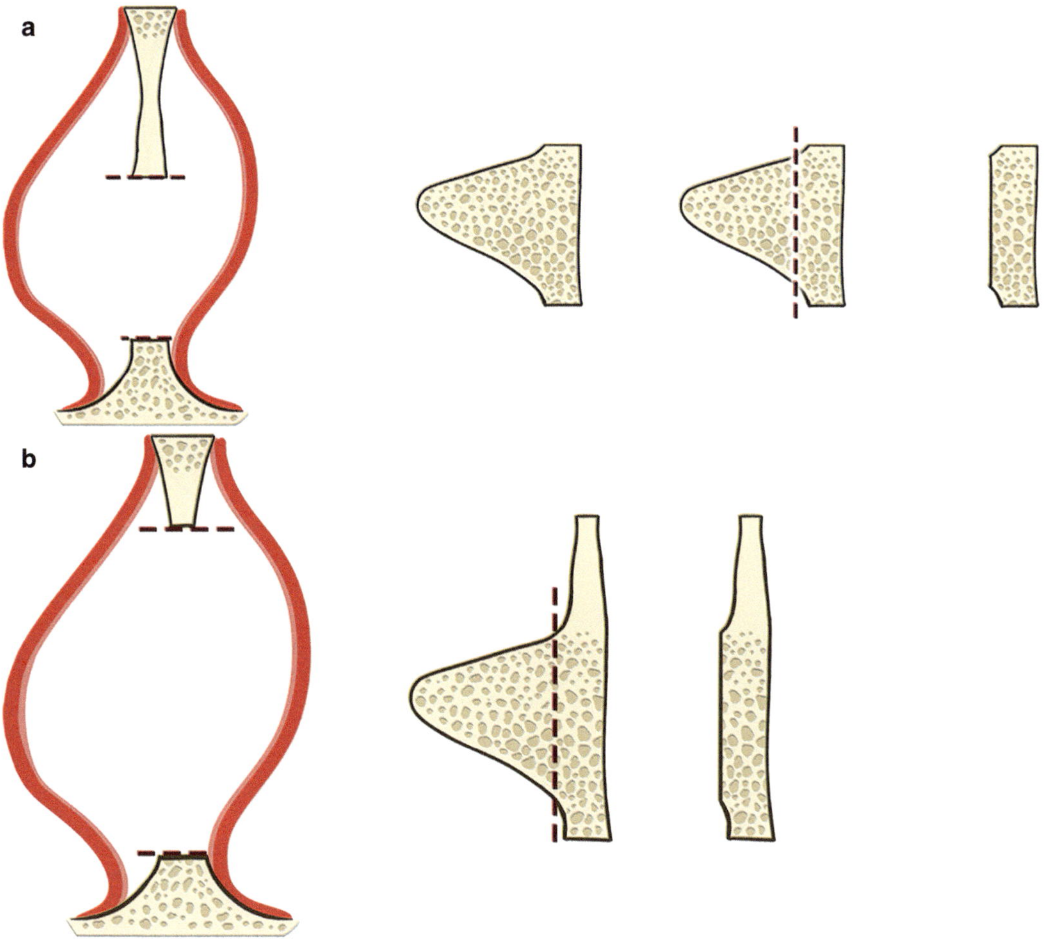

Fig. 12.9 A small (**a**) or a big graft (**b**) can be obtained from the bony septum depending on where it is cut

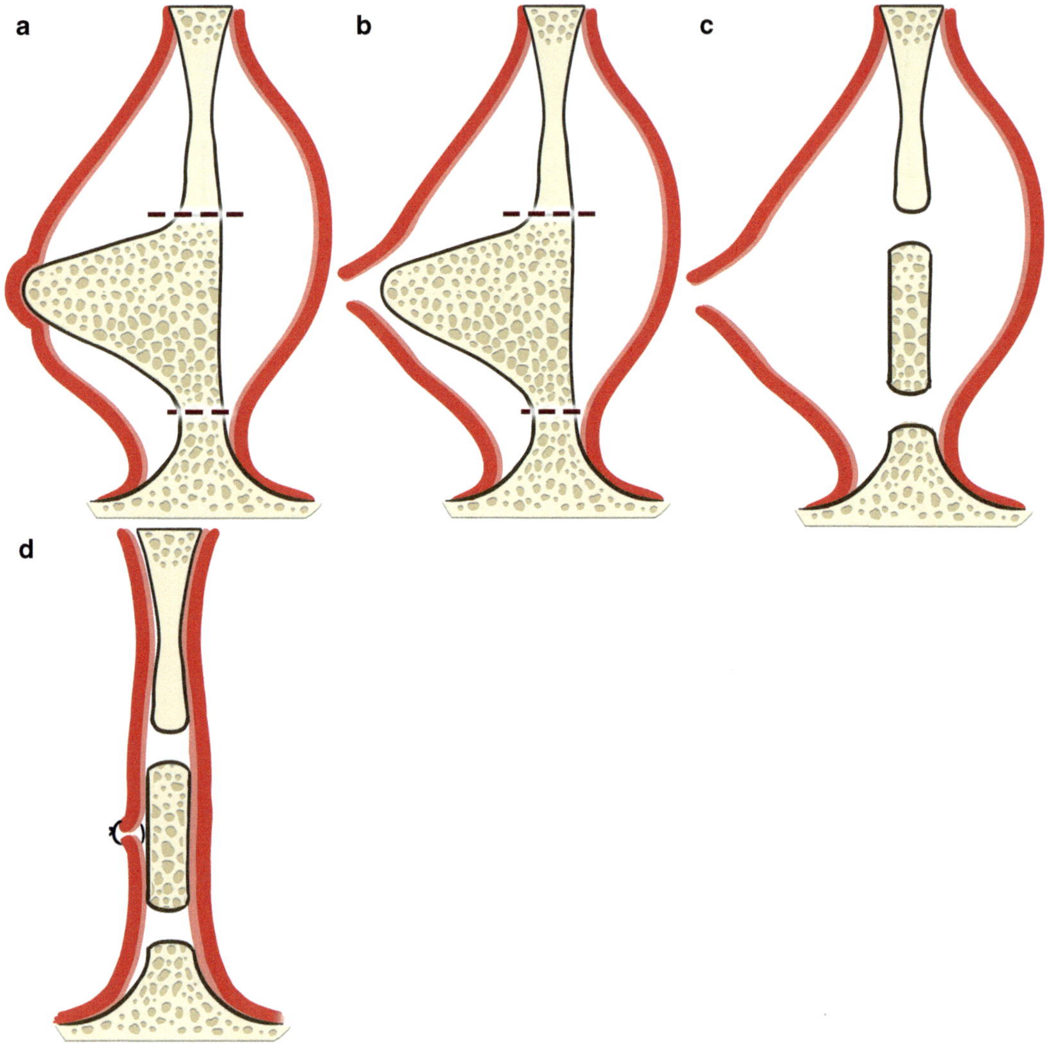

Fig. 12.10 When resecting a bony spur, the mucosa at the sharpest part is usually lacerated (**a**, **b**). When the bony implant is put back, the lacerated edges are tried to be sutured (**c**, **d**), or at least folded back and supported by silicone splints

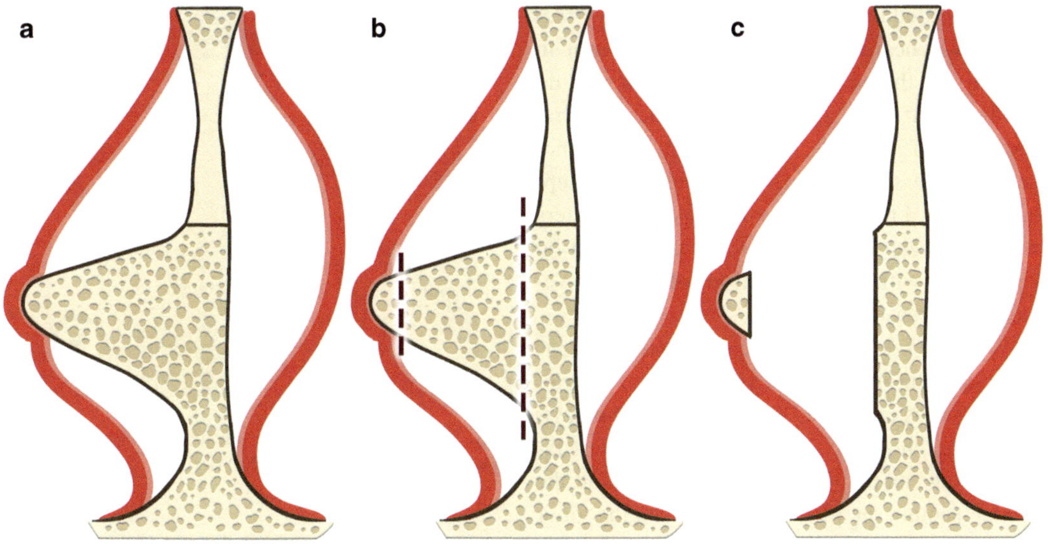

Fig. 12.11 When resecting a bony spur, the mucosa at the sharpest part can be spared with the help of Piezotome under endoscopic guidance. Precise cuts are possible with this setting (**a**, **b**, **c**)

12.5 Maxillary Crest

The maxillary crest houses the septal cartilage like a saddle. Sometimes the maxillary crest deviates as part of the septal deviation. I have been using osteotomes or chisels for a long time to resect or medialize deviations of the maxillary crest obstructing the airway. The downside of this method is that the entire maxillary crest is usually mobilized and resected. In recent years, I switched to using bone-cutting scissors and Piezotome to partially resect only the deviated portions of the maxillary crest. Both instruments work very effectively to maintain the main body of the maxillary crest in place. In these cases, either the deviated part is resected by bone-cutting forceps or Piezo, or by chisel, or it is fractured and medialized. In all these cases, care should be taken not to remove the anterior nasal spine. The resected pieces of bone can be used as filler implants between the mucoperichondrial flaps.

12.6 Anterior Nasal Spine

The anterior nasal spine is usually found in the midline. It should be kept in mind that it is part of the premaxilla and the most fragile part of the bony septum. So, when dealing with it surgically, the surgeon should be meticulous and avoid applying forceful maneuvers. In my opinion, it is a very important structure for two reasons: (1) It is the main anchor point of the caudal septum, i.e., its strong existence and firm relation with the caudal septum are very critical factors for obtaining stable long-term results in rhinoplasty. (2) It is the most important structure defining the subnasale; therefore, it should be kept intact to see a nice nasolabial angle. I heard in some meetings that some surgeons tended to sacrifice it when it was deviated. In my mind, this is a big mistake because it is easy to end up with a retracted subnasale and loss of projection. I have seen surgeons breaking the deviated anterior nasal spine and using a miniplate to fix it in the midline [12].

I never needed this kind of maneuver in my practice. I also heard some surgeons breaking it to bring it into the midline and leaving it there. I do not think that it is a good idea either because you end up with a mobile anchor point that cannot bear the pressure coming from the caudal septum. Surely, I respect the expertise of the masters who have been using these techniques, but I do not agree with them because of the above-mentioned reasons.

What do I do when the anterior nasal spine is deviated? The answer is easy for me. The anterior nasal spine is composed of two wings. The deviated wing should be resected, and the left-in-place wing can be used as a doorstop to hold the caudal septum in place after a swinging door maneuver. A second option is to reshape it with the help of a burr.

That is one more important message regarding the anterior nasal spine and the medial margin of the pyriform aperture adjacent to it. Sometimes, at the basal view, the footplates may look profoundly flaring. Please do not forget to palpate the bony structures, because not infrequently, the surgeon should shave the bony margins of these structures to be able to bring the footplates together.

12.7 The Use of Bony and Hybrid Grafts in the Nose

The bone and bony-cartilaginous pieces obtained from the septum can be used for many purposes [2]:

1. A filler material between the mucoperichondrial flaps: This is a known entity for more than 70 years. I do favor this technique very much. If the bony fragments are deviated, semi-fractures are created at curvature sites with great care in order not to disturb the integrity of the implant.
2. A splinting implant for supporting cross-hatched septal cartilage: the best material is a piece of thin ethmoid lamina or recycled vomer.
3. A splinting spreader graft in a crooked nose (Fig. 12.12).

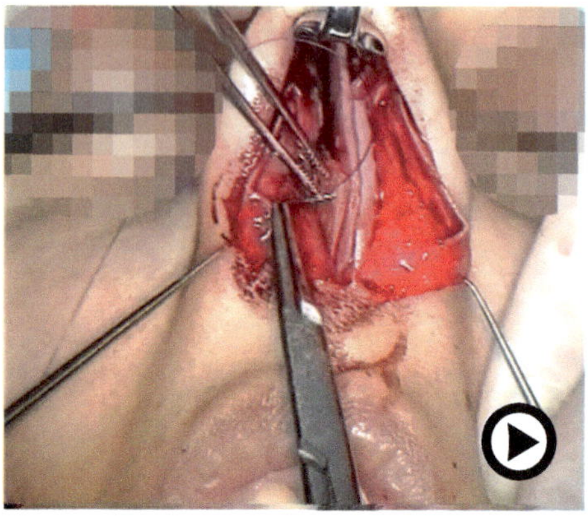

Fig. 12.12 Ethmoid bone was used as spreader graft (▶ https://doi.org/10.1007/000-dzj)

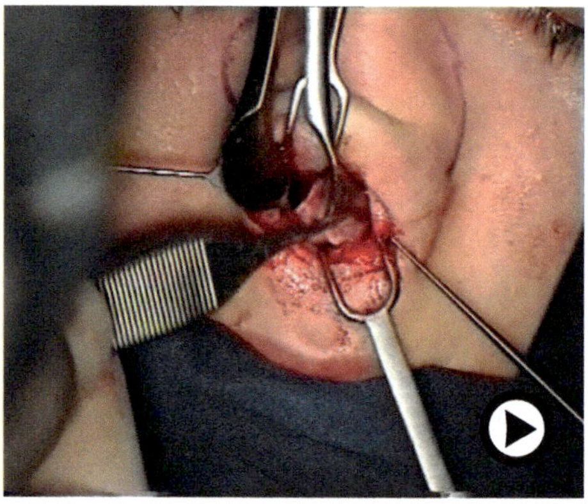

Fig. 12.13 A septal spur was resected and used as a bony premaxillary graft (▶ https://doi.org/10.1007/000-dzm)

4. A premaxillary graft (Fig. 12.13).
5. An L-strut graft to straighten the L-strut framework.
6. Subtotal septal reconstruction.

In conclusion, rhinoplasty surgeons tend to forget and then neglect the bony septum. However, it should be kept in mind that there is a bony septum in the nose, which can be helpful on many occasions as grafts.

References

1. Gray's anatomy. http://www.bartleby.com.
2. Apaydin F. Bone recycling in nasal septal reconstruction. Facial Plast Surg. 2013;29:473–8.

3. Foda HM. The role of septal surgery in management of the deviated nose. Plast Reconstr Surg. 2005;115(2):406–15.
4. Metzinger SE, Boyce RG, Rigby PL, Joseph JJ, Anderson JR. Ethmoid bone sandwich grafting for caudal septal defects. Arch Otolaryngol Head Neck Surg. 1994;120:1121–5.
5. Slavit DH, Bansberg SF, Facer GW, Kern EB. Reconstruction of caudal end of septum. A case for transplantation. Arch Otolaryngol Head Neck Surg. 1995;121:1091–8.
6. Kayabasoglu G, Yilmaz MS, Altundag A, Cayonu M, Varlı AF, Guven M. Bone grafts as a recyclable material in nasal surgeries. Auris Nasus Larynx. 2015;42:24–8.
7. Yao WC, Bleier BS. A simple, single stage technique to harvest optimal ethmoid bone grafts for caudal septal deflections. Int Forum Allergy Rhinol. 2015;5:622–5.
8. Sazgar AA. The bony cartilaginous unit: the missing graft in septorhinoplasty. Int J Oral Maxillofac Surg. 2016;45:1006–8.
9. Sazgar AA, Teimouri Y, Sazgar AK. Use of bone-cartilaginous unit in revision rhinoplasty. Aesthet Surg J. 2019;39:841–7.
10. Sazgar AA, Aalizadeh A, Sazgar AK, Golparvaran S, Saedi B. Outcome evaluation of using bone-cartilaginous units to correct deviated noses in rhinoplasty. Facial Plast Surg Aesthet Med. 2024;26(1):34–40.
11. Dupont C, Cloutier GE, Prevost Y. Autogenous vomer bone graft for permanent correction of the cartilaginous septal deviations. Plast Reconstr Surg. 1966;38:243–7.
12. Haack S, Hacker S, Mann S, Gubisch W. Bony fixation of the nasal framework. Facial Plast Surg. 2019;35:23–30.

13 Dorsum Preservation and the Nasal Septum

13.1 Introduction

Dorsum preservation techniques were initiated by Goodale and Lothrop more than 100 years ago [1, 2]. They were popularized again after extensive anatomical and surgical work by Saban, Palhazi, Çakır, and Daniel in recent years [3–5]. The nasal septum is a key anatomic structure in all of these techniques. However, the rhinoplasty surgeon should be thinking a bit differently in terms of the nasal septum because the principles and techniques are quite different from the structural or Joseph techniques.

The bony pyramid can be lowered in dorsum preservation techniques using foundation techniques, namely push down or let down, and surface techniques. There are four main approaches to the nasal septum to lower the bony-cartilaginous pyramid.

13.2 High Strip

This is the oldest approach of all, which was initiated by Goodale and Lothrop and then popularized by Saban in recent years [1, 2, 4]. As the name implies, an incision is made just under the dorsum, following the curvature of the dorsum. A second cut is then made to lower the cartilaginous dorsum. The ethmoid bone corresponding to the bony hump under the nasal bones is resected using thru-cutting forceps, baby rongeur, piezo, or burrs (Fig. 13.1). Having tried all of these, cut-through forceps are the most practical and easiest of all for me. The Piezotome with long tips is the most effective one in my opinion. It is even possible to make root osteotomy using Piezo from inside. I have been using a 2.5 wide-angle loupe with a light source on it, which helps to have good

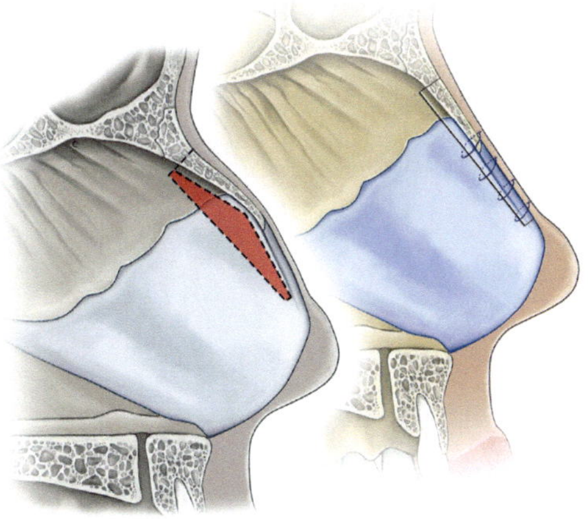

Fig. 13.1 High strip is resection of the cartilaginous hump without touching the nasal dorsum

Supplementary Information The online version contains supplementary material available at https://doi.org/10.1007/978-3-031-74734-2_13. The videos can be accessed individually by clicking the DOI link in the accompanying figure caption or by scanning this link with the SN More Media App.

© The Author(s), under exclusive license to Springer Nature Switzerland AG 2025

F. Apaydın, *Septal Surgery Challenges in Rhinoplasty*,
https://doi.org/10.1007/978-3-031-74734-2_13

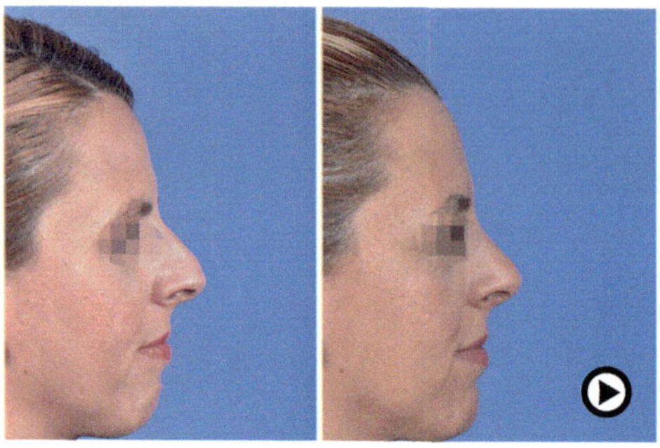

Fig. 13.2 A spare roof type B dorsal preservation rhinoplasty was performed (▶ https://doi.org/10.1007/000-dzp)

exposure. In my opinion, the best method is to use an endovision system. It is much easier to resect the bone under direct endoscopic vision by looking at the monitor as if performing endoscopic sinus surgery. The dorsum sits on the superior margin of the nasal septum, creating a new dorsum profile. In my opinion, this is the most effective method of the techniques listed in this chapter to obtain and maintain the desired profile. This is because the dorsum can easily be sutured to the nasal septum, which is a robust structure that helps the dorsum maintain its position. Another advantage of this method is that the surgeon can easily harvest septal cartilage by leaving an L-strut framework, as in traditional rhinoplasty.

Spare roof techniques (Type A and B [6, 7]) described by Ferreira also use a high strip technique. In addition, small triangles of bone are resected just lateral to the bony dorsum, and the lateral keystone area is dissected. Then the dorsum is sutured to the nasal septum. If needed, lateral osteotomies are done (Fig. 13.2). I have very limited experience with the type B spare roof technique, and I like using it in selected cases (Fig. 13.3) because the bony pyramid is not fully mobilized as in the let-down or push-down techniques, and it is a more predictable technique (Figs. 13.4 and 13.5).

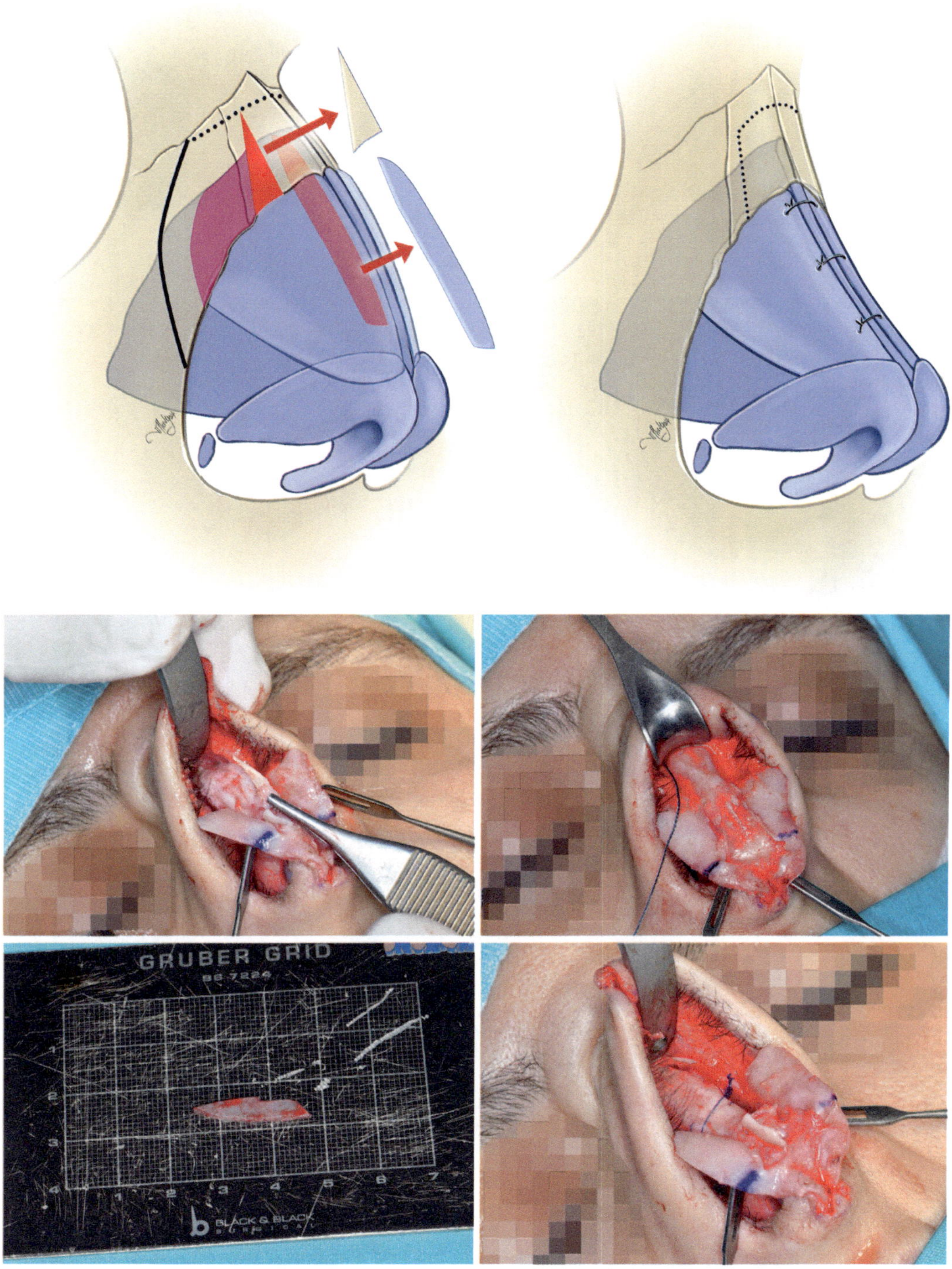

Fig. 13.3 In the Spare roof technique Type B, in addition to the high strip, small triangles of bone are resected just lateral to the bony dorsum, and the lateral keystone area is dissected. Then, the dorsum is sutured to the nasal septum. If needed, lateral osteotomies are done

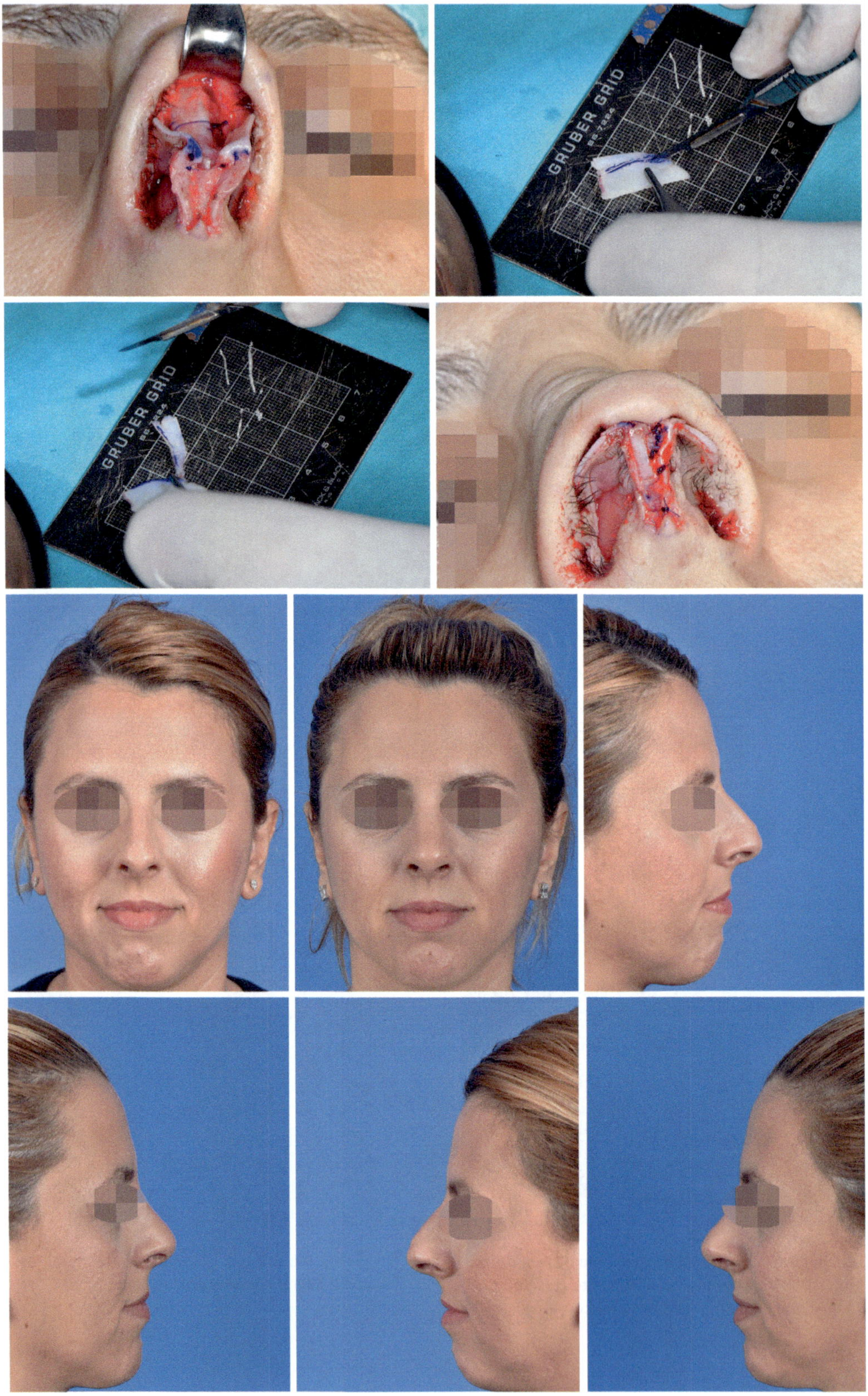

Fig. 13.3 (continued)

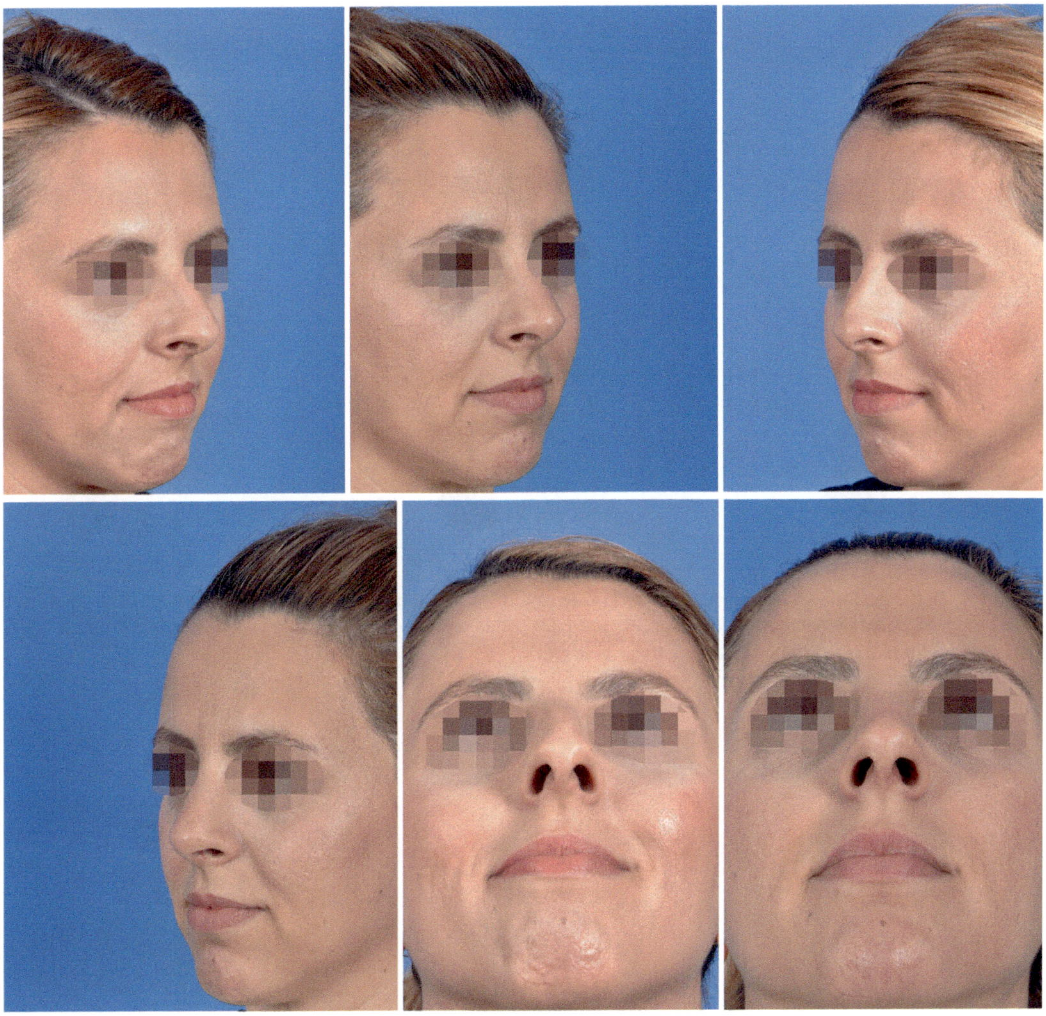

Fig. 13.3 (continued)

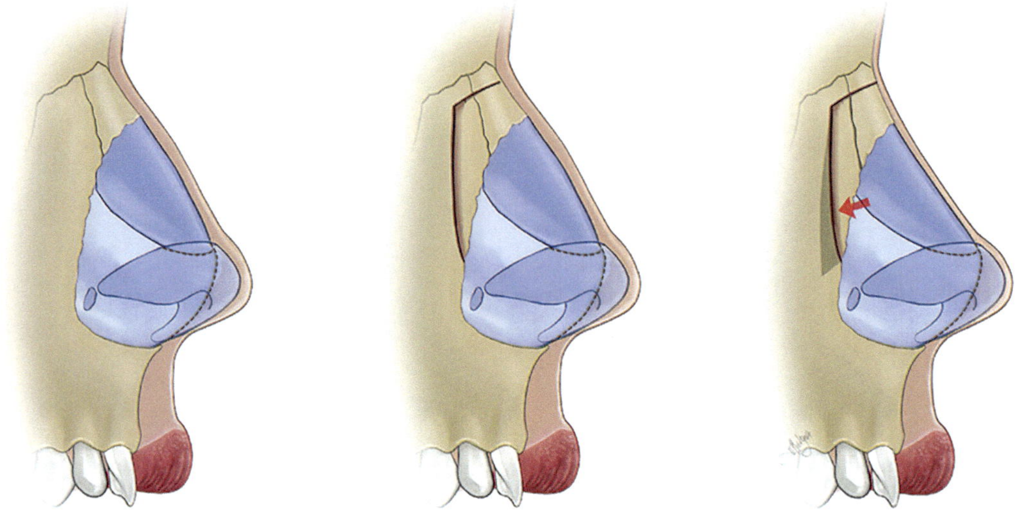

Fig. 13.4 In the push-down technique, the lateral osteotomies are performed perpendicular to the cheek, not parallel as in traditional osteotomies. After the transverse and root osteotomies, the bony pyramid is pushed down, and this type of osteotomy allows lowering the dorsum

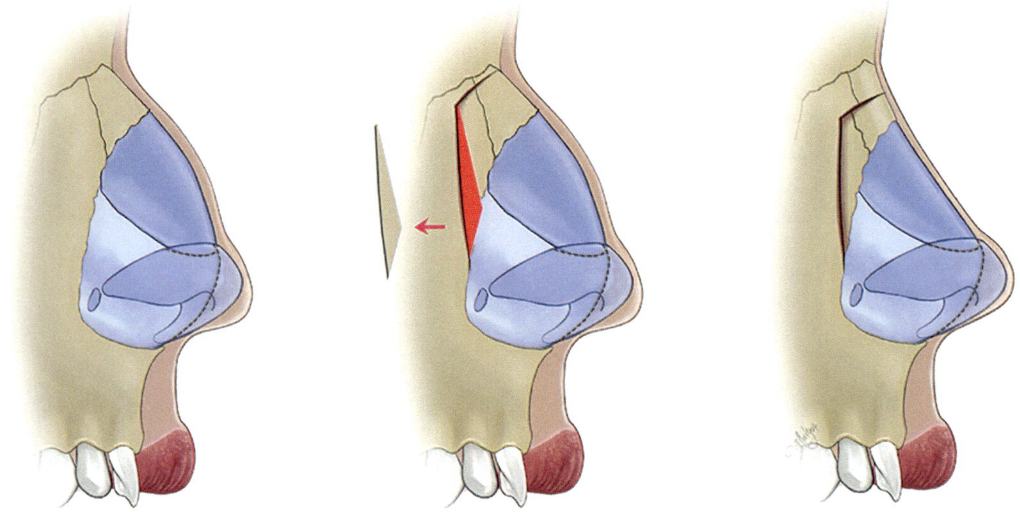

Fig. 13.5 In the let-down technique, the lateral osteotomies are performed perpendicular to the cheek, not parallel as in traditional osteotomies. After the transverse and root osteotomies, the bony pyramid is pushed down, and this type of osteotomy allows lowering the dorsum

13.3 Intermediate (Medium) Strip

In this method, 5–10 mm of septal cartilage is left attached to the upper lateral cartilages, and a strip of septal cartilage and a piece of ethmoid bone (except the Ishida method) are removed. There are some modifications to it:

13.3.1 Septal Strip Resection with Vertical Chondrotomy

In this technique, the superior cut is performed parallel to the cartilaginous dorsum by leaving a 7–10 segment of cartilage attached to the nasal dorsum. The incision is extended to the level of the transverse osteotomy (d). The inferior cut is planned and executed such that the cut line stays parallel to the planned dorsal profile line. The strip of cartilage between these two cuts is resected. A small triangle of ethmoid bone under the nasal bones must be resected to bring down the bony pyramid. Vertical chondrotomy is performed so that the dorsal hump can be straightened and does not bounce back. After the bony pyramid is mobilized, the mobilized upper and lower segments of the nasal dorsum are sutured to the septal cartilage using single or continuous sutures of eight [8] (Fig. 13.6). I have never tried this technique because it cuts the caudal septum, which in my opinion weakens the central pillar of the tip.

13.3.2 Segmental Tetris Concept

In this technique, a 5–8-mm-high rectangular block of cartilage with a base from the cartilaginous dorsum is designed between the junction of the upper lateral cartilages and nasal septum (WASA point) and the most prominent point of the dorsal hump. The amount of hump to be reduced is drawn and then resected just below the rectangular block. A triangular piece of cartilage and bone is resected just under the bony pyramid to the transverse osteotomy level. After the bony pyramid is mobilized, the dorsum is pushed down. The overlapping caudal border of the rectangular cartilaginous block is trimmed. The protruding position of the caudal septum in front of the WASA point is then trimmed [9] (Fig. 13.7). I find this technique very elegant; however, it is sometimes tricky to place the sutures exactly. The second downside is that the flap is thin and sits on a thin margin. In my experience, this can make the new construct more vulnerable and less stable. However, if the suture passes through the mucoperichondrium on one side, part of the suture will be in the nose and can create a bad

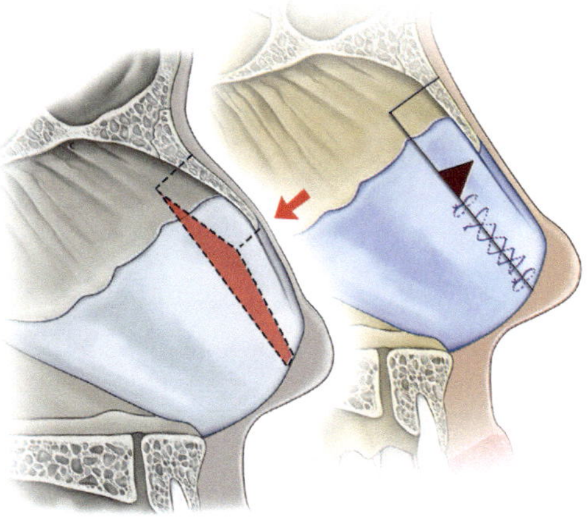

Fig. 13.6 Septal strip resection with vertical chondrotomy

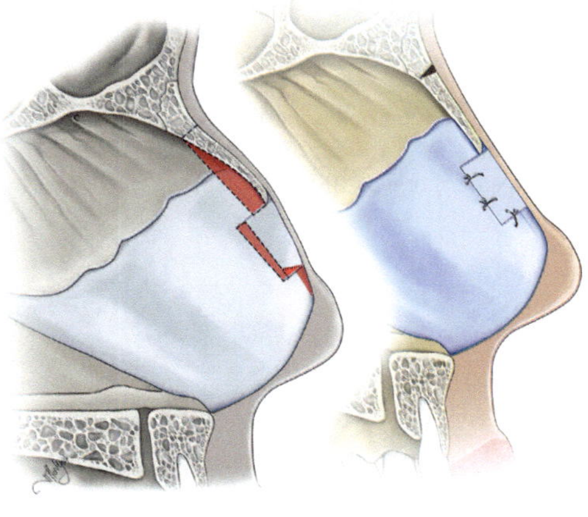

Fig. 13.7 Segmental Tetris concept

smell for some time, but it can be more stable. This technique works great in crooked noses because the superior flap is overlapped on the nasal septum to medialize the dorsum, suturing is much easier, and the construction is more stable.

13.3.3 Subdorsal Z-Flap

This is a modification of the Tetris technique in which the rectangular block takes the form of a Z-flap (Figs. 13.8 and 13.9). The original description states that this flap is sutured in an overlapping manner, so it can only be used in slightly crooked noses [10].

13.3.4 Modified Subdorsal Strip Method

This technique is an elegant modification of the two techniques described by Neves [8, 9]. In this technique, the caudal septum is preserved, and the incision starts from the WASA point and does not traverse the caudal septum as part of the lower incision. Therefore, the caudal septum is spared. An upper and lower cut is performed on the septal cartilage to remove a triangular piece and to bring the dorsum down [11]. It has been reported that a triangular portion could be resected from the ethmoid bone or a simple longitudinal cut on the ethmoid could be sufficient. The subdorsal strut connected to the dorsal cartilage is 3–5 mm. One or two vertical incisions are made into this strut to facilitate the downward movement of the nasal dorsum. The subdorsal cartilage is then sutured to the inferior cartilage (Fig. 13.10). I have no experience with this technique.

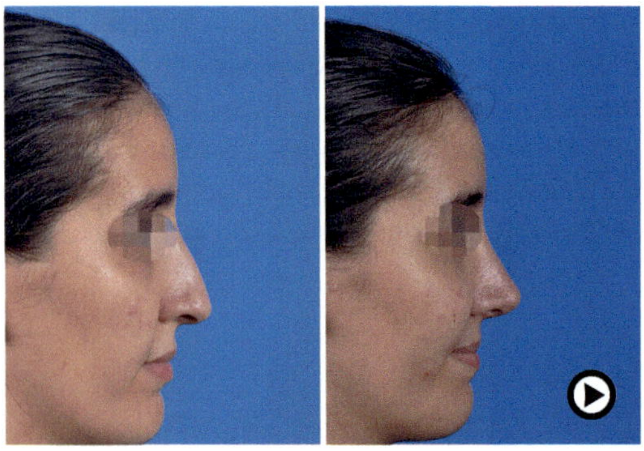

Fig. 13.8 A modified subdorsal Cottle technique was performed as a dorsal preservation rhinoplasty (▶ https://doi.org/10.1007/000-dzn)

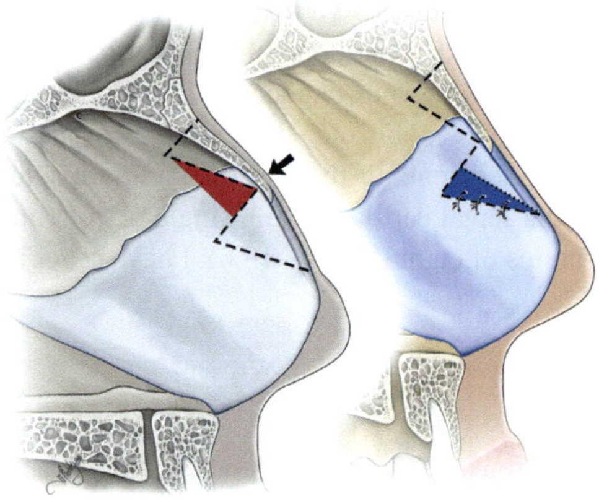

Fig. 13.9 Subdorsal Z-flap is another intermediate strip technique

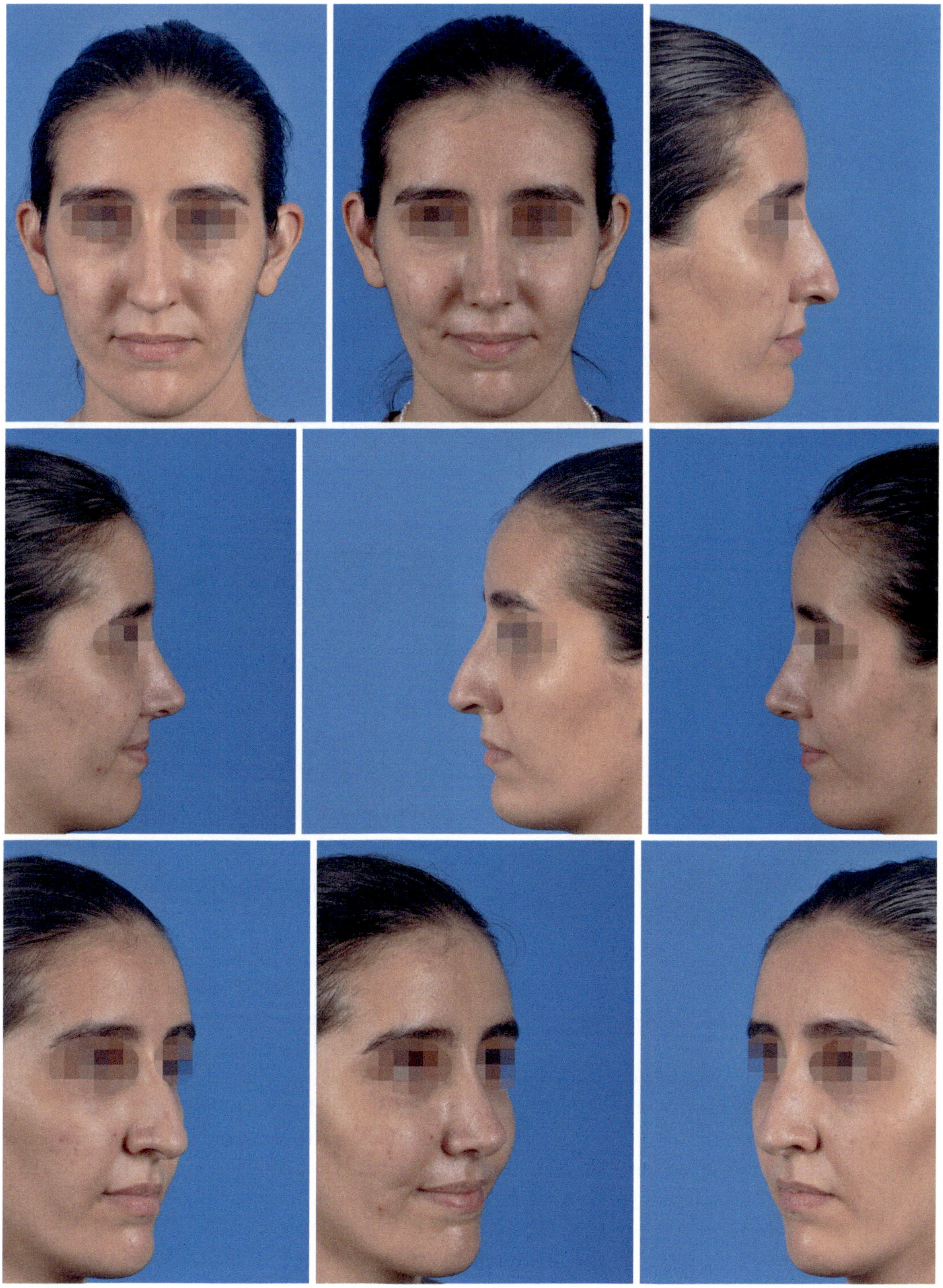

Fig. 13.9 (continued)

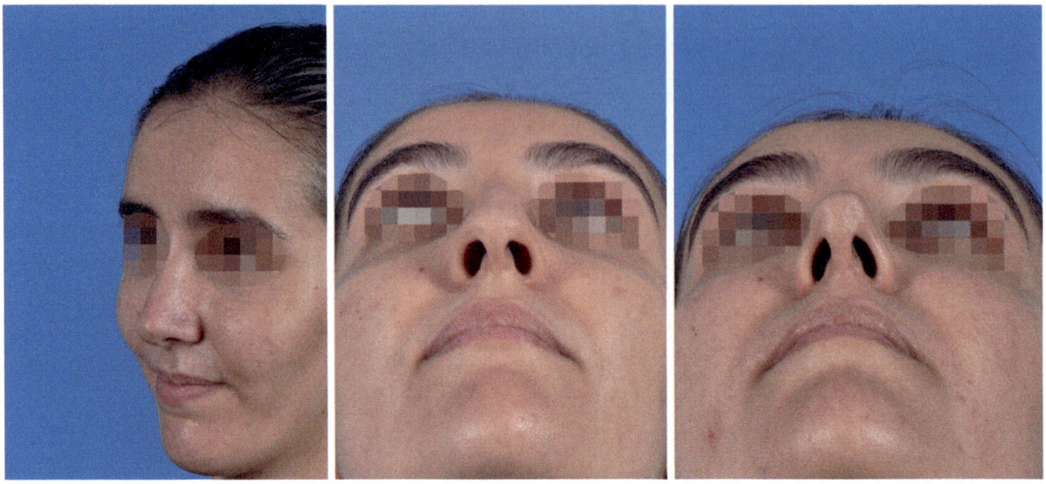

Fig. 13.9 (continued)

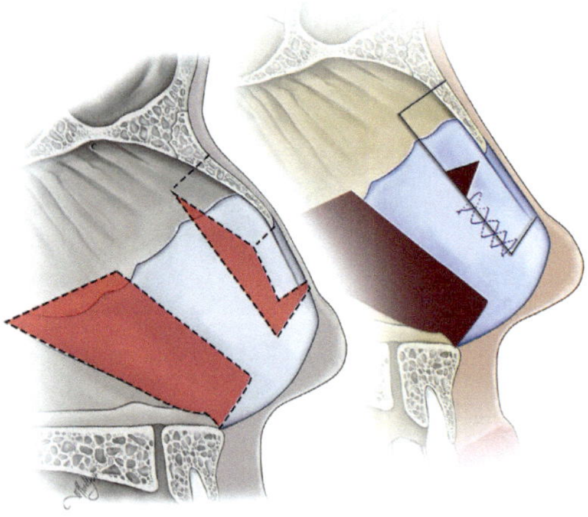

Fig. 13.10 Modified subdorsal strip method

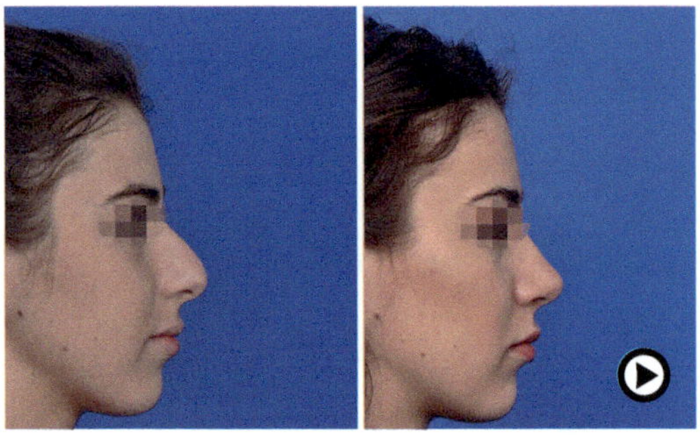

Fig. 13.11 A Cottle-type dorsal preservation was performed (▶ https://doi.org/10.1007/000-dzq)

13.4 Low Strip

As in the Cottle type of septoplasty, the operation starts with vertical chondrotomy at the level of the septal cartilage and ethmoid junction. However, the incision is raised to the keystone area, and a 4–5 mm strip of cartilage is removed just under the most prominent point of the dorsal hump. A triangular piece of bone is resected under the bony pyramid. After the bony pyramid is mobilized, the septal cartilage is freed from the maxillary crest and anterior nasal spine. The cartilage overlapping the bed of the maxillary crest is marked and resected incrementally in order not to end up with a short caudal segment. The lower part of the caudal septum is gently pulled posteriorly and downward and sutured to the anterior nasal spine and surrounding soft tissues [12]. If additional grafts are required, cartilage can be harvested by leaving the L-strut framework in place (Figs. 13.11 and 13.12).

This is my favorite technique for crooked noses for many reasons. First, it is technically much easier than the other techniques described in this chapter. Second, as an experienced ENT surgeon who performs septal surgery, it looks as if I am doing a Cottle-type septoplasty. Third, it is the most efficient technique for treating crooked noses with high septal deviations. For years, I have been

Fig. 13.12 Low strip technique is popularized by Cottle

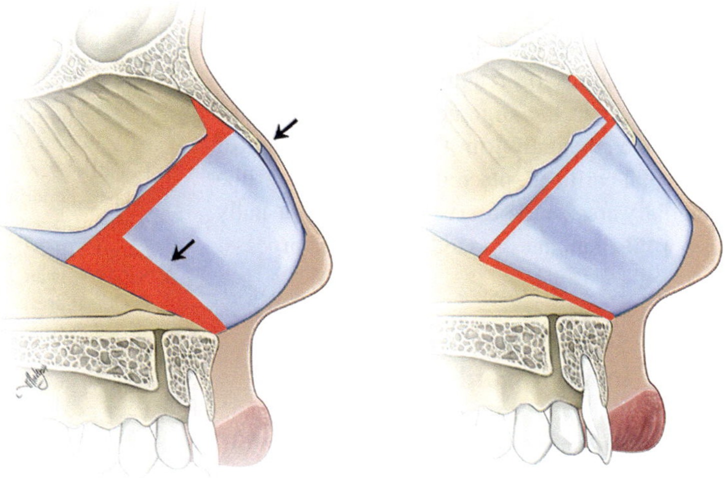

using splinting spreader grafts for this type of high septal deviation, and on some occasions, I have seen recurrences. I was always reluctant to use extracorporeal septoplasty in these types of cases, which could be a solution, especially in these types of noses. In traditional teaching, I was told to respect the junction of the ethmoid and septal cartilage under the keystone area and never disarticulate this junction. Because you end up saddling at the keystone area. If it occurs incidentally, it is not easy to correct it. When I first learned about the low strip of Cottle, I said to myself that it was completely contrary to everything I had learned. Therefore, I never used it. However, I have met many colleagues using this technique extensively in Mexico and Brazil. When the preservation techniques were revitalized, I decided to use them. My first experiences were surprisingly successful. I was pretty skeptical for three reasons. First, the overmobilization of the bony pyramid made me quite nervous. I asked myself, is this real preservation, or am I overkilling? Second, building the whole septum and the dorsum and a single anchoring suture on the anterior nasal spine seemed to be the weakest link in this method. Third, it was not easy to obtain the desired profile as I can obtain with precision in structural rhinoplasty. With experience, I learned to overcome these problems by listening to lectures, watching live surgeries, and operating cases.

How did I overcome the problem of overmobilization? I do not dissect the bony dorsum completely anymore. I only perform percutaneous transverse and root osteotomies. Therefore, the periosteum and the soft tissues on the bony dorsum keep the fractured segment in place.

Do I rely on one suture that also pulls the whole construct downward and inferiorly? I learned from very experienced surgeons who have been doing this kind of surgery for three decades that if you free the dorsum from blocking forces, this suture becomes just a simple suture fixing the nasal septum on the maxillary crest. Releasing the lateral keystone area to prevent bouncing back of the hump, cutting the cartilage vertically just under the most prominent portion of the dorsum, and performing osteotomies efficiently for let-down and push-down. My recent approach involves resecting the Webster triangle and pushing down the bony pyramid. I faced deviations of the bony pyramid laterally on some occasions with the let-down approach. I also want to share an important trick that I have been using while fixing the nasal septum to the anterior nasal spine. I do not skeletonize the maxillary crest unless I have a bony deviation, which is less likely in most cases. Therefore, after disarticulating the septal cartilage from the maxillary crest, excess cartilage is trimmed to align the profile. The caudal margin of the remaining cartilage sits in the groove of the maxillary crest. In addition to one or two strong mattress sutures fixing the caudal septum to the ANS, I try to embrace the inferior portion of the cartilage with soft tissues and sutures to strengthen the fixation.

What about the alignment of the dorsal profile? I incrementally trim the inferior margin of the septal cartilage, place it in the groove of the maxillary crest, and observe the profile. I usually use profile templates to guide me in this process.

13.5 Septal Strip Resection Involving only Cartilage

The Ishida technique involves cartilaginous push-down with bony cap preservation [13]. Bony hump reduction and osteotomies are performed as in traditional rhinoplasty. The nasal septum is undermined until the perpendicular plate of the ethmoid bone, and a strip of septal cartilage is resected parallel to the dorsum while keeping the ethmoid intact. This resection is usually performed on the more deviated portion. The resection can be low, mid-septal, or high, depending mainly on the location of the septal deviation (Fig. 13.13). When there is no or minimal septal deviation, the preferred spot for resection is approximately 3–4 mm below the dorsum.

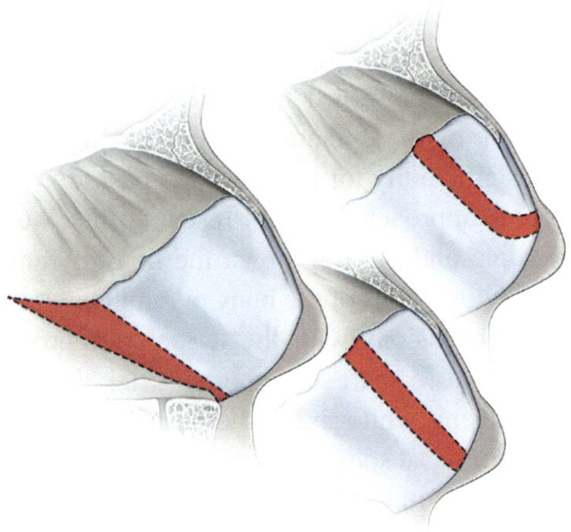

Fig. 13.13 Septal strip resection involving only cartilage by Ishida

References

1. Goodale JL. A new method for the operative correction of exaggerated Roman nose. Boston Med Surg J. 1899;140:112.
2. Lothrop OA. An operation for correcting the aquiline nasal deformity; the use of new instrument; report of a case. Boston Med Surg J. 1914;170:835–7.
3. Cakir B, Oreroğlu AR, Doğan T, Akan M. A complete subperichondrial dissection technique for rhinoplasty with management of the nasal ligaments. Aesthet Surg J. 2012;32:564–74.
4. Saban Y, Daniel RK, Polselli R, Trapasso M, Palhazi P. Dorsal preservation: the push down technique reassessed. Aesthet Surg J. 2018;38:117–31.
5. Daniel RK. The preservation rhinoplasty: a new rhinoplasty revolution. Aesthet Surg J. 2018;38:228–9.
6. Ferreira MG, Monteiro D, Reis C, Almeida e Sousa C. Spare roof technique: a middle third new technique. Facial Plast Surg. 2016;32:111–6.
7. Ferreira MG, Santos M. The barn doors greenstick fracture-a new 3D geometry for common osteotomies in rhinoplasty: the first 50 patients with 1-year follow-up. Facial Plast Surg. 2023;39:434–40.
8. Neves JC, Arancibia Tagle D, Dewes W, et al. The split preservation rhinoplasty: "the Vitruvian Man split maneuver". Eur J Plast Surg. 2020;43:323–33.
9. Neves JC, Arancibia-Tagle D, Dewes W, Ferraz M. The segmental preservation rhinoplasty: the split Tetris concept. Facial Plast Surg. 2021;37:36–44.
10. Kovacevic M, Veit JA, Toriumi DM. Subdorsal Z-flap: a modification of the Cottle technique in dorsal preservation rhinoplasty. Curr Opin Otolaryngol Head Neck Surg. 2021;29:244–51.
11. Patel PN, Abdelwahab M, Most SP. Dorsal preservation rhinoplasty: method and outcomes of the modified subdorsal strip method. Facial Plast Surg Clin North Am. 2021;29:29–37.
12. Cottle MH, Loring RM. Corrective surgery of the external nasal pyramid and the nasal septum for restoration of normal physiology. Ill Med J. 1946;90:119–35.
13. Ishida LC, Ishida J, Ishida LH, Tartare A, Fernandes RK, Gemperli R. Nasal hump treatment with cartilaginous push-down and preservation of the bony cap. Aesthet Surg J. 2020;40:1168–78.

Surgical Management of the Septal Perforation

14

14.1 Introduction

Septal perforations are one of the sequelae that are very difficult to manage. The main goal in the management of septal perforation is to restore the normal function and physiology to the nose. The surgeon should learn about the etiology of the perforation (Table 14.1), the size of the nasal septum, the location, and the size of the perforation before planning surgery [1, 2]. After deciding on the type of reconstruction, the options are discussed with the patient, such as the design of the endonasal mucosal flap, incorporation of an interposition graft, and the source of this graft, as well as the surgical approach [1–3].

The perforations can be classified according to the size. They can be accepted small when the diameter is less than or equal to 0.5 cm, medium between 0.5 and 2 cm, and bigger than 2 cm [4]. The perforations at the posterior part of the nasal septum and bigger ones are usually less problematic for the patients and do not need surgery because there is rapid humidification of the inspired air by the nasal mucosal lining and turbinates [1, 5, 6].

The techniques using flaps inside the nose are very helpful in replacing like with like. However, squamous metaplasia might still replace the normal mucosa and cause dryness inside the nose [1]. That is why skin grafts and flaps obtained

Table 14.1 Etiology of nasal septal peroration [1, 2]

1. Trauma
   (a) External
   - Fracture
   - Septal hematoma

   (b) Self-inflicted
   - Nose picking
   - Foreign bodies

   (c) Iatrogenic
   - Septoplasty
   - Rhinoplasty
   - Septal cauterization
   - Septal packing
   - Nasotracheal intubation
2. Nasal drug abuse
   (a) Cocaine
   (b) Vasoconstrictive nasal spray
   (c) Intranasal steroids
   (d) Smoking
3. Inflammatory
   (a) Granulomatosis with polyangiitis (Wegener's granulomatosis)
   (b) Eosinophilic granulomatosis with polyangiitis (Churg Strauss syndrome)
   (c) Systemic lupus erythematosus
   (d) Rheumatoid arthritis
   (e) Crohn's disease
   (f) Sarcoidosis
4. Infectious
   (a) Septal abscess
   (b) Syphilis
   (c) HIV
   (d) Invasive fungal infections
   (e) Tuberculosis
5. Neoplasms
6. Occupational exposure
   (a) Heavy metals (chromic acid)
   (b) Physical and chemical irritants

© The Author(s), under exclusive license to Springer Nature Switzerland AG 2025

F. Apaydın, *Septal Surgery Challenges in Rhinoplasty*,
https://doi.org/10.1007/978-3-031-74734-2_14

from the mouth and neighboring skin do not create areas with mucociliary transport and are not very popular [7, 8].

14.2 Preoperative Stage

During the preoperative consultation, thorough history taking is very important to identify the possible reasons for perforation (Table 14.1). The most important thing in decision-making is the condition of the patient. Does the patient have disturbing symptoms due to septal perforation? An endoscopic nasal examination can reveal the size and location of the perforation. After topical anesthetic application inside the nose, the surgeon can try to palpate the nasal mucosa to determine the osseocartilaginous support. For Alobid et al., the existence of this support is very critical in surgical decision-making [9].

14.3 Conservative Nonsurgical Approach

If the septal perforation is not disturbing the patient, is located posteriorly, and has well-healed edges, it is better to be conservative. The goal is to keep the nasal chambers moist, devoid of crusting and infection. Nasal douches with saline applied under pressure by a silicone pump are very effective. There are many different saline sprays available on the market. Some of them are hypertonic, and some of them include emollients. For decades, I asked patients to prepare custom-made hypertonic saline at home. I do not do it anymore because it is very difficult to obtain a standard therapy in each case. I also like prescribing saline gels to keep the nasal chambers moist for a longer time. If the patient has frequent epistaxis, it should be treated. If there is another cause creating the perforation, as mentioned in the etiology, and if it is possible to treat, it should be done as well.

If the conservative measures are not successful, silicone buttons can be suggested [10].

Unfortunately, the prostheses that are available commercially do not adequately fit larger perforations. In these cases, a custom-made silicone button can be designed by using the data obtained from CT images and printed out by 3D printers [11]. Some patients use these buttons without any problems for years. However, it is not the case for every patient, as they can sometimes cause crusting and irritation in the mucosa.

14.4 Surgical Management

14.4.1 Unilateral or Bilateral Septal Rotation and Transposition Flaps

Seiffert described an advancement flap after a relieving incision 1 cm away from the perforation margin to close small perforations [12] (Fig. 14.1a, b). Inferiorly and superiorly based rotation flaps were also reported for small defects [13] (Fig. 14.2a, b). Meyer described a flap of perichondrium and periosteum with a wide bipedicled bridge for small defects [14]. A unilateral rotation flap was brought up by Converse [15] (Fig. 14.3a–d). In the cross-stealing (Fig. 14.4a–c) technique of Mladina, contralateral inferiorly and superiorly based are created using the perforation margins as a hinge [16].

14.4.2 Free Tissue Grafts

Free tissue grafts, such as temporalis fascia [17, 18], split-thickness grafts [19], and composite grafts [20], have been reported for closing perforations. Tragal cartilage with perichondrium on both sides, which was sandwiched between the superficial and deep layers of temporal fascia, was also described with successful closure [21] (Fig. 14.5). The use of conchal cartilage with perichondrium on both sides was described in children [22]. Its use during external and endonasal rhinoplasty was also reported in adults [23, 24].

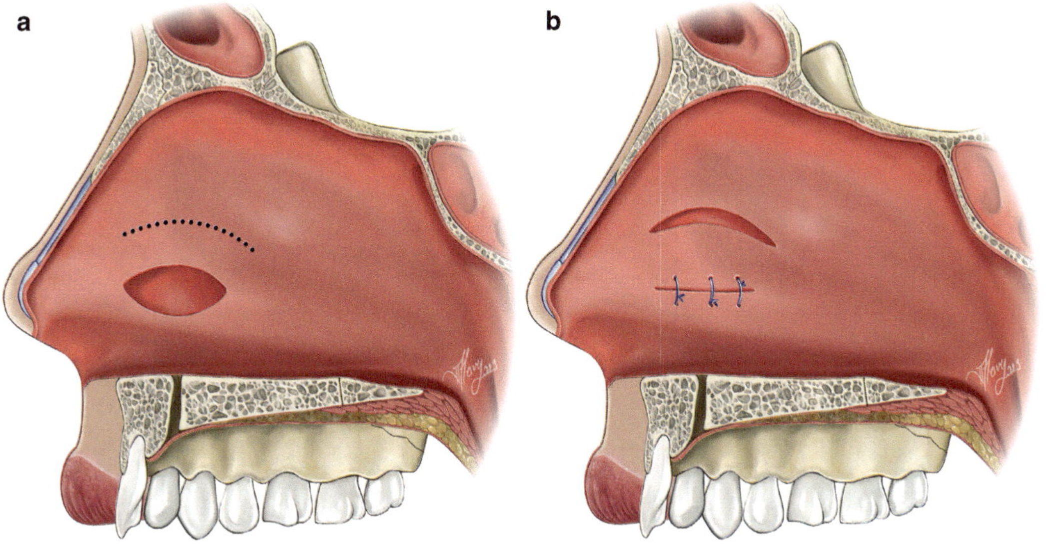

Fig. 14.1 In the case of a small perforation, an advancement flap can be used to close the perforation after a relieving incision 1 cm away from the perforation margin (**a**, **b**)

14.4.3 Inferior Turbinate Flap

Seiffert described closure by synechia formation with the inferior turbinate and a mucosal flap from the inferior turbinate to close the defect [12]. Friedman reported the successful utilization of a one-sided anteriorly based inferior turbinate flap [25] (Fig. 14.6a, b). An endoscopic closure of small or medium perforations was described using a rotation flap from the inferior turbinate and a cellular human dermal allograft (Alloderm, Life-Cell Corporation, Branchburg, NJ, USA) as an interposition graft. The major disadvantage of this flap is the need for a second stage [26].

14.4.4 Extensive Flaps

Seeley was one of the first to describe an extensive elevation and advancement of the endonasal mucosa in 1948 [27]. In 1980, Fairbanks reported bipedicled mucosal advancement flaps with temporalis fascia or pericranium as interpositional grafts, with a remarkable success of 95% in 20 patients [28]. He used an endonasal approach with full transfixion incisions. Goodman described the use of a similar technique to Fairbanks by an external rhinoplasty approach [29]. Kridel also reported that the external approach could facilitate wider exposure and easier access to the tissue planes for a tension-free closure by bipedicled flaps [30]. Romo introduced the midfacial degloving to gain access into the nose [31]. In order to get rid of flap deficiencies, especially to reconstruct big perforations, Romo reported the long-term nasal mucosal tissue expansion to increase the flap dimensions [32]. Hade et al. put importance on repairing the perforation by using differently designed bilateral intranasal flaps with nonopposing suture lines [33]. Similarly, Kridel [30] and Schultz-Coulon [34] made changes to the design of the bipedicled mucosal advancement flaps to prevent opposition of the suture lines (Fig. 14.7a–d).

Castelnuovo described the anterior ethmoidal artery septal flap, where the elevation of the flaps and the closure were all done endoscopically in anterior septal perforations with sizes of 10–25 mm, with success [35]. The posterior aspect of the perforation marks the anterior border of the superiorly based flap (Fig. 14.8a, b). The flap has been raised only on one side. Another

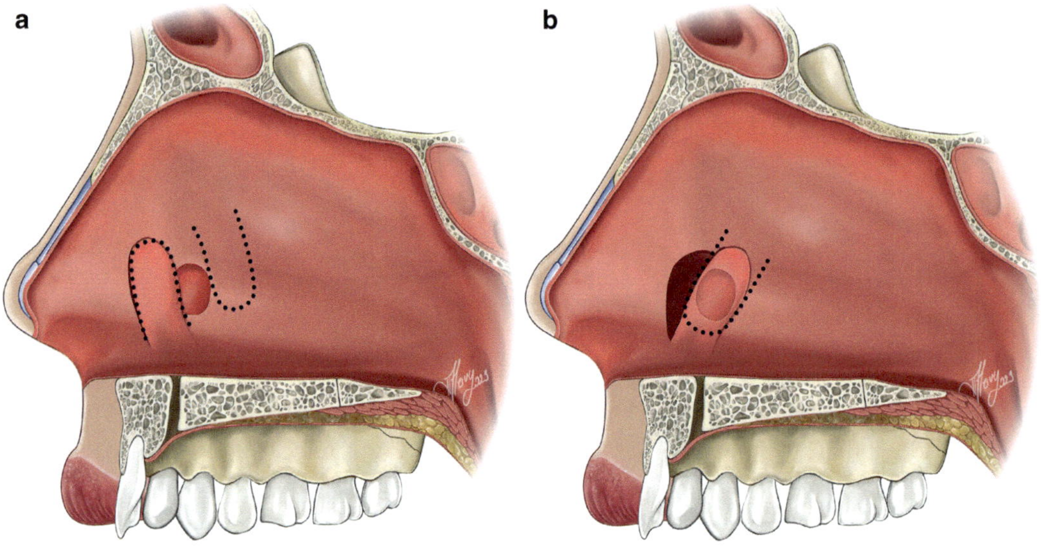

Fig. 14.2 Rotational flaps from both sides can be used to close a small defect

endoscopic method has been described by Morera et al. [36]. Bilateral mucosal flaps, posteriorly pedicled by the nasoseptal branch of the sphenopalatine artery, were used to close bigger septal perforations. Dissection on one side has gone into the subperichondrial/subperiosteal plane above the septal perforation, and on the other side, below the perforation. Each flap was covering above 50% of the septal perforation from opposite directions, with a small area of overlapping at the mid part (Fig. 14.9a–d). An interposition deep temporalis fascia graft has been used as an interpositional graft.

In recent years, Alobid et al. reflected their expertise in advanced endoscopic sinus surgery techniques in the management of septal perforations. The extended anterior ethmoidal artery flap is a modification of the flap described by Castelnuovo that allows the complete closure of perforations larger than 2 cm [37] . The greater palatine artery pedicled flap is based on the terminal branch of the greater palatine artery (Fig. 14.10). It is designed to repair anterior perforations smaller than 2 cm [38]. In fact, anterior perforations are always a big challenge for the surgeon, and this flap seems like a good solution to use without affecting the main steps of rhinoplasty. The nasal floor and inferior meatus flap is supplied by the inferior branch of the nasal septal artery. It can be used for repairing the perforations of the posterior portion of the nasal septum [39]. The lateral nasal wall pedicle flap can be used for perforations up to 3 cm. It can be used as anteriorly, receiving its blood supply from the anterior ethmoidal and facial arteries. The posteriorly based flap is nourished by branches of the posterolateral nasal artery. The major disadvantage is the necessity of a second stage to divide the pedicle [40]. The middle turbinate pedicle flap is supplied by lateral branches of the sphenopalatine artery and anterior ethmoidal artery [2]. The pericranial flap seems to me the impossible flap to apply as a rhinoplasty surgeon. It should be used only by rhinoplasty surgeons who have vast experience in advanced endoscopic skull base surgeries. It is indicated in cases of very large or total perforations and receives blood supply from deep branches of the supraorbital and supratrochlear arteries [41]. Alobid has already started coupling cross-steal flaps with extended anterior ethmoidal artery flaps or greater palatine artery flaps to create two-layer closures instead of one [2].

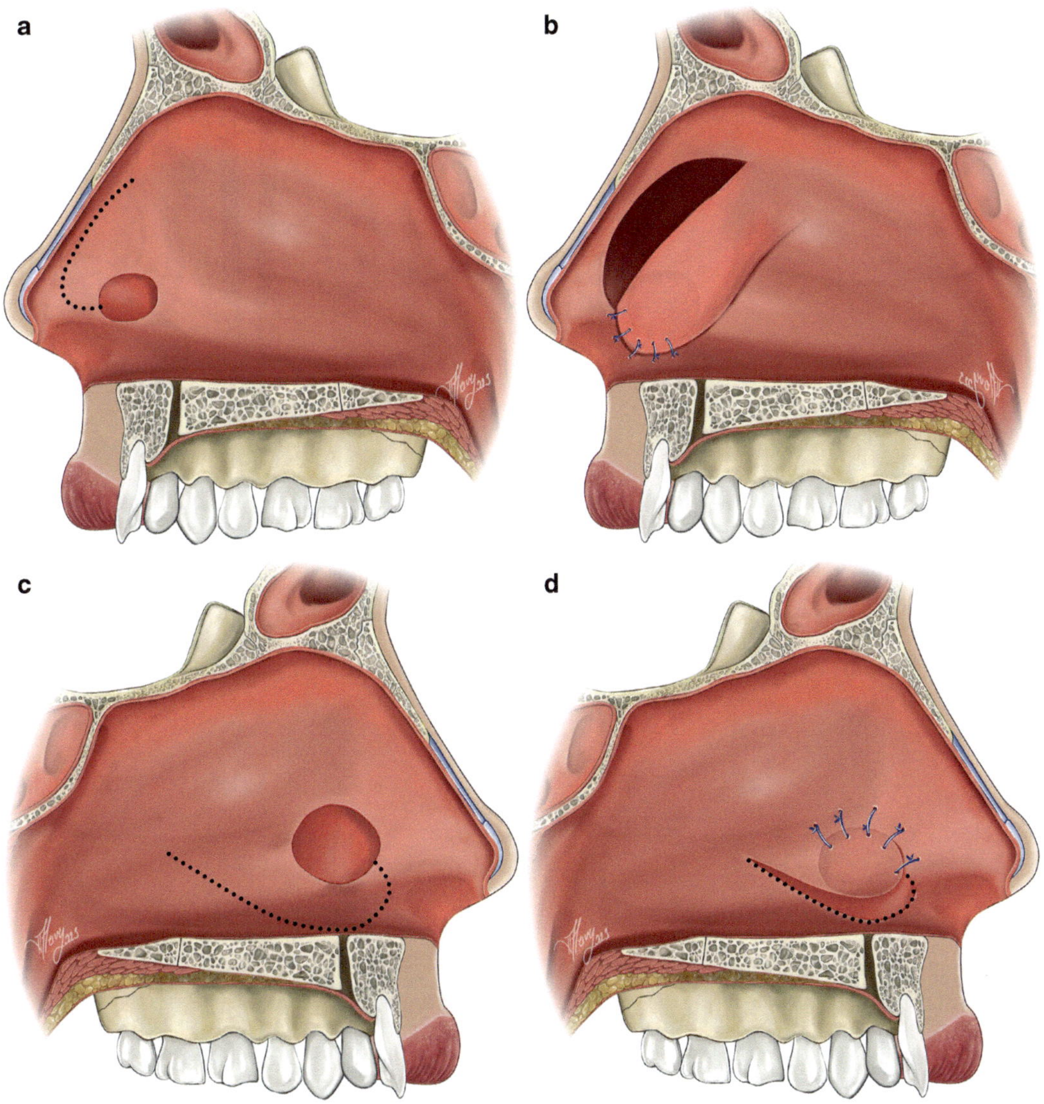

Fig. 14.3 Unilateral rotation flaps can be taken from the mucosa adjacent to the upper (**a**, **b**) or lower (**c**, **d**) part of the perforation in the case of a small perforation

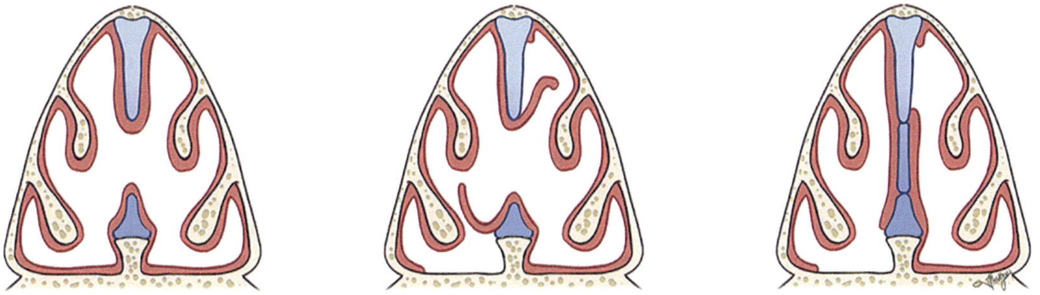

Fig. 14.4 Cross-stealing technique is an elegant technique. The perforation borders are kept as a hinge while elevating a flap from the contralateral side, one superiorly based and one inferiorly based

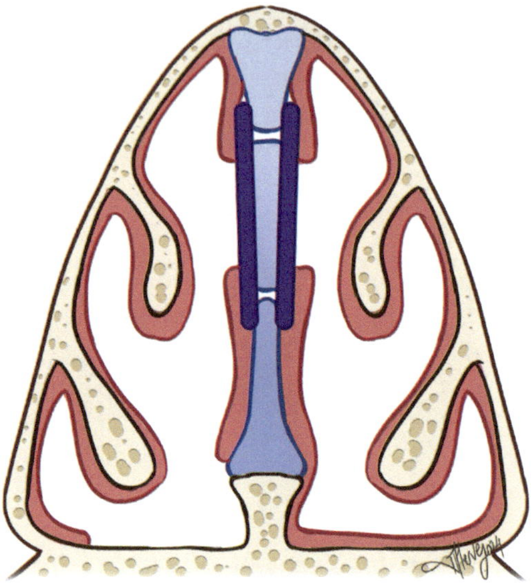

Fig. 14.5 Tragal cartilage with perichondrium on both sides can be used to cover a perforation like the butterfly-graft technique in tympanoplasty

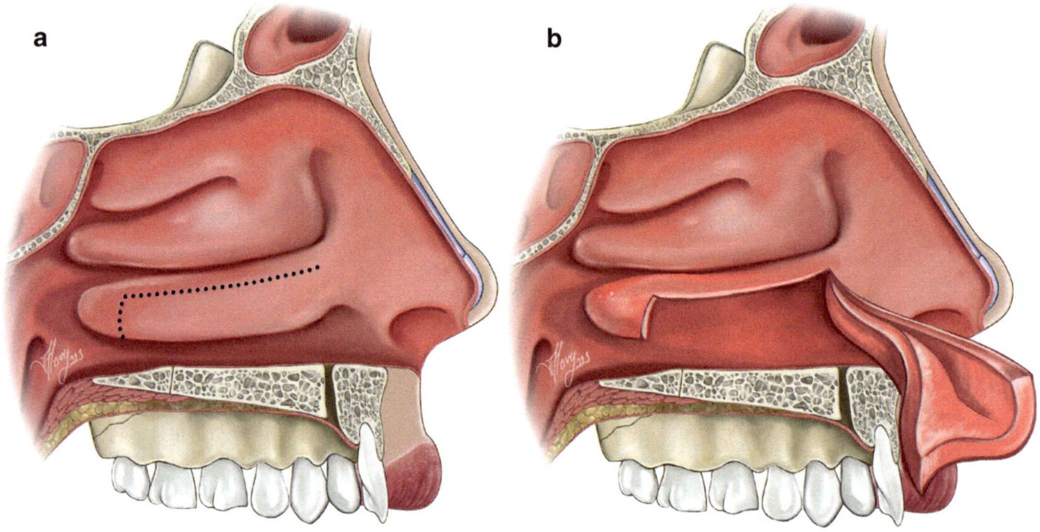

Fig. 14.6 An anteriorly based inferior turbinate flap can also be used to close small to medium-sized perforations (**a**, **b**)

14.4.5 Interpositional Grafts

Interpositional grafts are used to maximize the success of the closure. They can support one-sided flap deficiencies, flap dehiscences, and reduce the likelihood of reperforation [1].

A local cartilage graft can be used between the mucoperichondrial planes in small perforations when most of the septal cartilage is present. Fairbanks et al. stated that the long-term success of using temporalis fascia could be due to its low vascular requirement and its action as a framework for fibroblast growth [28]. Cartilage grafts from the septum, auricle, or rib have also been reported to be successfully used [34]. Toriumi reported that costal perichondrium was thicker and had a more robust fibrous structure than temporalis fascia, with a high affinity for vascular ingrowth [42].

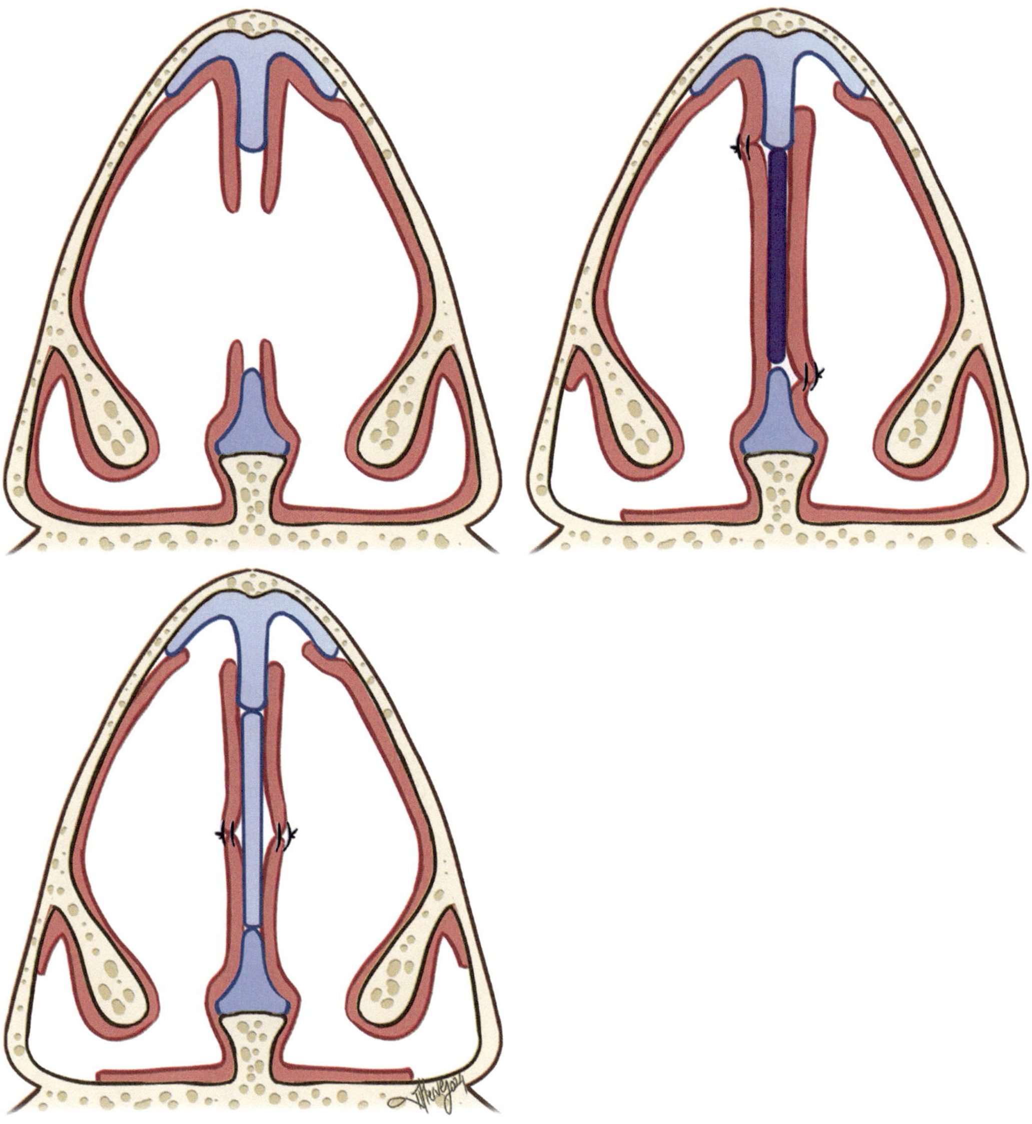

Fig. 14.7 Bipedicled mucosal advancement flaps can be designed in different ways depending on the situation and experience of the surgeon. They can both be advanced from below or above the perforation after making a relieving incision just under the inferior turbinate or at the upper part of the nose

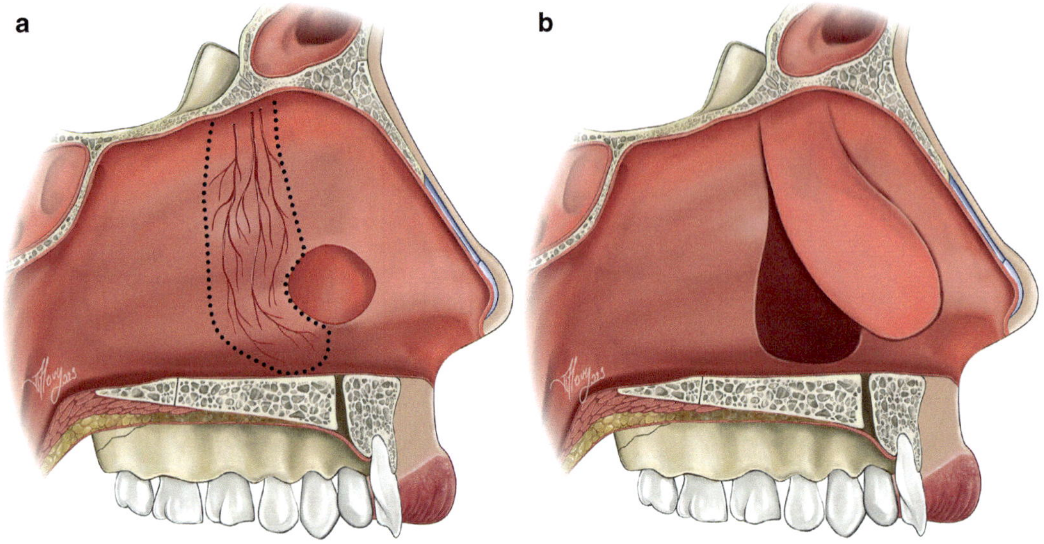

Fig. 14.8 A one-sided superiorly based flap nourished by the anterior ethmoid artery can also be used to close small- to medium-sized anterior perforations

The closure of septal perforation is a great challenge for the surgeon. The success is not only dependent on the technique but also on the experience of the surgeon. There are a lot of techniques, and it is impossible for a surgeon to try all. It should also be kept in mind that some of the techniques presented in this chapter require experience in endoscopic sinus and skull base surgery. Therefore, the surgeon should choose the technique depending on his experience or should refer these patients to more experienced colleagues.

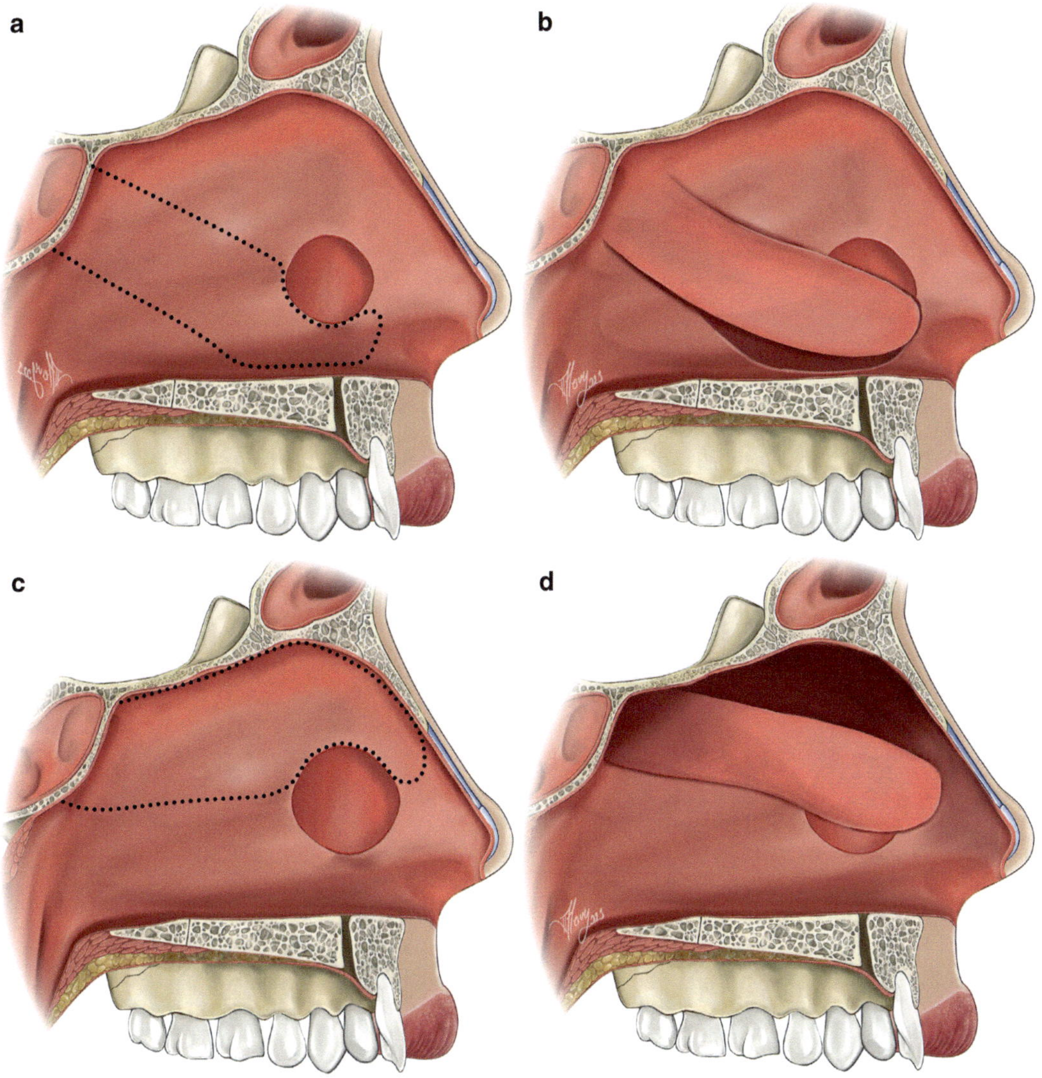

Fig. 14.9 Bilateral mucosal flaps posteriorly pedicled by the naso septal branch of the sphenopalatine artery can be used to close bigger septal perforations

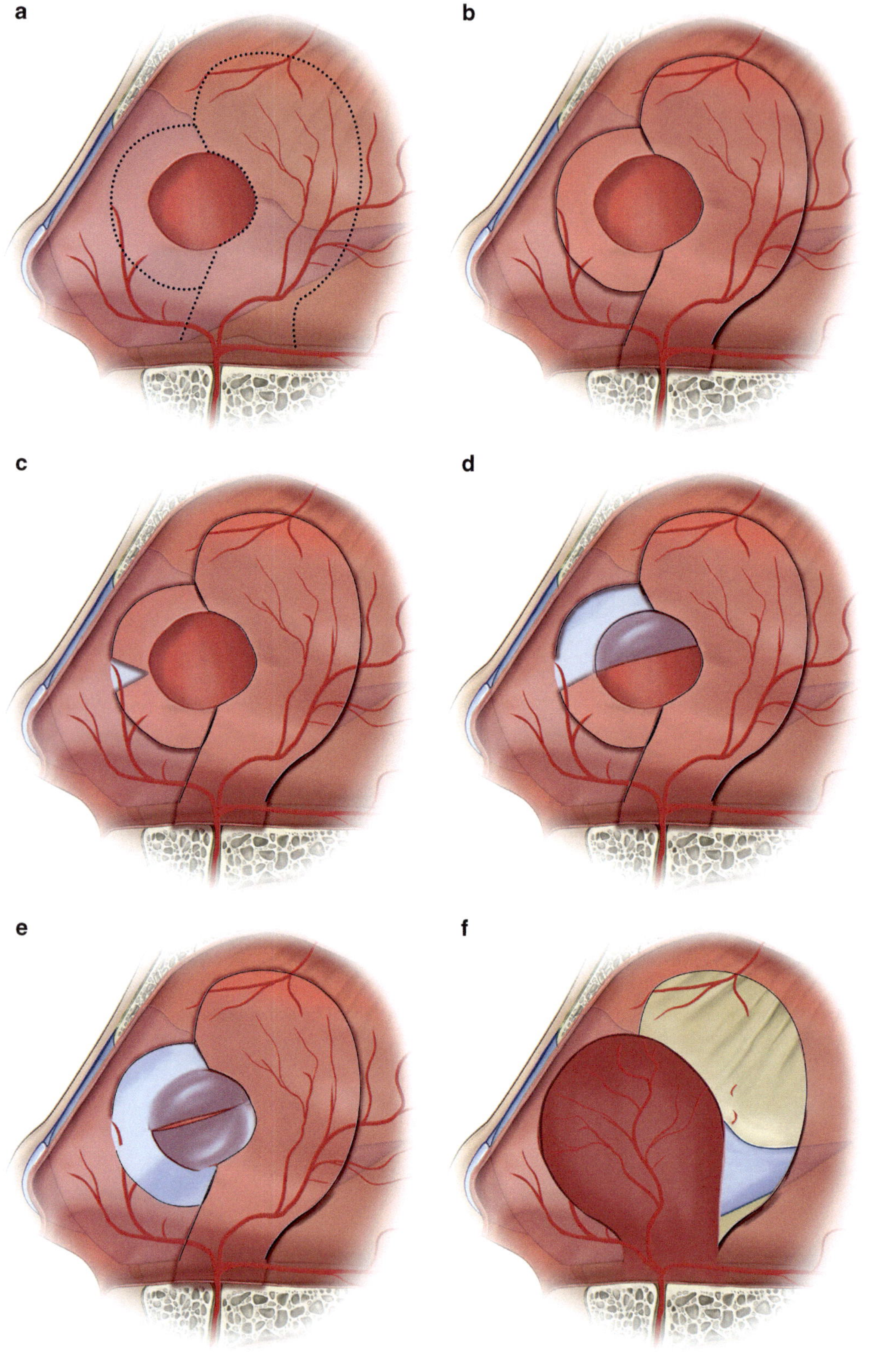

Fig. 14.10 Greater palatine artery pedicled flap is based on the terminal branch of the greater palatine artery and designed to repair anterior perforations smaller than 2 cm (**a**, **b**). The edges of the perforation can be cut 5–6 mm away from the perforation edges and can be used to close the contralateral defect as in the cross-stealing technique (**c**, **d**, **e**, **f**)

References

1. Kridel RW. Considerations in the etiology, treatment, and repair of septal perforations. Facial Plast Surg Clin North Am. 2004;12:435–50.
2. Garaycochea O, Santamaría-Gadea A, Alobid I. State-of-the-art: septal perforation repair. Curr Opin Otolaryngol Head Neck Surg. 2023;31:11–6.
3. Goh AY, Hussain SS. Different surgical treatments for nasal septal perforation and their outcomes. J Laryngol Otol. 2007;121:419–26.
4. Younger R, Blookmanis A. Nasal septal perforations. J Otolaryngol. 1985;14:126–31.
5. Cogswell LK, Goodacre TE. The management of nasoseptal perforation. Br J Plast Surg. 2000;53:117–20.
6. Teichgraeber JF, Russo RC. The management of septal perforations. Plast Reconstr Surg. 1993;91:229–35.
7. Tipton JB. Closure of large septal perforation with a local labiobuccal flap. Plast Reconstr Surg. 1970;46:514–5.
8. Ohlsén L. Closure of nasal septal perforation with a cutaneous flap and a peri-chondrocutaneous graft. Ann Plast Surg. 1988;21:276–88.
9. Santamaría-Gadea A, Mariño-Sánchez F, Arana-Fernández B, Mullol J, Alobid I. Innovative surgical techniques for nasal septal perforations: management and treatment. Curr Allergy Asthma Rep. 2021;5(21):17.
10. Beekhuis GJ, Eisenstein B. Repair of nasal septal perforation with a silicone button. Laryngoscope. 1977;87:635–7.
11. Stokken JK, Pallanch JF. The emerging role of 3-dimensional printing in rhinology. Otolaryngol Clin N Am. 2017;50:583–8.
12. Seiffert A. Die Operation an Nase, Mund und Hals. Leipzig: Barth; 1936. p. 146–8.
13. Schultz-Coulon HJ. Three-layer repair of nasoseptal defects. Otolaryngol Head Neck Surg. 2005;132:213–8.
14. Denecke HJ, Meyer R. Plastic surgery of the head and neck. In: Corrective and reconstructive rhinoplasty. New York: Springer Verlag; 1967. p. 137–40.
15. Converse JM. Corrective rhinoplasty. In: Converse JM, editor. Reconstructive plastic surgery. Toronto: WB Saunders Co.; 1977. p. 1150–2.
16. Mladina R, Heinzel B. "Cross-stealing" technique for septal perforation closure. Rhinology. 1995;33:174–6.
17. Levine LA. The closure of symptomatic septal perforation. Laryngoscope. 1980;90:1238–9.
18. Gerhardt HJ. Zum plastischen Verschluss von Septumperforationen. Laryngol Rhinol. 1968;47:392–5.
19. Heermann J. Behandlung grosser Septumperforationen mit Ohrmuschel-, Haut-, Knorpel-Hauttransplantaten, 2-Wochen-Tamponade, Hautabstanzung. Laryngol Rhinol. 1974;53:935–8.
20. McCollough EG. An approach to repair of septal perforations. ORL Digest. 1976;38:13.
21. Hussain A, Murthy R. Modified tragal cartilage temporoparietal and deep temporal fascia sandwich graft technique for repair of nasal septal perforations. J Laryngol Otol. 1997;111:435–7.
22. Chua DY, Tan HK. Repair of nasal septal perforations using auricular conchal cartilage graft in children: report on three cases and literature review. Int J Pediatr Otorhinolaryngol. 2006;70:1219–24.
23. Yenigun A, Meric A, Verim A, Ozucer B, Yasar H, Ozkul MH. Septal perforation repair: mucosal regeneration technique. Eur Arch Otorrinolaringol. 2012;269:2505–10.
24. Ozturan O, Yenigun A, Senturk E, et al. Endoscopic endonasal repair of septal perforation with interpositional auricular cartilage grafting via a mucosal regeneration technique. Otolaryngol Head Neck Surg. 2016;155:714–7.
25. Friedman M, Ibrahim H, Ramakrishnan V. Inferior turbinate flap for repair of nasal septal perforation. Laryngoscope. 2003;113:1425–8.
26. Ayshford CA, Shykhon M, Uppal HS, et al. Endoscopic repair of nasal septal perforation with acellular human dermal allograft and an inferior turbinate flap. Clin Otolaryngol Allied Sci. 2003;28:29–33.
27. Seeley RC. Repair of septal perforations. Laryngoscope. 1949;59:130–46.
28. Fairbanks DN. Closure of nasal septal perforations. Arch Otolaryngol. 1980;106:509–13.
29. Goodman WS, Strelzow VV. The surgical closure of nasoseptal perforations. Laryngoscope. 1982;92:121–4.
30. Kridel RW, Appling WD, Wright WK. Septal perforation closure utilizing the external septorhinoplasty approach. Arch Otolaryngol Head Neck Surg. 1986;112:168–72.
31. Romo T 3rd, Foster CA, Korovin GS, et al. Repair of nasal septal perforation utilizing the midface degloving technique. Arch Otolaryngol Head Neck Surg. 1988;114:739–2.
32. Romo T 3rd, Jablonski RD, Shapiro AL, et al. Long-term nasal mucosal tissue expansion use in repair of large nasoseptal perforations. Arch Otolaryngol Head Neck Surg. 1995;121:327–31.
33. André RF, Lohuis PJ, Vuyk HD. Nasal septum perforation repair using differently designed, bilateral intranasal flaps, with nonopposing suture lines. J Plast Reconstr Aesthet Surg. 2006;59:829–34.
34. Schultz-Coulon HJ. Experiences with the bridge-flap technique for the repair of large nasal septal perforations. Rhinology. 1994;32:25–33.
35. Castelnuovo P, Ferreli F, Khodaei I, et al. Anterior ethmoidal artery septal flap for the management of septal perforation. Arch Facial Plast Surg. 2011;13:411–4.
36. Morera Serna E, Ferrán de la Cierva L, Fernández MT, Canut SQ, Mesquida JA, Purriños FJG. Endoscopic closure of large septal perforations with bilateral Hadad-Bassagasteguy flaps. Eur Arch Otorrinolaringol. 2017;274:1521–5.

37. Santamaría-Gadea A, Langdon C, Alobid I. Extended anterior ethmoidal artery flap: novel endoscopic technique for large septal perforation. Laryngoscope. 2022;132:298–300.
38. Santamaría-Gadea A, Vaca M, de Los SG, Alobid I, Mariño-Sánchez F. Greater palatine artery pedicled flap for nasal septal perforation repair: radiological study and case series. Eur Arch Otorrinolaringol. 2021;278:2115–21.
39. Santamaria-Gadea A, Lopez-Chacon M, Langdon C, Van Gerven L, Valls-Mateus M, Bernal-Sprekelsen M, Alobid I. Modified nasal floor and inferior meatus flap for septal perforation repair. Extension and limits. Rhinology. 2018;56:386–92.
40. Alobid I, Mason E, Solares CA, Prevedello D, Enseñat J, De Notaris M, Prats-Galino A, Bernal-Sprekelsen M, Carrau R. Pedicled lateral nasal wall flap for the reconstruction of the nasal septum perforation. A radio-anatomical study. Rhinology. 2015;53:235–41.
41. Alobid I, Langdon C, López-Chacon M, Enseñat J, Carrau R, Bernal-Sprekelsen M, Santamaría A. Total septal perforation repair with a pericranial flap: radio-anatomical and clinical findings. Laryngoscope. 2018;128:1320–7.
42. Toriumi DM, Cappelle QM, Chung V. Use of costal perichondrium as an interpositional graft for septal perforation closure. JAMA Facial Plast Surg. 2017;19:121–7.

15 Surgery of the Nasal Valve

15.1 Introduction

Rhinoplasty is an operation that changes the form and function of the nose. Nasal obstruction can easily be caused by the surgeon in reduction rhinoplasty if an underlying problem is missed or new problems are created during rhinoplasty by the surgeon. It can be due to mucosal, skeletal, and cartilaginous abnormalities of the nose.

15.2 Definition and Anatomy

The human nose has a septal valve (nasal septum), a turbinal valve (inferior turbinates), an internal valve, and an external valve [1]. This was a statement that I heard from Eugene Kern almost 30 years ago, and I had the chance to experience how right he was until today. However, the rhinoplasty surgeon tends to think that there are two valves in the nose: the external and internal valves. The internal valve area is surrounded by the caudal septum, the caudal end of the upper lateral cartilages (ULCs), the head of the inferior turbinate, and the remaining tissues surrounding the pyriform aperture (Fig. 15.1). The external valve is the area around the lateral crura, starting from the nasal entrance to the internal valve, including the alar rim and nasal floor [2] (Fig. 15.2).

© The Author(s), under exclusive license to Springer Nature Switzerland AG 2025

F. Apaydın, *Septal Surgery Challenges in Rhinoplasty*,
https://doi.org/10.1007/978-3-031-74734-2_15

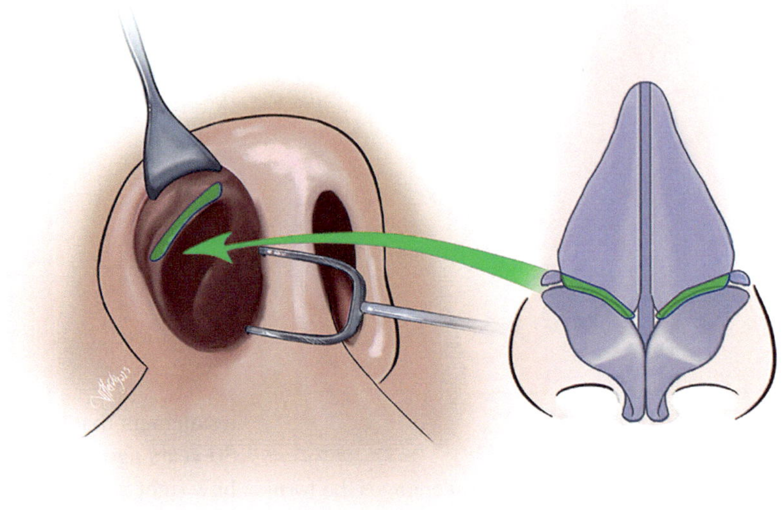

Fig. 15.1 The internal valve area is surrounded by the caudal septum, the caudal end of the upper lateral cartilages (ULCs), the head of the inferior turbinate, and the floor of the nasal cavity

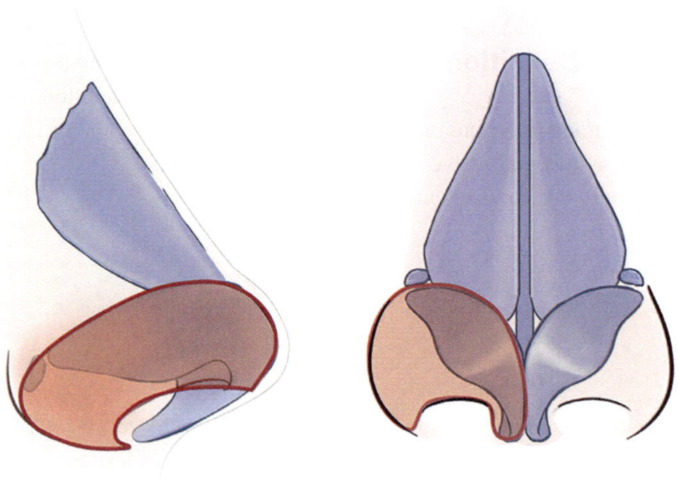

Fig. 15.2 The external valve is the area around the lateral crura, starting from the nasal entrance to the internal valve, including the alar rim and nasal floor

15.3 Management of the Internal Nasal Valve Problems

The internal nasal valve is accepted as a regulator of airflow and resistance, and it is the most flexible and narrowest portion of the nasal airway [1]. The problems causing nasal obstruction can be due to the anatomic structures composing the internal nasal valve (Fig. 15.3). The details of examination and pathologies that can be seen in this region are written in Chap. 4 (Fig. 15.4). There are many surgical techniques to solve these problems, and the most important ones are listed in detail in this chapter.

15.3.1 Spreader Grafts

These grafts are detailed in Chap. 10. Some surgeons claim that spreader grafts are not useful in widening or opening the internal valve during meetings. I have experienced in my cases over the last 25 years that when spreader grafts are used thick enough to splint and widen the valve area alone or together with spreader flaps, they work well. This fact was reflected in the patient-reported outcome measures of my patients [3].

There are two main points that the surgeon should know about the usage of spreader grafts for the internal nasal valve: (1) They work best to widen the internal nasal valve when the middle vault is intact, and the spreader grafts are popped in the tight pocket opened under the middle vault (Fig. 15.5). (2) They should be thick enough to spread and widen the internal nasal valve angle. The optimum thickness should be 1.5–2 mm. If it is thicker, it can cause widening of the middle vault and the tip (Fig. 15.6).

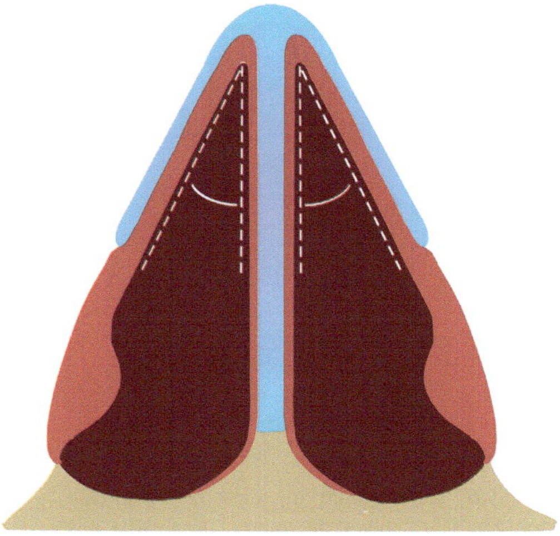

Fig. 15.3 Internal nasal valve angle is 10–15° in Caucasians

15.3.2 Spreader Flaps

Spreader flaps were first reported by Fomon in 1950 to correct a collapsed ala [4]. Then the first reports on these flaps appeared again in the 1990s [5, 6]. Since then, the popularity of these flaps has been increasing. I started using these flaps in 2010 and was very impressed with their versatility in reduction rhinoplasty. They have become my workhorse for middle vault reconstruction and for keeping the internal nasal valve open in primary reduction rhinoplasties.

I have already published a classification of my own for spreader flaps [7]. I recently revisited this classification after using it on many patients. In this classification, there are six types: the first three only as spreader flaps, and the latter three as a combination of spreader flaps and grafts.

Type 1: Suturing of ULCs to the septum after hump removal (Fig. 15.7). This type is used in cases where there is a limited hump of 1–2 mm at the key area that does not reach the lower half of the middle vault. In these cases, the mucoperichondrium of the nasal septum and the lower portion of the upper lateral cartilages are not dissected. After elevating the perichondro-periosteal flap (PPF), the surgeon can see a groove in the midline and shoulders laterally, causing the hump and dorsal widening at the keystone area [8]. The first action should be to remove the bony hump using the Piezotome. The shoulders on both sides of the midline groove become more prominent after bony hump removal. A limited resection of these prominent shoulders can solve the whole problem in these patients. In cases where there is a need for a 2–3 mm reduction, incremental resection of the nasal septum at the keystone

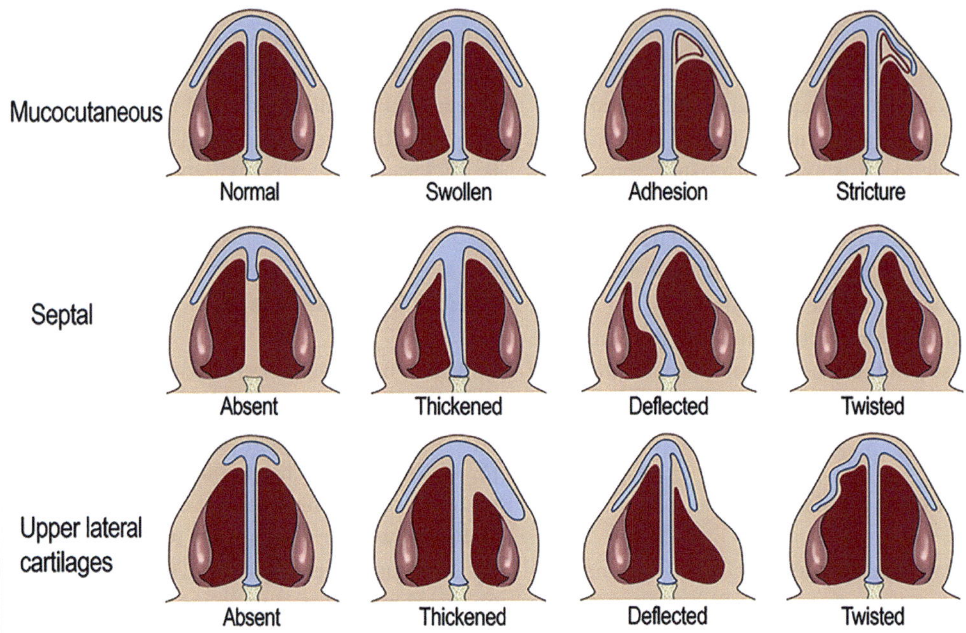

Fig. 15.4 Pathologies of the internal nasal valve are depicted in this illustration. The nasal valve can be narrowed or obstructed due to mucocutaneous, septal and upper lateral cartilage pathologies

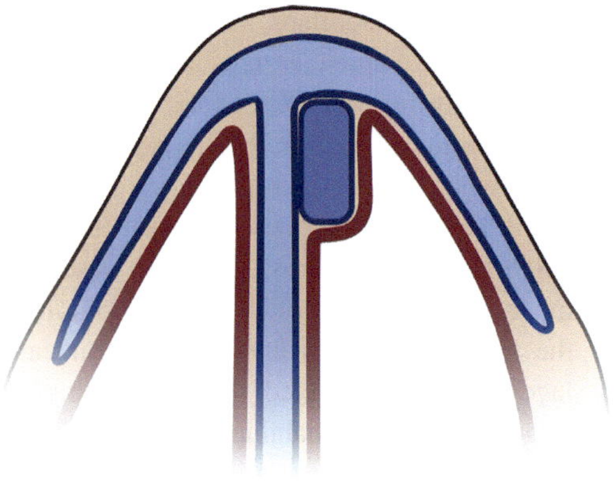

Fig. 15.5 The spreader grafts work best when the middle vault is intact, and the spreader grafts are popped in the tight pocket opened under the middle vault

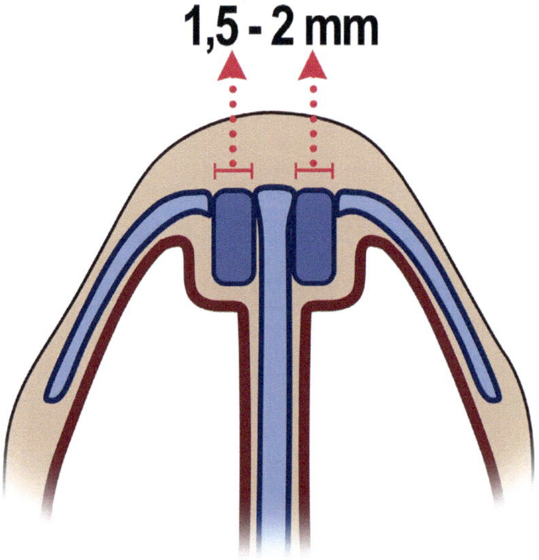

Fig. 15.6 The optimum thickness of the spreader graft should be 1.5–2 mm at the internal nasal valve angle

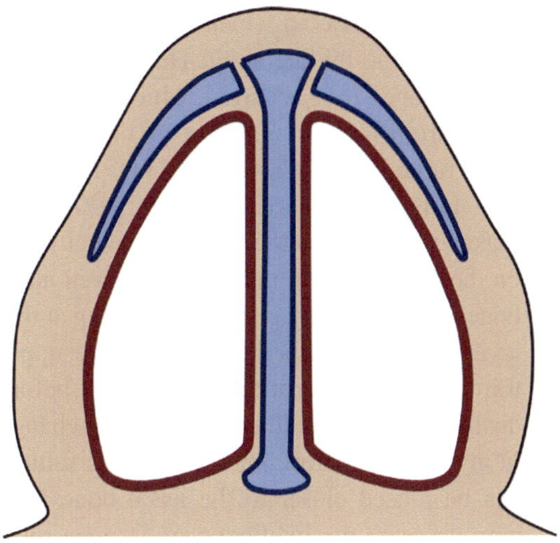

Fig. 15.7 Type 1 spreader flaps

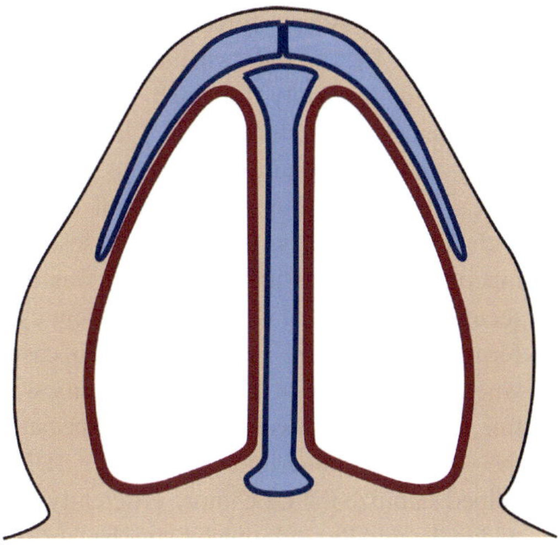

Fig. 15.8 Type 2 spreader flaps

area to remove the hump should be performed. In these cases, the mucoperichondrium under the cartilaginous vault is intact. At the end of these refinements, the ULCs should be sutured to the nasal septum, but in some cases, this is not necessary because the intact mucoperichondrium acts like a suture holding the nasal septum and the ULCs together and like a soft tissue spreader.

I also found that when a 1–3 mm hump is resected, especially at the keystone area, the nasal septum shows a thicker portion. Cottle described this situation in 1958 in his article and proposed the term "processus lateral dorsales" [9]. Recently, it was named as "septal T" by Robotti [10]. This thicker portion of the nasal septum prevents collapse of the middle vault when using type 1 spreader flaps.

Type 2: Suturing of the ULCs over the septum after septal hump removal (Fig. 15.8): I find this technique very elegant and anatomical in cases with a slight hump of 1–2 mm and no need for narrowing the bony vault. After rasping the bony hump, a very limited excision of the ULCs medially with some septal cartilage is performed. The internal valve is not disturbed. Then, the medial edges of the ULCs are simply sutured together, slightly narrowing the cephalic part of the middle vault. In addition, the nasal septum and the intact mucoperichondrium under the sutured ULC act as a fulcrum to keep the middle vault in the desired shape [11].

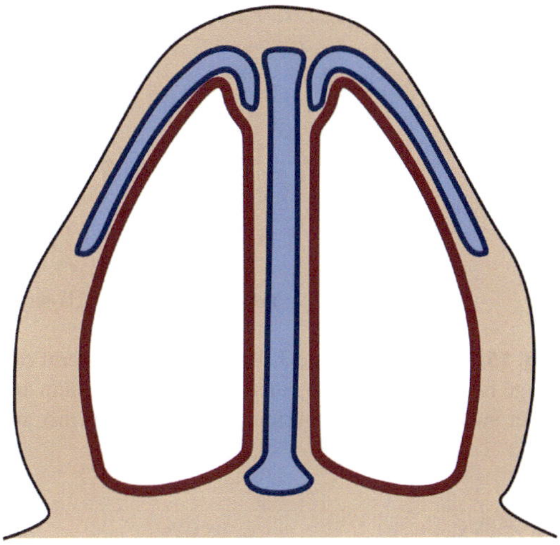

Fig. 15.9 Type 3 spreader flaps

Type 3: Turn-in spreader flaps (Fig. 15.9): This is the most traditional flap design described for spreader flaps [4, 5, 12, 13]. In my daily practice, I have been using this type for big humps. After hump removal, the use of turn-in spreader flaps is very efficient in reconstructing the normal anatomy of the middle vault. When I started using these flaps in 2010, this flap was the only technique I used. In earlier cases, Brown–Adson forceps were used to turn in the ULCs, and two mattress sutures were used separately for each side, which were then sutured to the septum. I later started using straight mosquito forceps to turn the ULCs in and fix them on the nasal septum with longer needles. In earlier cases, the mucoperichondrium under the ULC was dissected away from the cartilage to prevent cyst formation under the sutured ULC. In cases where the ULC was thick enough, this was fine, but later, this was used less often because the mucoperichondrium under the ULC helped stabilize the ULC more efficiently and widen the middle vault much better because of the double-layer existence of mucoperichondrium under the ULCs (Fig. 15.10). For some years, I was against making an incision on the turned-in ULC in order not to lose the spring effect of the ULC to widen the internal nasal valve and the middle vault. However, in one case, an open roof occurred, which seemed to result from the spring effect of the cephalically turned-in ULCs (Fig. 15.11). I learned two things from this case: (1) it is better to make an incision on the ULC cephalically and on the ULC, staying under the removed nasal bones to remove any possible widening at this level, and (2) finish the work on the upper third, that is, perform the osteotomies before dealing with the middle third. By this change in my surgical algorithm, the cephalic sutures can be placed closer to the nasal bones and help decrease the likelihood of an open roof, giving more stability to the caudal edge of the bony pyramid. Moreover, I started using partial small incisions on the ULCs to reshape the middle vault more precisely and to relieve

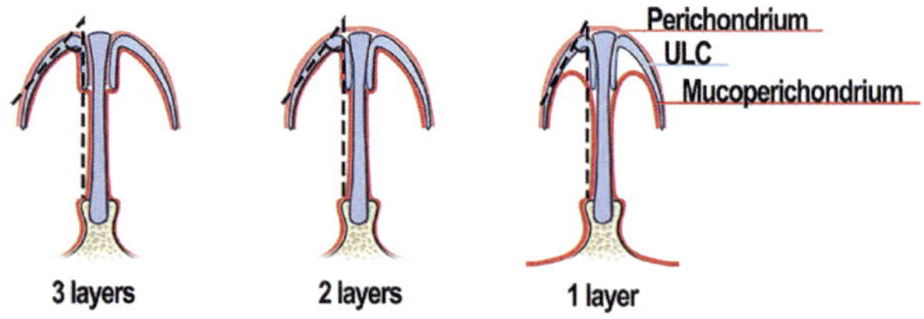

Fig. 15.10 Layers of type 3. When the upper lateral cartilage is turned in with the outer intact perichondrium and inner intact mucoperichondrium, it stays much firmer and stronger, and the valve angle becomes wider. The valve angle becomes the narrowest when both layers are dissected away from the upper lateral cartilage

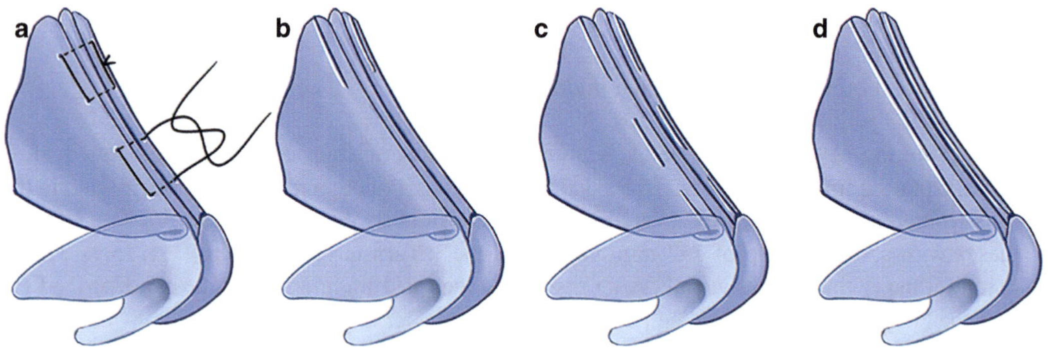

Fig. 15.11 Subtypes of type 3 spreader flap. In subtype (**a**), the upper lateral cartilage is simply turned in and the folded medial portions are sutured to the upper margin of the nasal septum. In subtype (**b**), a relieving incision is performed at the keystone area to break the resiliency of the cartilage, so the folded upper lateral cartilage will not create an open roof. In rare cases, multiple relieving partial incisions can be done on the ULCs to create the dorsal aesthetic lines (**c**). In subtype (**d**), a longitudinal cut is done along the upper lateral cartilage to prevent wide dorsum

excessive tension on the middle vault, which proved to be very valuable in some selected cases. After reading publications mentioning that incising ULCs vertically throughout their lengths did not cause internal valve stenosis, I started using this technique, especially in the endonasal approach, which seemed to be easier and work well [14] (Fig. 15.11). The elevation of the perichondro-periosteal flap before dividing the ULCs from the nasal septum has also been routinely used in recent years [8].

Type 4: Suturing of ULCs to the septum and over the spreader grafts (Fig. 15.12): I started using this technique in crooked noses approximately 15 years ago when there was a need to splint the dorsal segment of the cartilaginous septum and not to widen the middle vault. In addition, the spreader grafts act as a fulcrum to avoid inferomedial collapse of the ULCs. The thickness of the spreader grafts can be modified, helping to reshape the middle third and maintain the brow-tip esthetic lines [15]. This type has recently been one of my favorite techniques for rebuilding the middle vault in cases of crooked noses. In addition, I can still use spreader grafts under the intact middle third for splinting the existing deviations and splinting the caudal septal extension grafts.

Type 5: Suturing of ULCs over the septum and spreader grafts (Fig. 15.13). I started using this technique first when I needed an augmentation of 1–2 mm at the middle third. As in the previous technique, the spreader grafts act as a fulcrum to prevent the inferomedial collapse of the ULCs. When the edges are properly aligned in the midline by sutures, it is much easier to obtain a straight and smooth profile on the middle third [11].

Type 6: Turn-in flaps sutured to the spreader grafts (Fig. 15.14). According to my experience, this is the most powerful technique for widening the middle third and internal nasal

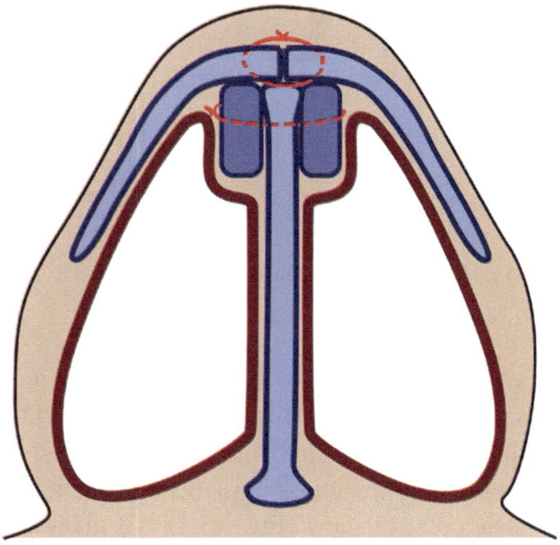

Fig. 15.13 Type 5 spreader flaps

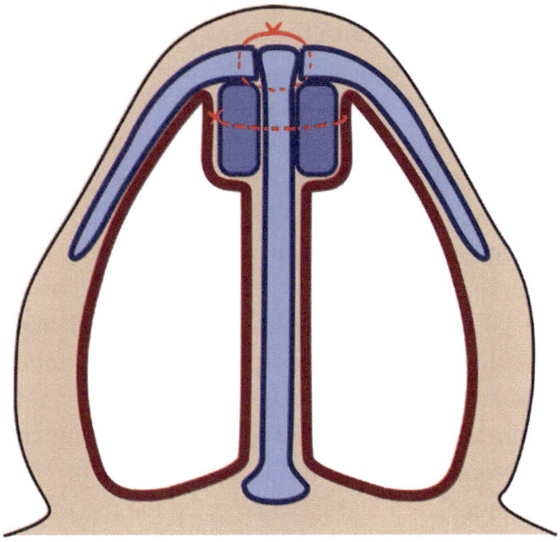

Fig. 15.12 Type 4 spreader flaps

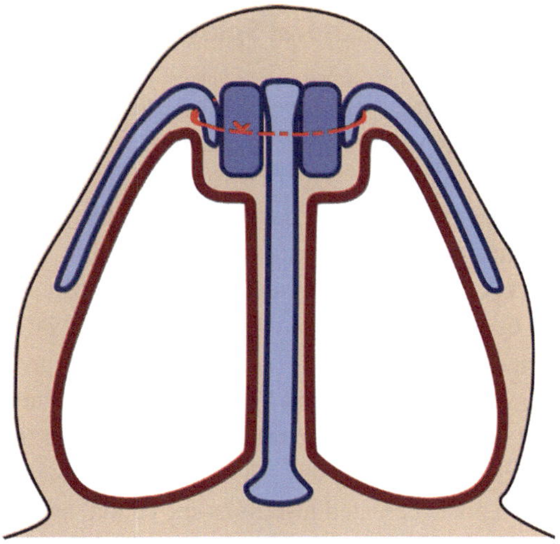

Fig. 15.14 Type 6 spreader flaps

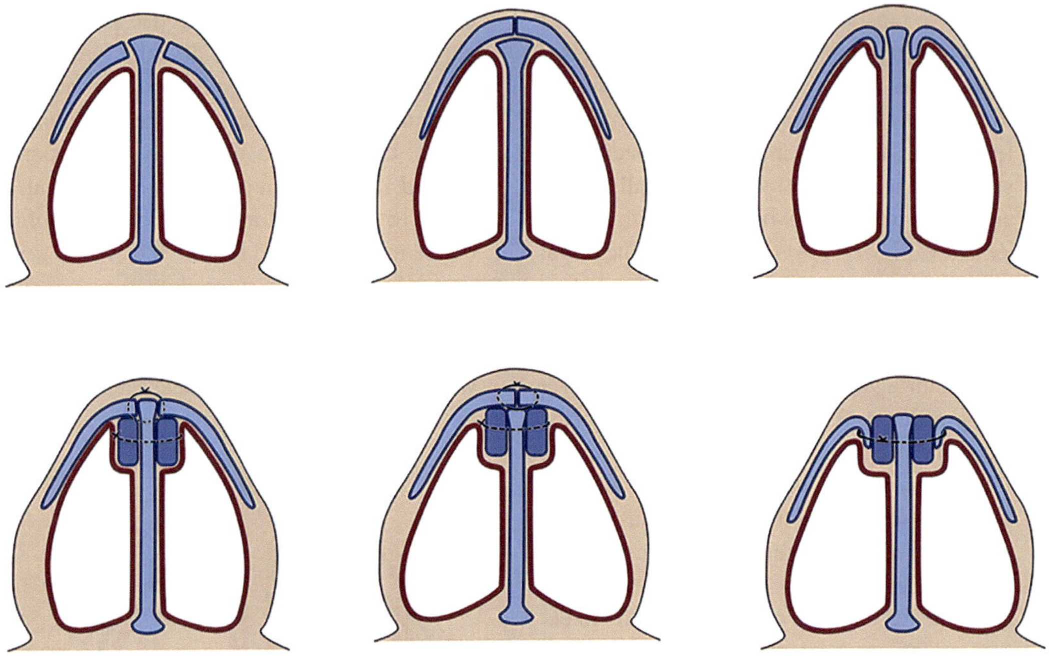

Fig. 15.15 Apaydin classification of spreader flaps

valve in very narrow noses. Therefore, it is seldom used except for a very narrow middle third that requires maximum widening [7].

This is a very practical classification from my standpoint of view (Fig. 15.15). It gives the surgeon all the solutions for middle vault reconstruction.

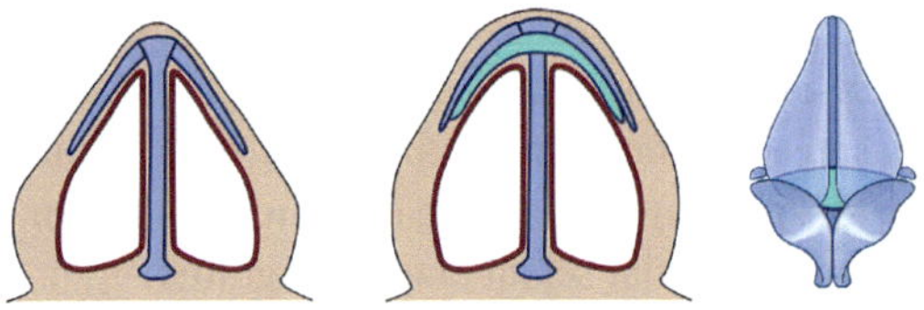

Fig. 15.16 Upper lateral splay graft

15.3.3 Upper Lateral Splay Graft

Middle vault collapse can be the result of the surgical reduction of the nasal dorsum. This is usually caused by the loss of structural integrity or support of the ULCs. Overresection of the dorsal septum, excessive resection of the ULCs, full-thickness mucocartilaginous transection of each ULC, and mucosal scarring with internal valve synechia are the main reasons [16]. Guyuron reported that the natural "T" of the upper lateral and septal cartilages could be achieved using the upper lateral splay graft [17]. This graft is inserted into a pocket created just under the caudal half of the ULCs (Fig. 15.16). The use of conchal cartilage is more desirable because of its shape and spring effect, which can provide the necessary splay action. Islam et al. used a modified splay graft technique in 11 patients [18]. They opened a window in the septal cartilage just under the caudal end of the ULCs without detaching them from the nasal septum. The graft was prepared according to the need and was passed through the window in a way that the perichondrium would be at the top and placed in pockets opened under the ULCs. With this modification, they claimed that the use of the endonasal approach, limited dissection plane, septal cartilage with perichondrium on one side, and no need for suturing created some additional advantages over the original technique. Sen and Iscen reported the use of two layers of sutured convex cartilages obtained from alar cartilage resection as a spring graft [19].

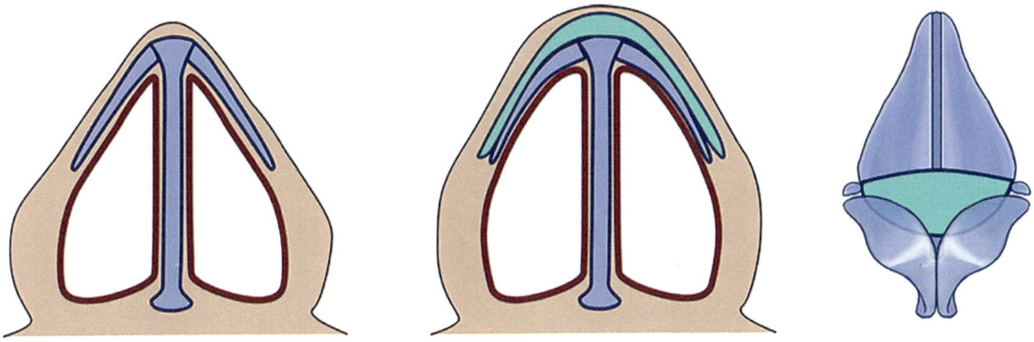

Fig. 15.17 Butterfly graft

15.3.4 Butterfly Graft

Clark and Cook reported the use of a conchal cartilage "butterfly" graft in 72 secondary rhinoplasty patients with a minimum of 2 years of follow-up [20]. They preferred to use the ascending portion of the conchal bowl as the optimal site because of its smooth curvature. Most grafts are approximately 2.5 cm in length by 1.2 cm in width in men and 2.2 cm in length by 0.9 cm in width in women. This graft is placed using either a closed or open approach. The butterfly graft is placed symmetrically over the nasal dorsum with the central "V-shaped portion pointing caudally (Fig. 15.17). The graft is then secured with a 5-0 PDS (Ethicon Inc., Somerville, NJ) suture laterally on each side. The Titanium Breathe-Implant (Heinz Kurz GmbH, Dusslingen, Germany) was designed like a butterfly graft to stabilize the internal nasal valve by Wengen [21].

15.3.5 Flaring Sutures

Flaring sutures have been reported by Park to widen the nasal valve angle [22]. After a 4-0 PDS mattress suture is placed from the caudal/lateral border of one ULC, across the nasal dorsum, and through the contralateral ULC, its tightening pulls the ULCs laterally, opening the nasal valve angle. It has also been shown that these sutures can be more effective with the use of spreader grafts [23] (Fig. 15.18).

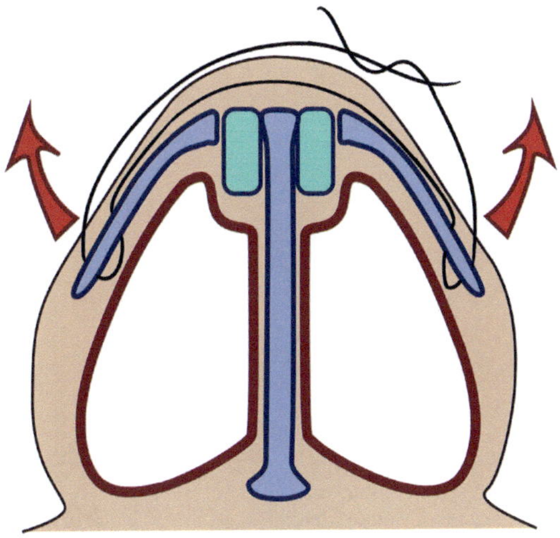

Fig. 15.18 Flaring sutures

15.3.6 M-Plasty

After the intercartilaginous incision, the caudal aspect of the ULC is freed from the skin dorsally and from the mucosa ventrally. A 2–3-mm section of the caudal end of the ULC is resected horizontally, and an additional medial triangle of the ULC can be removed submucosally after detachment from the septum. After the excess mucosa is trimmed, the incision is closed, leaving an "M" shape or linear line [1] (Fig. 15.19a, b).

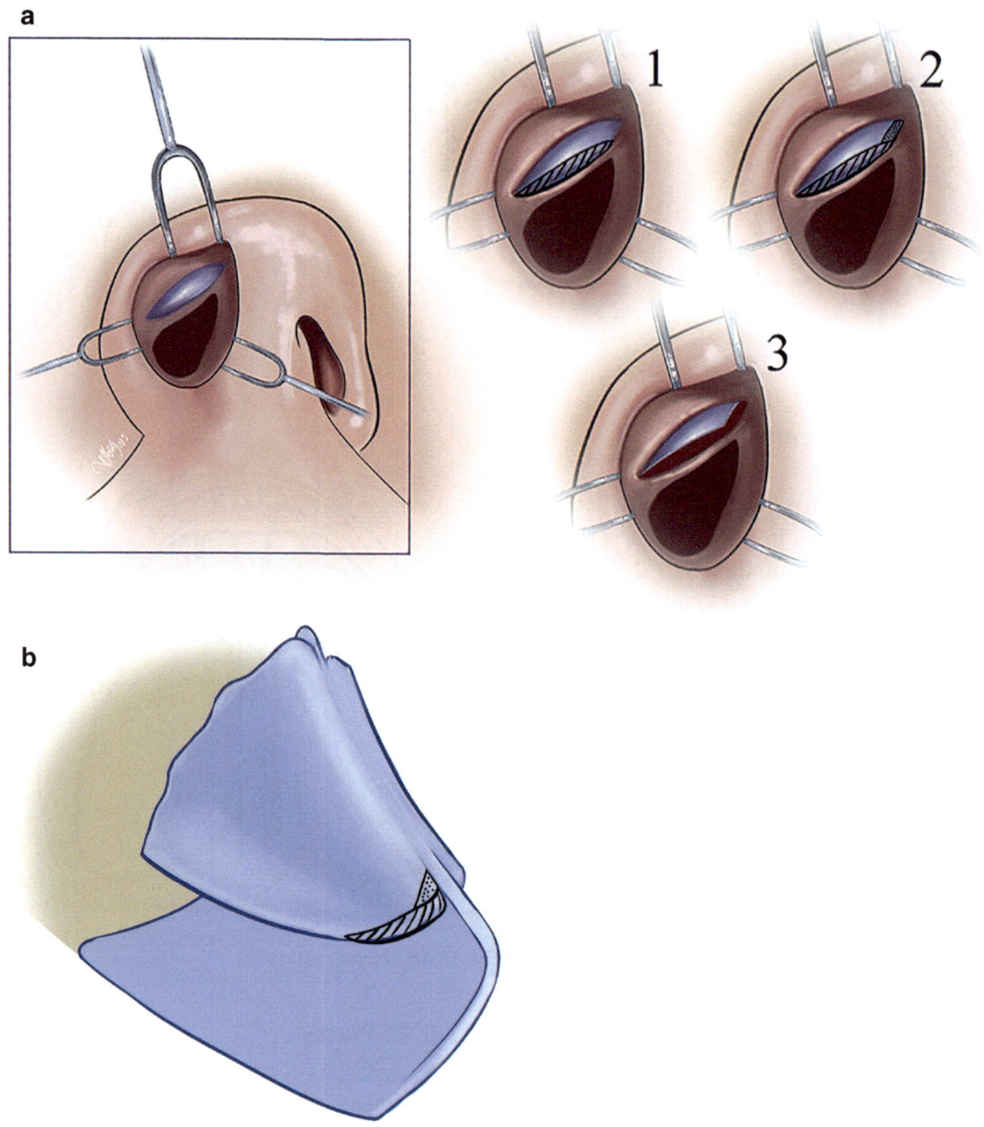

Fig. 15.19 M-plasty, the caudal portion of the upper lateral cartilage is resected to widen the internal valve angle (**a**, **b**)

15.3.7 Z-Plasty

Intranasal Z-plasty can be used to lateralize and lengthen the scroll region, especially in revision cases [24] (Fig. 15.20a–g). Besides, the internal nasal valve angle can be opened.

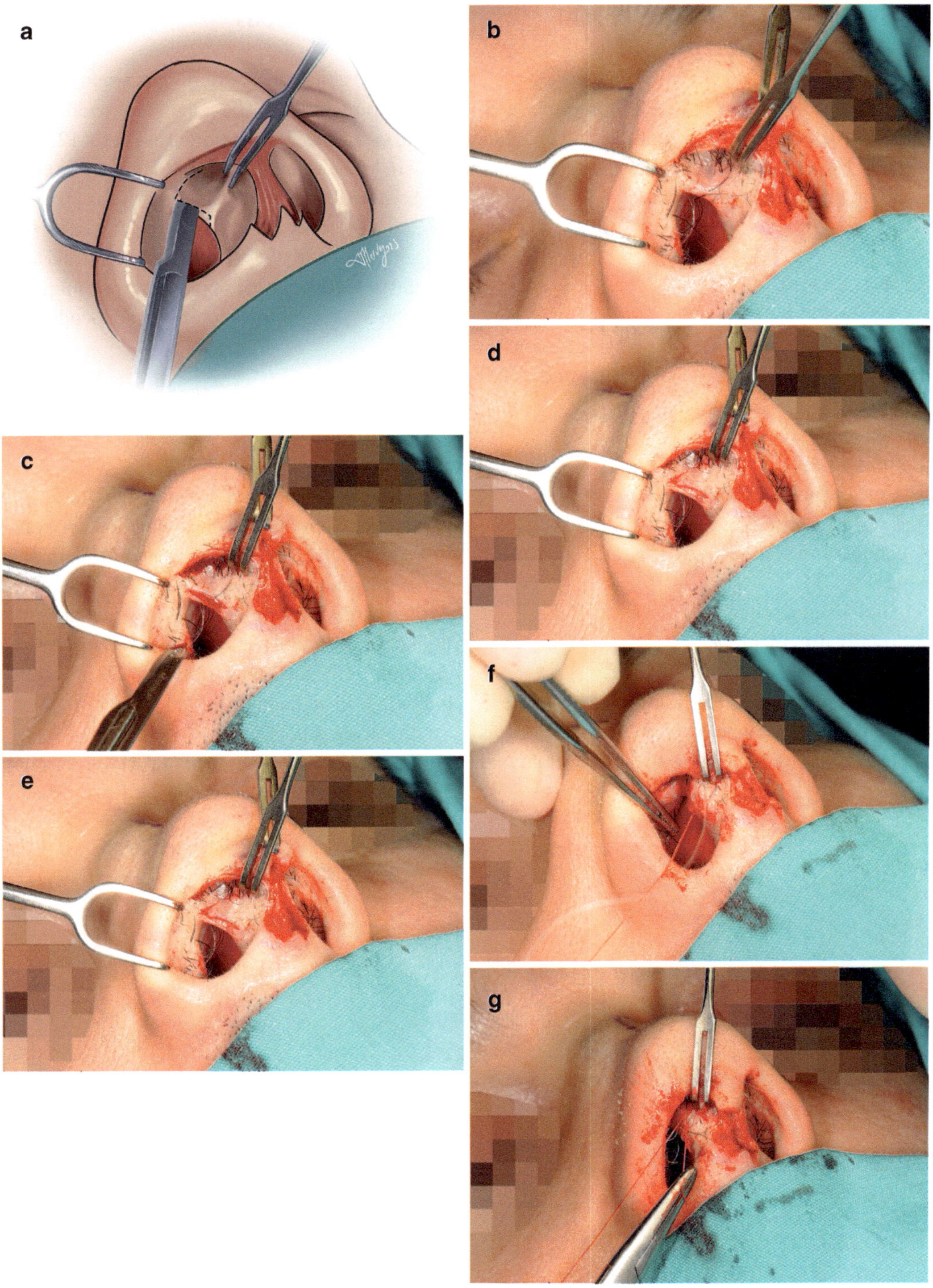

Fig. 15.20 Z-plasty can be very helpful in widening the airway at the internal valve area (**a**–**g**)

15.4 Management of External Valve Problems

The lateral crura are the most important anatomic structure for the external valve. They should be evaluated for shape, dimensions, strength, orientation, and axis.

15.4.1 Shape

Zelnik has described the following variations in the form of the lateral crus in his study [25] (Fig. 15.21):

1. Smooth convex (10%)
2. Convex medial, concave lateral (30%)
3. Concave medial, convex lateral (25%)
4. Concave medial, convex central, concave lateral (25%)
5. Smooth concave (25%)
6. Totally irregular (5%)

It is very clear from this study, which is quite in harmony with my clinical experience, that there is not one recipe for the management of lateral crura in rhinoplasty.

15.4.2 Dimensions

The dimensions are very important when it comes to reshaping the ala. The length and width of the lateral crura have been reported as 23.1 × 12.8 mm [25] in Caucasians, 17.9 × 10 mm in Koreans [26], 18 × 12 mm in African-Americans [16], and 15.2 × 10.4 mm in Black South-Africans [27] (Fig. 15.22). With these data in mind, the surgeon should select the most appropriate technique to reshape or support the lateral crura depending on ethnicity.

15.4.3 Cartilage Strength

The strength of the lateral crura is an underrated parameter. They should be meticulously examined by palpation and functional examination before any surgery and continue to be examined during surgery as well. It is proportional to the thickness of the lateral crus. It was measured as 0.5 mm in Caucasians [28] and Asians [29], 0.88–0.96 in Indians [30], and 0.9 mm in Black South Africans [27].

The weakness of the cartilage or overresection are two main reasons for alar collapse. That is

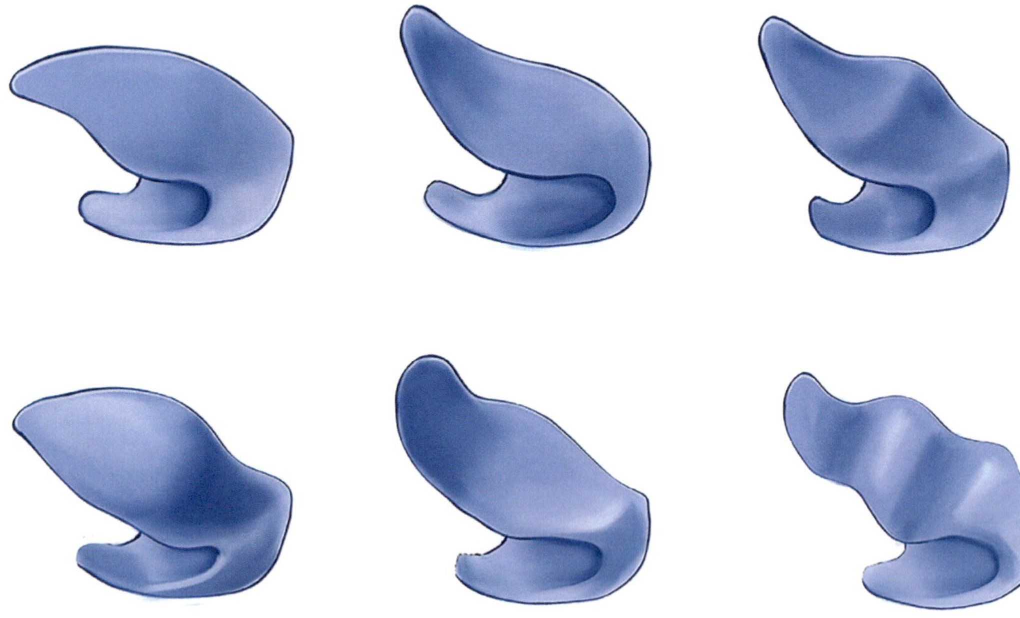

Fig. 15.21 Six different shapes of lateral crus as described by Zelnik. The figures are placed from left to right starting from above. (1) Smooth convex; (2) convex medial, concave lateral; (3) concave medial, convex lateral; (4) concave medial, convex central, concave lateral; (5) smooth concave; (6) totally irregular

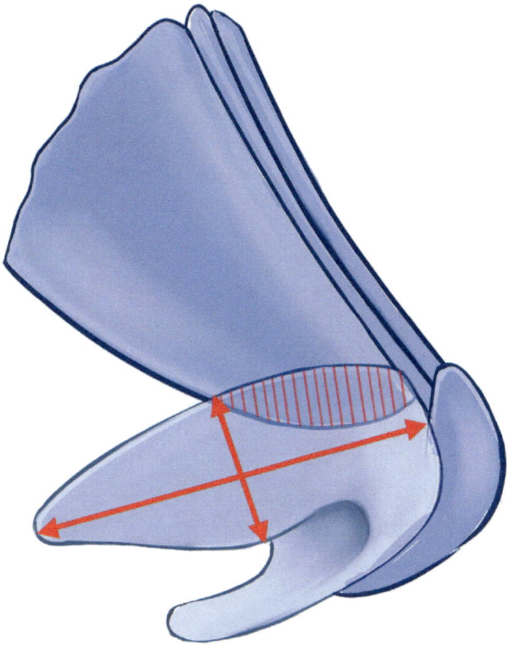

Fig. 15.22 The horizontal and vertical dimensions of the lateral crura should be evaluated thoroughly during rhinoplasty. The surgeon should always keep in mind that they are the main supporting structures of the external valve

why preoperative functional examination during quiet breathing is very important to diagnose the strength of the lateral crus.

Subperichondrial dissection of the lower lateral cartilages has been popular recently as part of the preservation rhinoplasty concept [31]. Having tried this technique in some cases, I experienced that the cartilage strength decreased so much that it was very difficult to manipulate the lateral crura, pass sutures through them, and reshape them due to increased fragility.

When the lateral crura are weak, it is better to choose a reinforcement method such as flaps or grafts instead of solely sutures.

15.4.4 Orientation

The orientation of the lateral crus is defined by the transverse axis lateral to the dome. If it is toward the lateral canthus of the ipsilateral eye, it is called an orthotopic lateral crus. However, if it runs toward the ipsilateral medial canthus, it is called malpositioned. It was first described by Sheen as malpositioned or parenthesis tip [32]. Toriumi published that, especially in a bulbous nasal tip, if the transverse axis of the lateral crus is 30° from the midline, it is called cephalic malposition [33] (Fig. 15.23a–c).

15.4.5 Axis

Toriumi suggested that the most esthetic appearance could be obtained when the caudal border was higher than the cephalic border [33]. This concept has been quite popular in recent years, and the tendency among prominent surgeons is to create this condition, including myself. While creating this position, the anatomic situation of the scroll area is also critical. There are many variations in the scroll area (Fig. 15.24). Therefore, the surgeon cannot handle this area with the same technique all the time.

15.4.6 Surgical Procedures

15.4.6.1 Lateral Crural Dissection and Repositioning

This method can be applied in two different ways [34]. The lateral crura can be inwardly concave with a pinched appearance. In this case, they are dissected free from the surrounding soft tissues, cut just lateral to the dome, reversed, and sutured back to their beds again. Therefore, the concavity turns out to be convex (Fig. 15.25a). A modification of this technique is to suture the resected lateral crura contralaterally (Fig. 15.25b).

In a situation where the lateral crura are cephalically oriented, they can be freed from the investing soft tissues and repositioned in more anatomically desirable beds. The detached lateral crura can be supported by lateral crural strut grafts to guarantee support and a better shape [34].

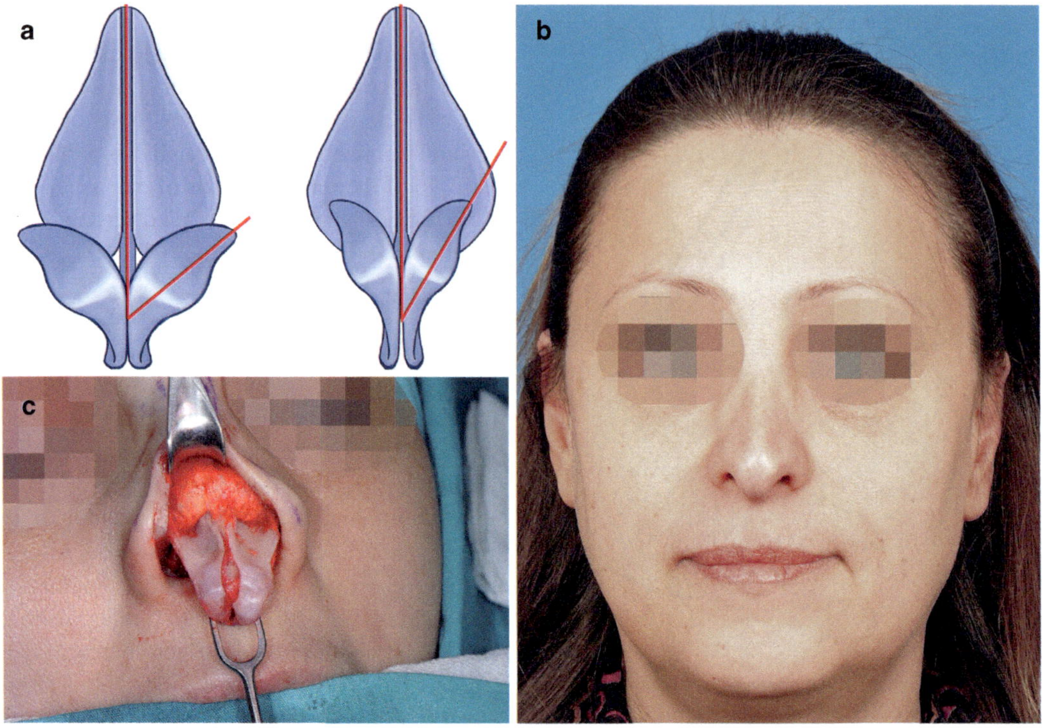

Fig. 15.23 Orthotopic lateral crura are toward the lateral canthi, and their transverse axis is higher than 30° from the midline. Malpositioned lateral crura are toward the medial canthi and less than 30° from the midline (**a**). Frontal view (**b**) and intraoperative view (**c**) of a patient with malpositioned lateral crura

Fig. 15.24 Scroll area and its variations

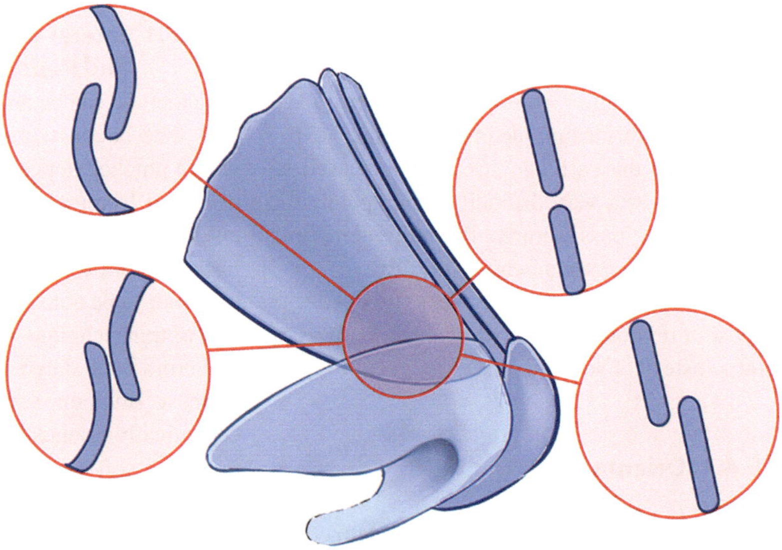

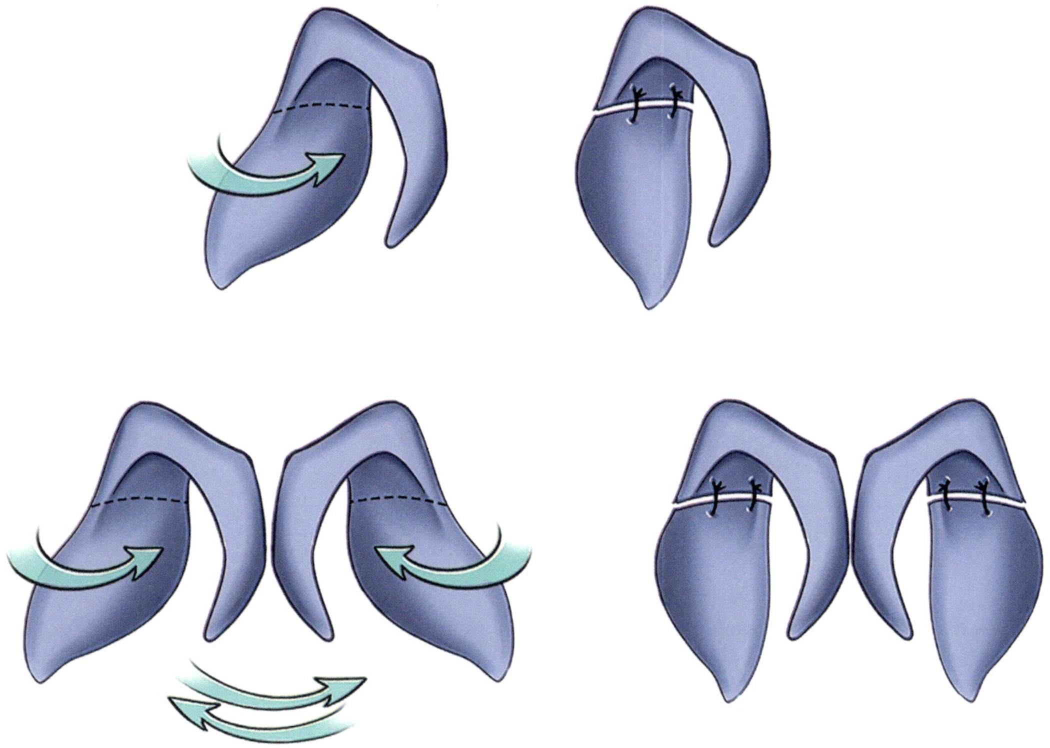

Fig. 15.25 Lateral crural dissection and repositioning. When the lateral crura are concave, they can be dissected free from the underlying mucosa, resected 2–3 mm lateral to the dome, flipped horizontally, and then sutured near the ipsilateral or contralateral dome

15.4.6.2 Lateral Crural Strut Grafts

These grafts are described by Gunter and are usually placed via an open rhinoplasty approach [35]. After a cephalic trim of the lateral crura is performed, the vestibular skin is undermined from above, keeping it adhered to the lateral crura at the caudal border. Sometimes, I perform dissection from the caudal margin and keep the vestibular skin adhered cephalically. In most revision cases and in some primary cases, my preference is to completely release the lateral crura. The linear axis of the pocket should be designed for maximum support of the lateral crura (Fig. 15.26). These grafts are usually obtained from the nasal septum and are 3–4 mm in width and 15–25 mm in length. They are placed into the pockets under the lateral crura and fixed in place using PDS mattress sutures. In cases of malpositioned lateral crura, alar retraction, and severe cases of alar collapse, a longer strut going beyond the pyriform aperture is indicated. There are two options regarding the length of these grafts. In these situations, I try to keep the length of these grafts at 30–35 mm to place the lateral portion of these grafts on the pyriform aperture. Therefore, the external valve is very strongly supported. Gunter reported using them for reshaping, repositioning, or reconstructing the lateral crura [35].

15.4.6.3 Alar Battens

Alar batten grafts are curvilinear cartilage grafts that are placed into a precise pocket at the point of maximal lateral wall collapse or supra-alar pinching [36]. The use of alar battens has been reported for the correction of both internal and external nasal valve collapse (Fig. 15.27). They were described as 10–15 mm in length and 4–8 mm in width. It was also noted that larger grafts could be used in patients with severe collapse or thicker skin [37]. My preference is usu-

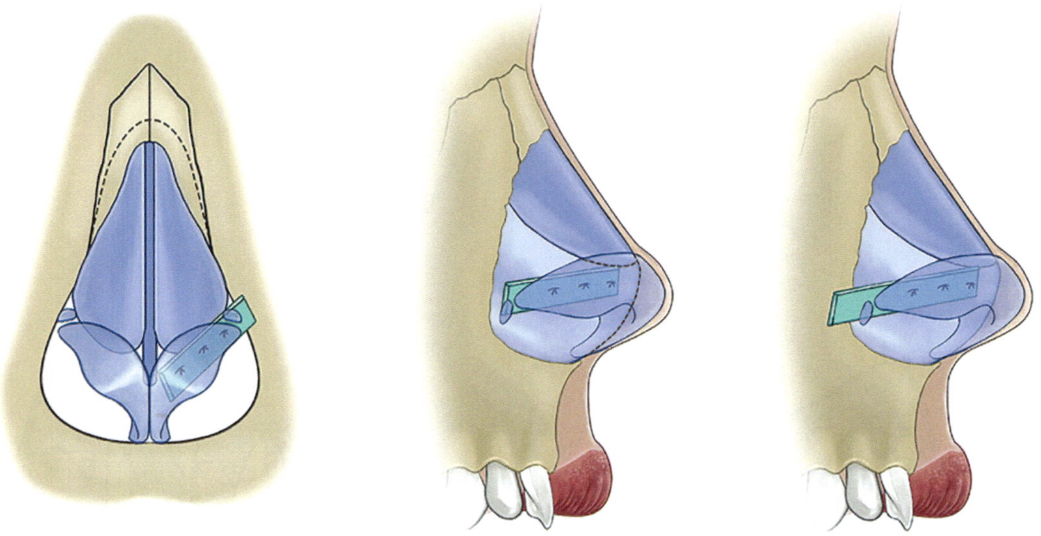

Fig. 15.26 Lateral crural strut grafts. These grafts are placed under the lateral crura, either short to cover throughout the lateral crus or longer, reaching over the piriform aperture. They were described to be used for reshaping, repositioning, or reconstructing the lateral crura

ally to use larger grafts placed in a tight pocket whose tail usually exceeds the pyriform aperture. Regardless of the approach, I also prefer suturing them to the lateral crura for fixation. When these grafts are used for the external valve, which is usually the case on many occasions, they are usually placed on and under the lateral half or two-thirds of the lateral crura. I do not prefer to use them for internal valve problems because the skin is thinner, and patients can suffer from the bulk of the grafts in the long term.

15.4.6.4 Lateral Crural Flaps

15.4.6.4.1 Lateral Crural Turn-in Flap

Tellioglu and Cimen used turn-in folding of the cephalic portion of the lateral crus to support the alar rim [38]. Murakami et al. have also reported the same technique to reinforce the alar cartilage after cephalic trimming [39].

I started using this method with some modifications in 2008 after reading the article by Tellioğlu and Cimen. Starting with the first case, I modified the original description [40]. Instead of cutting and turning in the medial two-thirds of the lateral crura, a partial linear cut was made along the horizontal axis of the lateral crus, leaving a 7-mm caudal segment (Fig. 15.28a). This method aimed to support the lateral crus on all parts and to have a splinting effect throughout the remaining lateral crus. It worked well in dealing with concave lateral crura when the lateral crura were thick and strong enough to counter opposing forces applied to each other obtained by turning in and suturing in a sandwich fashion. However, when the lateral crura were weak, it solely acted as an additional support to the remaining cartilage. After the sixth case, I made one more modification to simultaneously support both external and internal valves. After injecting 1:1 diluted 1% lidocaine with 1:100,000 adrenaline under the lateral crus for hydrodissection, a pocket was created under the lateral crus cephalically, starting near the dome (Fig. 15.28c–j). While opening this pocket along the lateral crus, a 2-mm caudal part was not detached, and the scroll area was not disturbed (i.e., the caudal part of the ULC stayed attached to the cephalic lateral half of the lateral crus). When the partially cut cephalic segment was turned into the pocket, a double layer of cartilage was created by suturing three 5-0 PDS mattress sutures (the first one close

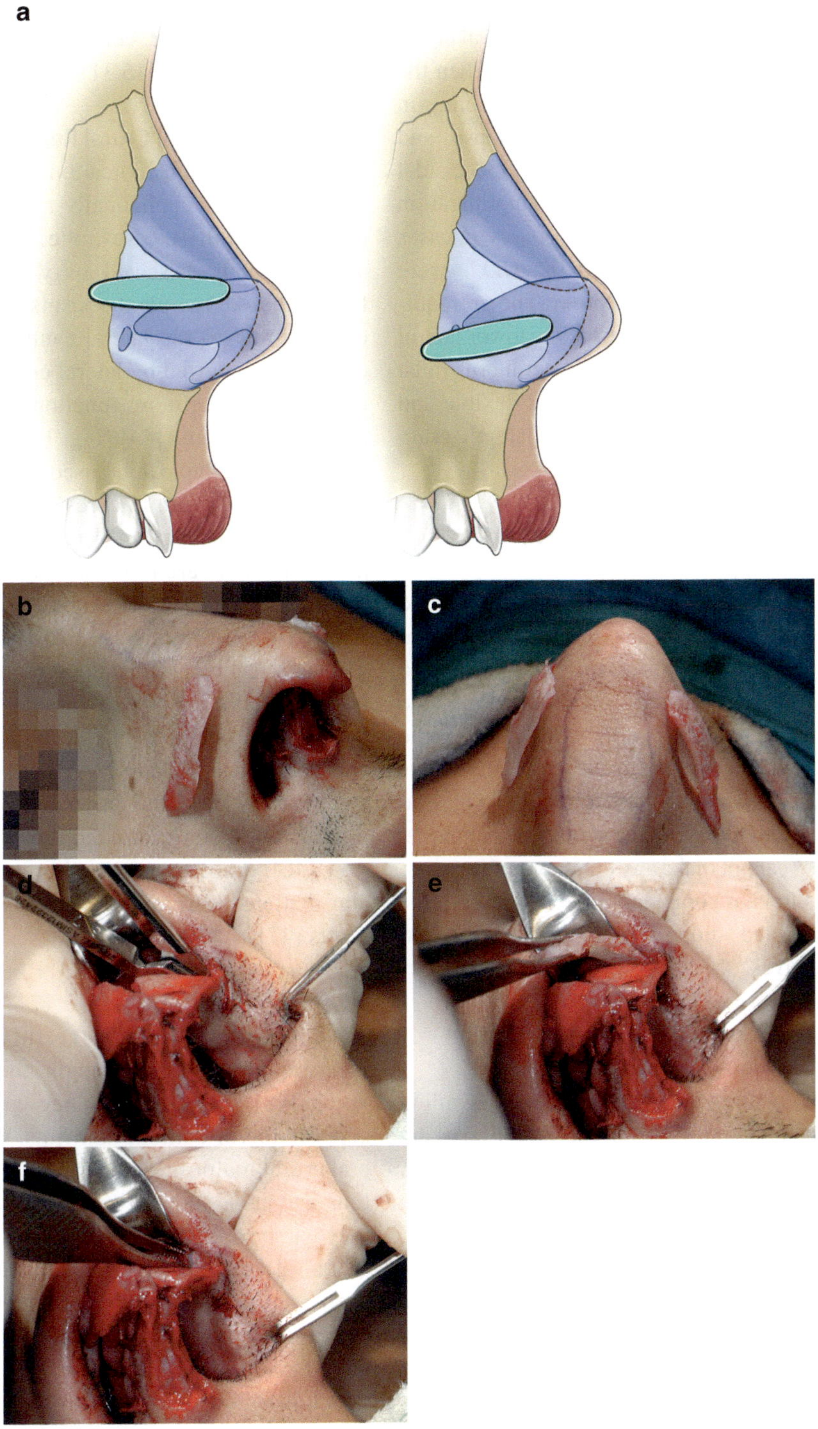

Fig. 15.27 Alar batten grafts: Alar batten grafts are curvilinear cartilage grafts that are placed into a precise pocket at the point of maximal lateral wall collapse or supra-alar pinching, either through an endonasal or external approach. If positioned above the lateral crura, they are used to support the internal nasal valve (**a**). If the position is below the lateral crura, they support the external valve (**a**). They are usually carved from septal cartilage and they are usually used to support external valve (**b**, **c**). A precise pocket is opened by using scissors (**d**) and the graft is inserted in this precise pocket (**e**) and then sutured to secure its place (**f**)

to the dome, the second one at the midline, and the third one to the lateral part of the lateral crus), leaving the knot on the lateral surface. When the scroll area was left undisturbed, this turning-in and suturing prevented inward collapse and sometimes helped lateral pull-up of the caudal part of the ULCs (Fig. 15.28k). This modification was found to be very helpful, especially in cases where a hump was taken and the ULCs were freed away from the nasal septum. The prerequisite is to have a complete strip of the lower lateral cartilages, and the height of the lateral crus must be at least 12 mm. This flap is very flexible and can be used in all shapes of lateral crura (Fig. 15.28l).

15.4.6.4.2 Sliding Alar Cartilage (SAC) Flap

In this technique, the cephalic trim is performed in the usual manner by leaving a 6-mm lateral crus in place. The trimmed cartilage is inserted into the pocket created after dissecting the mucosa under the lateral crus while keeping the scroll attachment intact (Fig. 15.29). This flap is then sutured to support the lateral crus [41]. I do not have enough experience with this technique; therefore, I cannot make any comments. However, it appears to be a good technique to preserve the scroll area and support both the internal and external valves.

15.4.6.4.3 Superior-Based Transposition Flap

After the cephalic trim, the trimmed part is pulled downward and sutured over the lateral crus by preserving the scroll attachment [42] (Fig. 15.30). This technique looks like an elegant technique that supports the internal and external valves. However, I do not have any experience to make detailed comments. This flap seems to be the most powerful for rotating the lateral crus on a horizontal axis, bringing the cephalic margin down.

15.4.6.4.4 Turn-Over Flap

This flap is described for similar indications as the aforementioned flaps. The cephalic cartilage (5–7 mm) is cut and turned over the remaining caudal portion after cutting it away from the scroll area [43] (Fig. 15.31).

15.4.6.4.5 Lateral Crural Repositioning

The most common indication for lateral crural repositioning is cephalically malpositioned lateral crura. In these cases, after the lateral crura are completely dissected away from the underlying mucosa, recipient pockets are opened and directed toward the lateral canthi. If the lateral crura are supported by lateral crural strut grafts, they may have a more functional benefit in the external valve area [44] (Fig. 15.32). The lateral crural turn-in flap can be used while repositioning the lateral crura in cases where the surgeon is short of cartilage [45] (Fig. 15.33a–t). The key points here are to be meticulous in opening the recipient pockets as symmetrically as possible and to use thinner and longer strut grafts. This is a technically challenging technique and is not suitable for novice surgeons. Honestly, I do not need to use this technique too often because in droopy and boxy tips, lateral crural steal is very powerful in changing the orientation of the lateral crura and removing malposition [46]. Another easier alternative is to use alar battens [36] and/or articulated alar rim grafts [47].

15.4.6.5 Alar Rim Grafts

Alar rim grafts are thin, soft cartilage grafts that measure 12–15 mm in length and 2–3 mm in width [48] (Fig. 15.34). They can be used to support and/or contour alar rims, namely in lateral crural malposition, alar retraction, alar contour anomaly, and alar collapse [49]. Although they can be used as a single entity, they are usually used as an adjunct to one of the major supportive grafts, such as alar battens or lateral crural strut grafts. They can be sutured to the lateral crura to act more like a structural graft, which is called an articulated alar rim graft [47] (Fig. 15.35). This modification supports the soft triangle much better and helps to get rid of medial alar retractions.

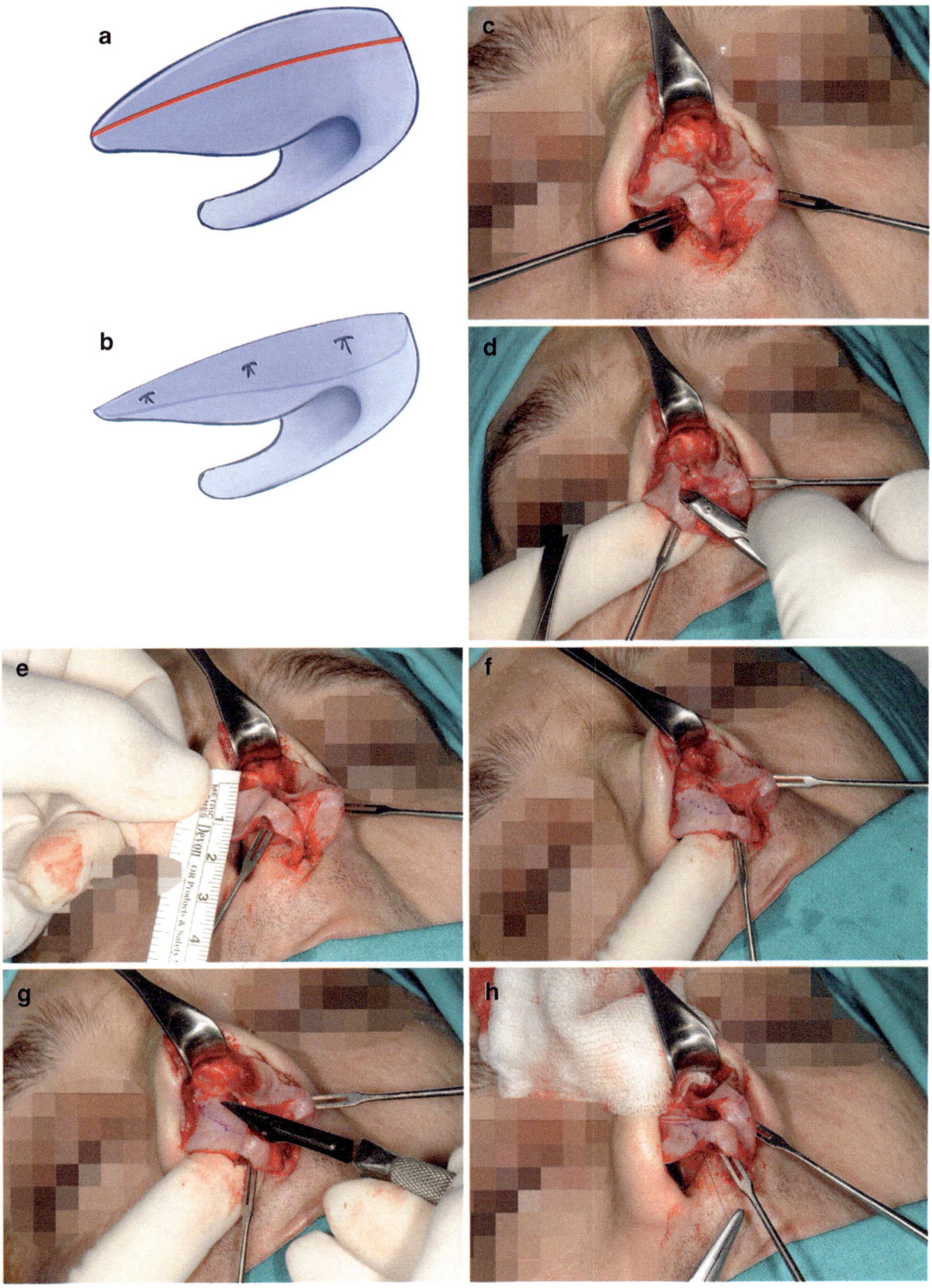

Fig. 15.28 Lateral crural turn-in flap is used when the width of the lateral crus is about 12 mm or more. The 7 mm caudal portion of the lateral crus is left in place and the cephalic portion is turned in after a partial cut and sutured like a sandwich (**a**, **b**). Concave lateral crura were exposed during surgery in a case (**c**). The skin under lateral crus is dissected away by leaving a 2 mm caudal part intact (**d**). The height of the lateral crus is measured (**e**). Then a partially and linearly cut cephalic portion is turned in and sutured like a sandwich (**f**–**j**). The biggest advantage of this technique is that two opposing surfaces of the lateral crus meet each other and end up with a favorable shape and stronger structure. Besides, if the scroll area is kept intact, this flap supports both the external and internal valve as well (**k**). It can be used with all shapes of lateral crura (**l**)

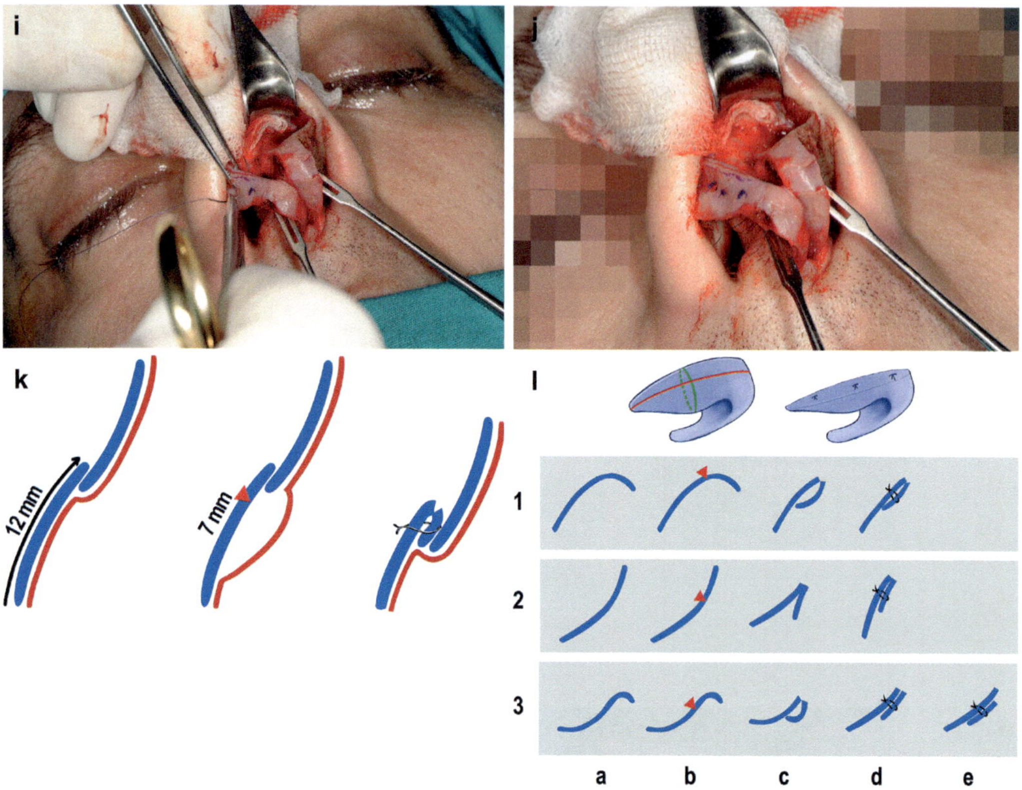

Fig. 15.28 (continued)

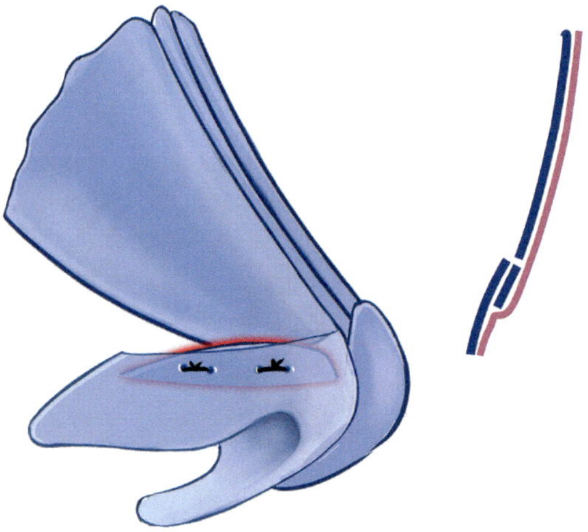

Fig. 15.29 Sliding alar cartilage (SAC) Flap. In the sliding alar cartilage flap, the cephalically trimmed portion is inserted in the pocket created after dissecting the mucosa under the lateral crus while keeping the scroll attachment intact and then sutured to the lateral crus

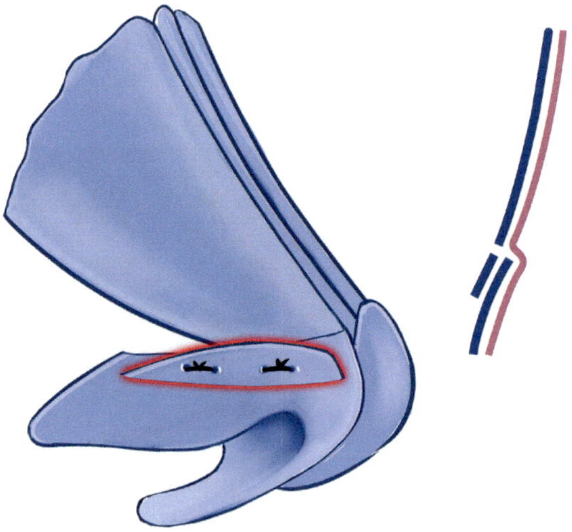

Fig. 15.30 Superior-based transposition flap. To create a superior-based transposition flap, the cephalically cut part is pulled downward and sutured over the lateral crus by preserving the scroll attachment

Fig. 15.31 Turn-over flap. A turn-over flap is obtained by simply folding the cephalically cut portion of the lateral crus outward on the lateral crus and then sutured in place. The scroll area needs to be cut as well

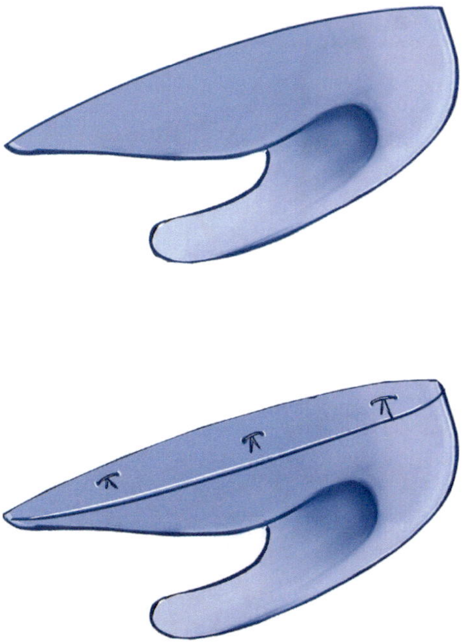

Fig. 15.32 Lateral crural repositioning and lateral crural strut graft. When the lateral crural are malpositioned, one of the techniques is to reposition them into an orthotopic position. In primary cases, septal cartilage can be used as the material of choice. However, in revision cases, rib cartilage can be the best source

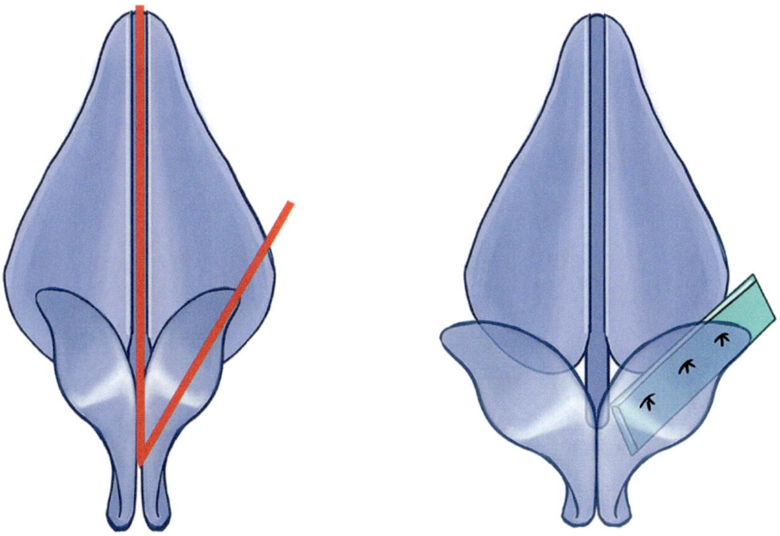

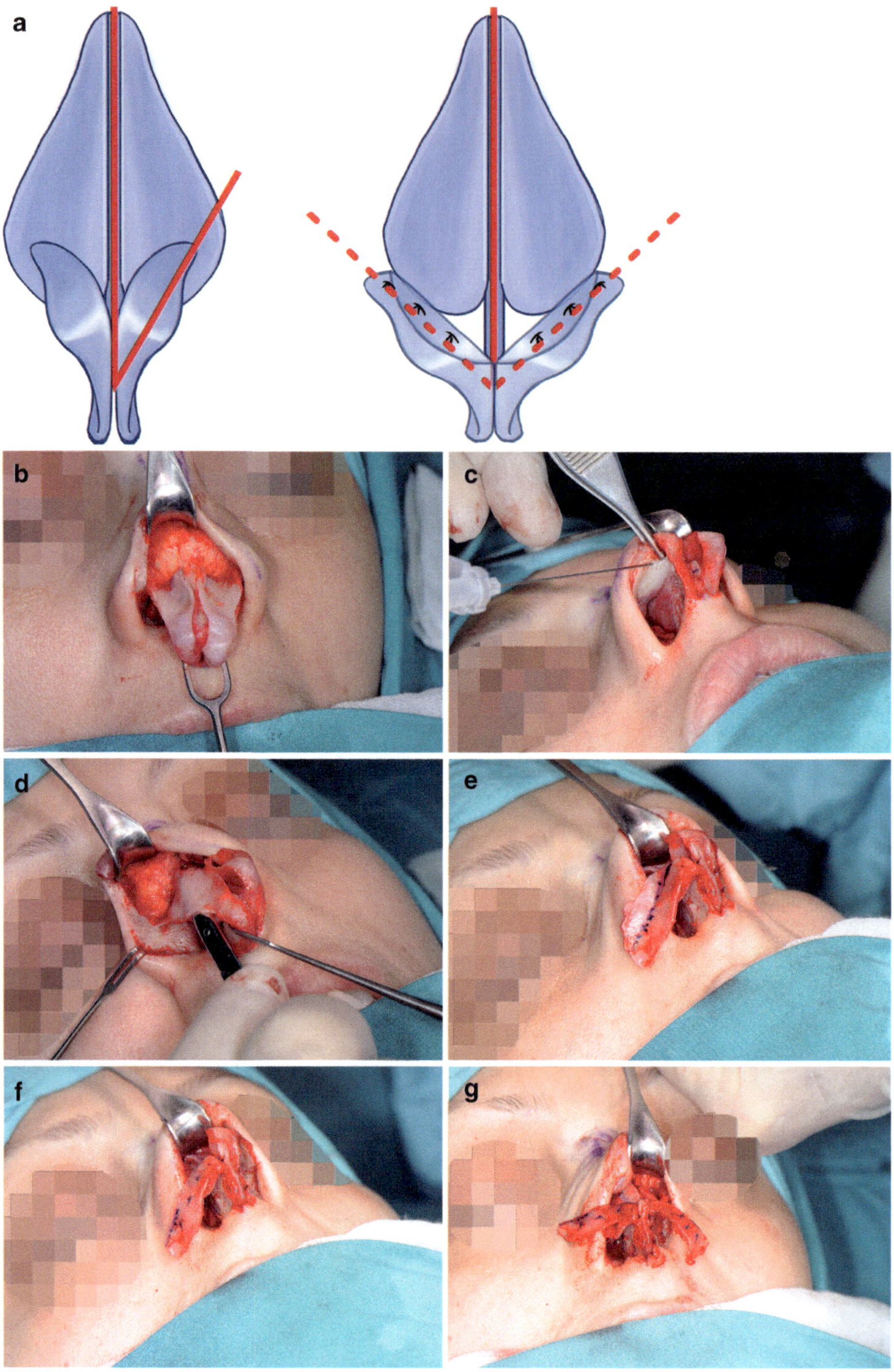

Fig. 15.33 Lateral crural repositioning and lateral crural turn-in flap. When there is not enough material to use as lateral crural strut grafts, the repositioned lateral crura can be supported by lateral crural turn-in flaps (**a**). The cephalically rotated lateral crura were released from their original positions (**b**–**e**). A medial crural steal of 4 mm was used first to deproject the tip (**e**). The cephalic portions of the lateral crura were partially cut and turned in to create the double layer flap (**f**, **g**). They were positioned in their newly created pockets towards to lateral canthi. After three years, the preoperative and postoperative pictures showed the efficacy of this technique (**h**–**s**)

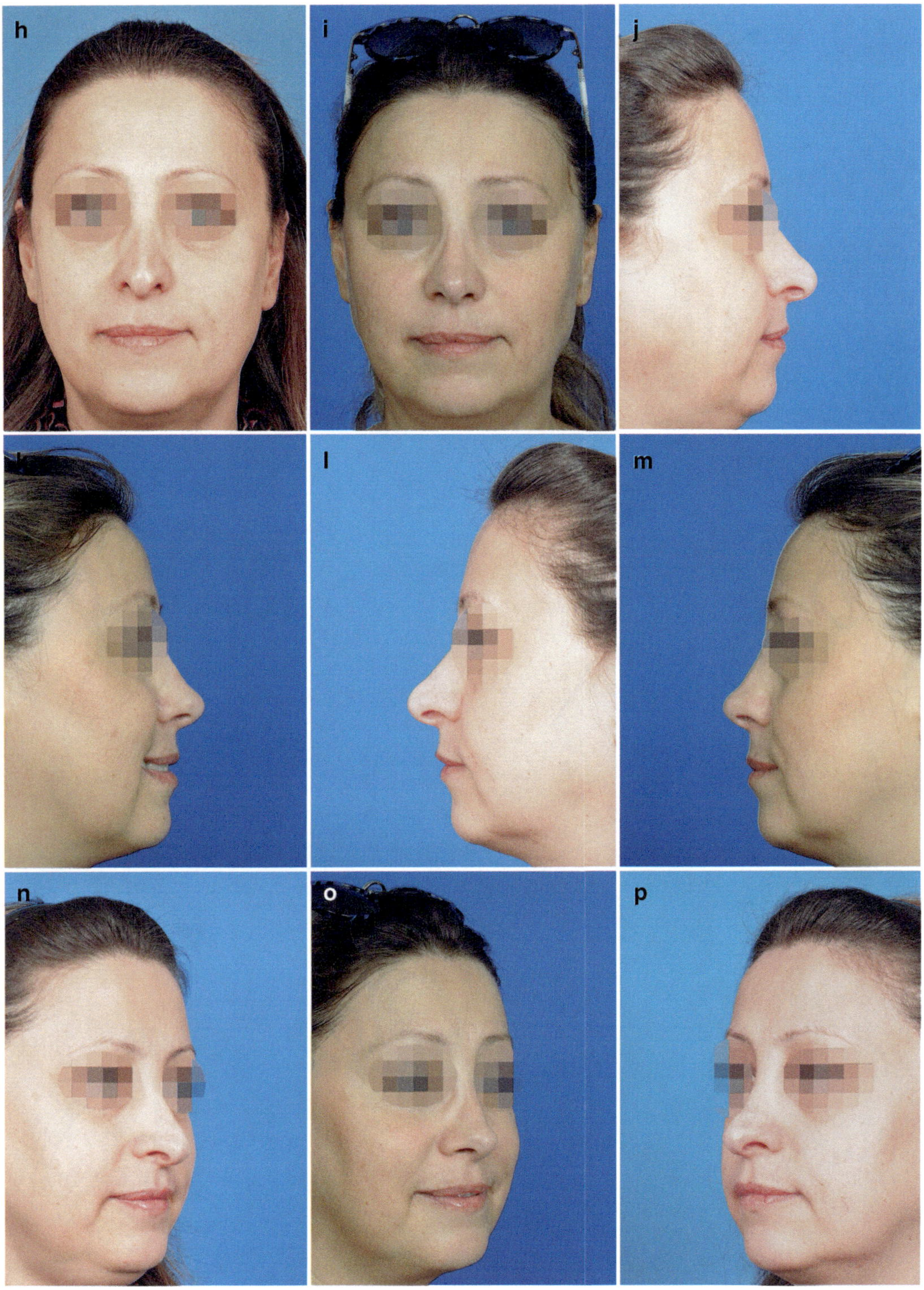

Fig. 15.33 (continued)

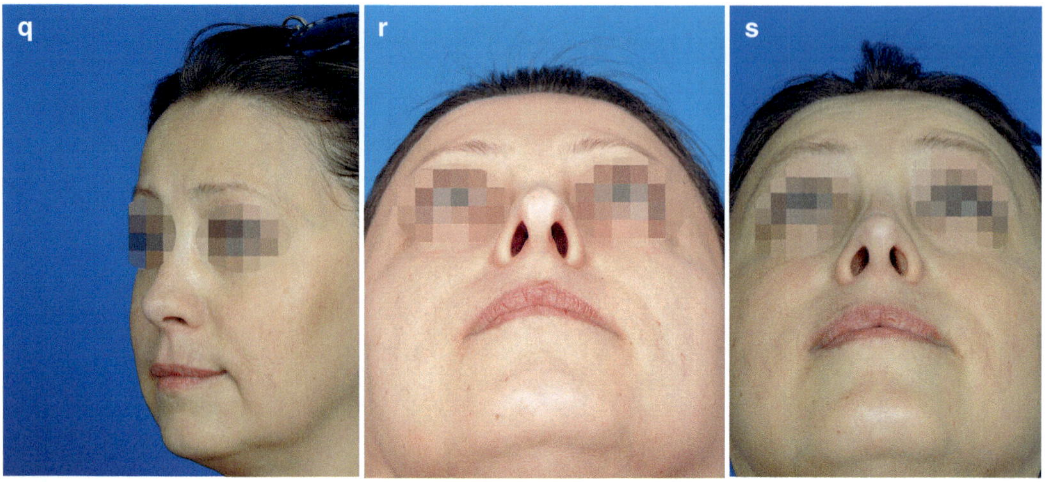

Fig. 15.33 (continued)

Fig. 15.34 Alar rim grafts can be used to provide structural support to the nasal rim and valve area

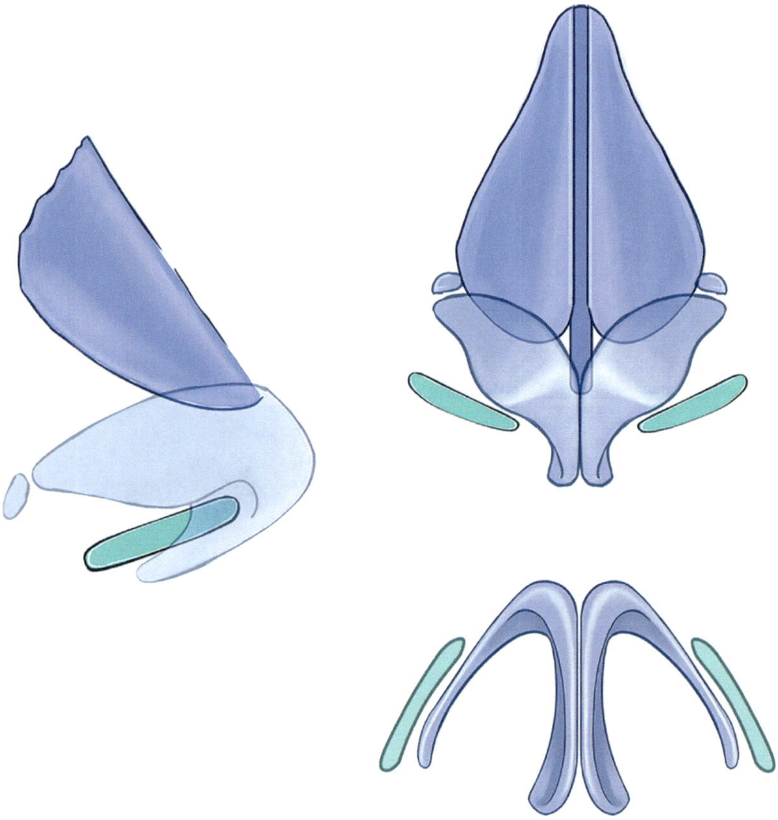

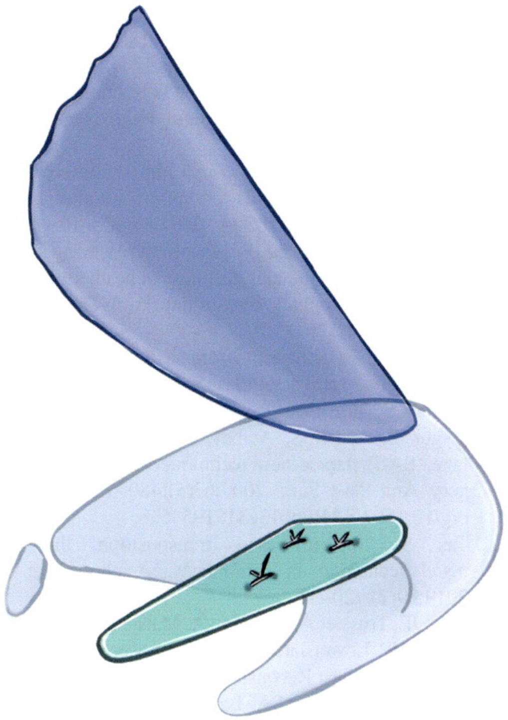

Fig. 15.35 Articulated alar rim grafts are sutured to the caudal portion of the lateral crura

15.5 Conclusion

Nasal valves have been neglected by many rhinoplasty surgeons for the sake of obtaining more esthetically pleasing noses. In particular, within the past two decades, many techniques have been presented to overcome the problems around the nasal valves. To perform functional rhinoplasty, a surgeon should pay attention to the nasal valves and do his or her best to reconstitute the nasal valve function using one or some of the techniques described in this article.

References

1. Kasperbauer JL, Kern EB. Nasal valve physiology. Implications in nasal surgery. Otolaryngol Clin N Am. 1987;20:699–719.
2. Most SP. Analysis of outcomes after functional rhinoplasty using a disease-specific quality-of-life instrument. Arch Facial Plast Surg. 2006;8:306–9.
3. Gode S, Ozturk A, Sahin M, Berber V, Apaydin F. Turkish validation of the standardized cosmesis and health nasal outcomes survey. Facial Plast Surg. 2019;35:397–9.
4. Fomon S, Gilbert JG, Caron AL, Segal S. Collapsed ala: pathologic physiology and management. Arch Otolaryngol. 1950;51:465–84.
5. Seyhan A. Method for middle vault reconstruction in primary rhinoplasty: upper lateral cartilage bending. Plast Reconstr Surg. 1997;100(7):1941–3.
6. Oneal RM, Berkowitz RL. Upper lateral cartilage spreader flaps in rhinoplasty. Aesthet Surg J. 1998;18(5):370–1.
7. Apaydin F. Rebuilding the middle vault in rhinoplasty: a new classification of spreader flaps/grafts. Facial Plast Surg. 2016;32:638–45.
8. Cerkes N. Concurrent elevation of the upper lateral cartilage perichondrium and nasal bone periosteum for management of dorsum: the perichondro-periosteal flap. Aesthet Surg J. 2013;33:899–914.
9. Cottle MH, Loring RM, Fischer GG, Gaynon IE. The maxilla-premaxilla approach to extensive nasal septum surgery. AMA Arch Otolaryngol. 1958;68:301–13.
10. Robotti E, Choc IS, Jaber O. Use of the "septal T" as a spacer and conformer for a properly contoured nasal tip in rhinoplasty. Aesthet Surg J. 2017;37:122–7.
11. Ashrafi AT. Management of upper lateral cartilages (ULCs) in rhinoplasty. World J Plast Surg. 2014;3(2):129–37.
12. Byrd HS, Meade RA, Gonyon DL Jr. Using the auto-spreader flap in primary rhinoplasty. Plast Reconstr Surg. 2007;119:1897–902.
13. Gruber RP, Park E, Newman J, Berkowitz L, Oneal R. The spreader flap in primary rhinoplasty. Plast Reconstr Surg. 2007;119:1903–10.
14. Saedi B, Amali A, Gharavis V, Yekta BG, Most SP. Spreader flaps do not change early functional outcomes in reduction rhinoplasty: a randomized control trial. Am J Rhinol Allergy. 2014;28(1):70–4.
15. Gwanmesia I, Couto R, Papay F. A cadaveric study comparing the efficacy of the Sheen spreader graft and the fulcrum spreader graft: part 1. Plast Reconstr Surg. 2015;136(4):669–76.
16. Ofodile FA, James EA. Anatomy of alar cartilages in blacks. Plast Reconstr Surg. 1997;100:699–703.
17. Guyuron B, Michelow BJ, Englebardt C. Upper lateral splay graft. Plast Reconstr Surg. 1998;102:2169–77.
18. Islam A, Arslan N, Felek SA, Celik H, Demirci M, Oguz H. Reconstruction of the internal nasal valve: modified splay graft technique with endonasal approach. Laryngoscope. 2008;118:1739–43.
19. Sen C, Iscen D. Use of the spring graft for prevention of midvault complications in rhinoplasty. Plast Reconstr Surg. 2007;119:332–6.
20. Clark JM, Cook TA. The 'butterfly' graft in functional secondary rhinoplasty. Laryngoscope. 2002;112:1917–25.

21. Wengen DF. www.breathe-implant.com. Accessed 12 Sept 2010.
22. Park SS. The flaring suture to augment the repair of the dysfunctional nasal valve. Plast Reconstr Surg. 1998;101:1120–2.
23. Schlosser RJ, Park SS. Surgery for the dysfunctional nasal valve. Cadaveric analysis and clinical outcomes. Arch Facial Plast Surg. 1999;1:105–10.
24. Dutton JM, Neidich MJ. Intranasal Z-plasty for internal nasal valve collapse. Arch Facial Plast Surg. 2008;10:164–8.
25. Zelnik J, Gingrass RP. Anatomy of the alar cartilage. Plast Reconstr Surg. 1979;64:650–3.
26. Dhong ES, Han SK, Lee CH, Yoon ES, Kim WK. Anthropometric study of alar cartilage in Asians. Ann Plast Surg. 2002;48:386–91.
27. McIntosh CN, van Wyk FC, Joubert G, Seedat RY. Lower lateral cartilages: an anatomic and morphological study in noses of black southern Africans. Aesthet Surg J. 2017;37:276–82.
28. Daniel RK, Palhazi P, Gerbault O, Kosins AM. Rhinoplasty: the lateral crura-alar ring. Aesthet Surg J. 2014;34:526–37.
29. Kim CH, Jung DH, Park MN, Yoon JH. Surgical anatomy of cartilaginous structures of the Asian nose: clinical implications in rhinoplasty. Laryngoscope. 2010;120:914–9.
30. Kasliwal A, Belaldavar B. Anthropometric overview of lower alar cartilage: an Indian perspective. Indian J Otolaryngol Head Neck Surg. 2018;70:538–43.
31. Cakir B, Oreroğlu AR, Doğan T, Akan M. A complete subperichondrial dissection technique for rhinoplasty with management of the nasal ligaments. Aesthet Surg J. 2012;32:564–74.
32. Sheen JH, Sheen AP. Aesthetic rhinoplasty. 2nd ed. St. Louis: Mosby; 1987.
33. Toriumi DM. New concepts in nasal tip contouring. Arch Otolaryngol. 2006;8:156–85.
34. Tardy ME. Rhinoplasty: the art and the science, Sculpture of the nasal tip, vol. II. Philadelphia, PA: Saunders; 1996.
35. Gunter JP, Friedman RM. Lateral crural strut graft: technique and clinical applications in rhinoplasty. Plast Reconstr Surg. 1997;99:943–52.
36. Tardy ME, Garner ET. Inspiratory nasal obstruction secondary to alar and nasal valve collapse: technique for repair using autologous cartilage. Oper Tech Otolaryngol Head Neck Surg. 1990;1:215–8.
37. Toriumi DM, Josen J, Weinberger M, Tardy ME Jr. Use of alar batten grafts for correction of nasal valve collapse. Arch Otolaryngol Head Neck Surg. 1997;123:802–8.
38. Tellioglu AT, Cimen K. Turn-in folding of the cephalic portion of the lateral crus to support the alar rim in rhinoplasty. Aesth Plast Surg. 2007;31:306–10.
39. Murakami CS, Barrera JE, Most SP. Preserving structural integrity of the alar cartilage in aesthetic rhinoplasty using a cephalic turn-in flap. Arch Facial Plast Surg. 2009;11:126–8.
40. Apaydin F. Lateral crural turn-in flap in functional rhinoplasty. Arch Facial Plast Surg. 2012;14(2):93–6.
41. Ozmen S, Eryilmaz T, Sencan A, Cukurluoglu O, Uygur S, Ayhan S, Atabay K. Sliding alar cartilage (SAC) flap: a new technique for nasal tip surgery. Ann Plast Surg. 2009;63(5):480–5. https://doi.org/10.1097/SAP.0b013e31819538a8.
42. Taş S. Superior-based transposition flap: a novel technique in rhinoplasty. Aesthet Surg J. 2019;39(7):720–32.
43. Janis JE, Trussler A, Ghavami A, Marin V, Rohrich RJ, Gunter JP. Lower lateral crural turnover flap in open rhinoplasty. Plast Reconstr Surg. 2009;123:1830–41.
44. Toriumi DM, Asher SA. Lateral crural repositioning for treatment of cephalic malposition. Facial Plast Surg Clin North Am. 2015;23(1):55–71.
45. Apaydin F. Projection and Deprojection techniques in rhinoplasty. Clin Plast Surg. 2016;43:151–68.
46. Kridel RW, Konior RJ, Shumrick KA, Wright WK. Advances in nasal tip surgery. The lateral crural steal. Arch Otolaryngol Head Neck Surg. 1989;115:1206–12.
47. Ballin AC, Kim H, Chance E, Davis RE. The articulated alar rim graft: reengineering the conventional alar rim graft for improved contour and support. Facial Plast Surg. 2016;32:384–97.
48. Troell RJ, Powell NB, Riley RW, Li KK. Evaluation of a new procedure for nasal alar rim and valve collapse: nasal alar rim reconstruction. Otolaryngol Head Neck Surg. 2000;122:204–11.
49. Boahene KD, Hilger PA. Alar rim grafting in rhinoplasty: indications, technique, and outcomes. Arch Facial Plast Surg. 2009;11:285–9.

16 Surgery of the Nasal Turbinates

16.1 Introduction

Turbinates play a crucial role in the function of the nose. However, they can sometimes be a reason for nasal obstruction. Depending on the development of the nose and nasal airways during childhood and in later years, the turbinates usually tend to adjust to the shape of the nasal septum. The aerodynamics of the nose are so special that the nasal airways should neither be too wide nor too narrow. When there is a need for surgery, the condition of the nasal airways should be thoroughly examined.

16.2 Inferior Turbinate Anatomy and Physiology

The inferior, middle, and superior turbinates are composed of thin bony structures adhered to the medial wall of the maxilla. They are covered by the mucoperiosteum. The mucosal layer is covered by pseudostratified ciliated columnar respiratory epithelium, except for the anterior tip of the inferior turbinate, which is covered by stratified squamous epithelium [1] (Fig. 16.1).

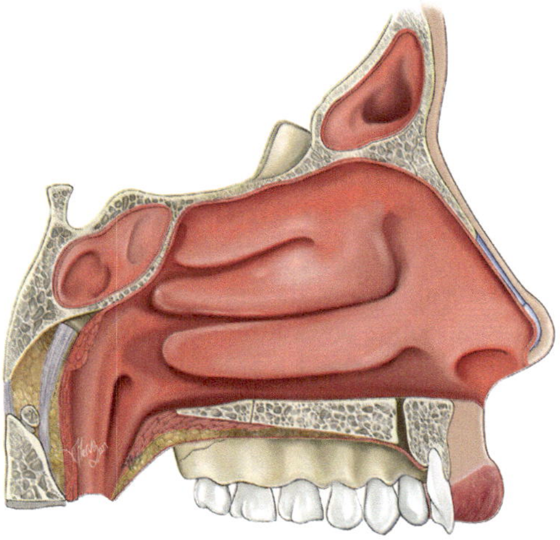

Fig. 16.1 The inferior, middle, and superior turbinates are composed of thin bony structures adhered to the medial wall of the maxilla and covered by the mucoperiosteum

The turbinates contribute to inspiratory resistance, which is essential for breathing through the entire airway system. As part of the valve area, they help to change the inspiratory lamellar airstream into a turbulent flow. Turbulence in the outer layers of air increases the interaction between air and nasal mucosa, which helps inhaled air to be humidified, warmed, and cleansed. They are also important for mucociliary transport and humoral and cellular defense [2].

Supplementary Information The online version contains supplementary material available at https://doi.org/10.1007/978-3-031-74734-2_16. The videos can be accessed individually by clicking the DOI link in the accompanying figure caption or by scanning this link with the SN More Media App.

© The Author(s), under exclusive license to Springer Nature Switzerland AG 2025

F. Apaydın, *Septal Surgery Challenges in Rhinoplasty*,
https://doi.org/10.1007/978-3-031-74734-2_16

16.3 Etiology of Inferior Turbinate Hypertrophy

Inferior turbinate hypertrophy can be due to disorders of the nasal mucosa, such as allergic and vasomotor rhinitis, or enlargement of the bony turbinate. It should be kept in mind that inferior turbinates have sinusoidal erectile tissue, and mucosal disorders should be treated with medical management, such as antihistamines, sympathomimetics, anticholinergics, and steroids. In cases where medical management is not adequate, surgical intervention will be necessary. However, in the majority of cases, hypertrophy is usually compensatory in cases of contralateral septal deviation.

16.4 Surgical Reduction of Inferior Turbinates

Intervention on the inferior turbinates is almost a routine procedure for many rhinoplasty surgeons, even though the turbinates are normal in shape and size. The justification is that in reduction rhinoplasty, the airway is reduced, and the turbinates can be a reason for nasal obstruction. In fact, I was trained by master rhinologists not to touch the inferior turbinates under any condition. Their teaching was that if the underlying cause, such as septal deviation, valve problems, or polyps, could be treated adequately, the inferior turbinates would normalize over time. After focusing more intensively on rhinoplasty, I witnessed that this was not always the case in many patients. Therefore, I have been making an intervention on turbinates in most of the cases.

I like to think of the inferior turbinate in three portions: anterior, middle, and posterior (Fig. 16.2). The anterior portion is part of the internal nasal valve, which is the narrowest portion of the respiratory tract. Therefore, its management is the most critical during rhinoplasty. However, I have frequently witnessed isolated hypertrophy of the middle and mostly posterior portions that did not obstruct the airway. Therefore, I highly recommend routinely examining the nasal airway with the help of an endoscope at the beginning of rhinoplasty. In many cases, rhinoplasty surgeons do not examine the

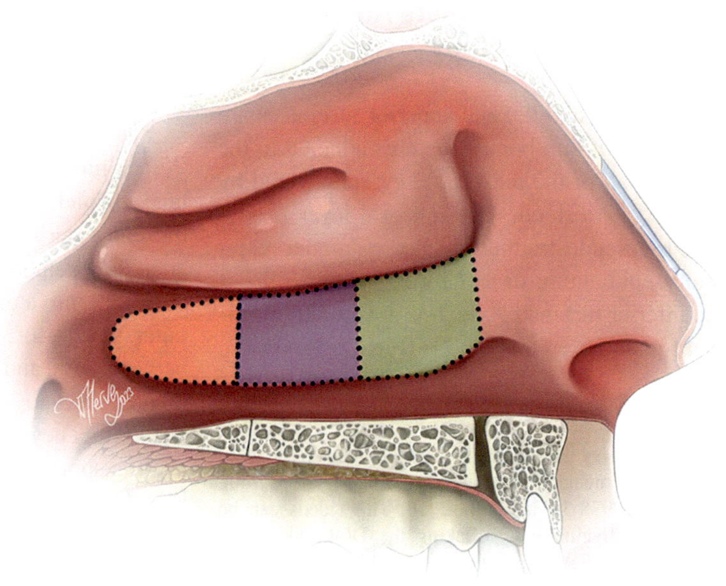

Fig. 16.2 The inferior turbinate can be divided into three zones: anterior, middle, and posterior

a

b

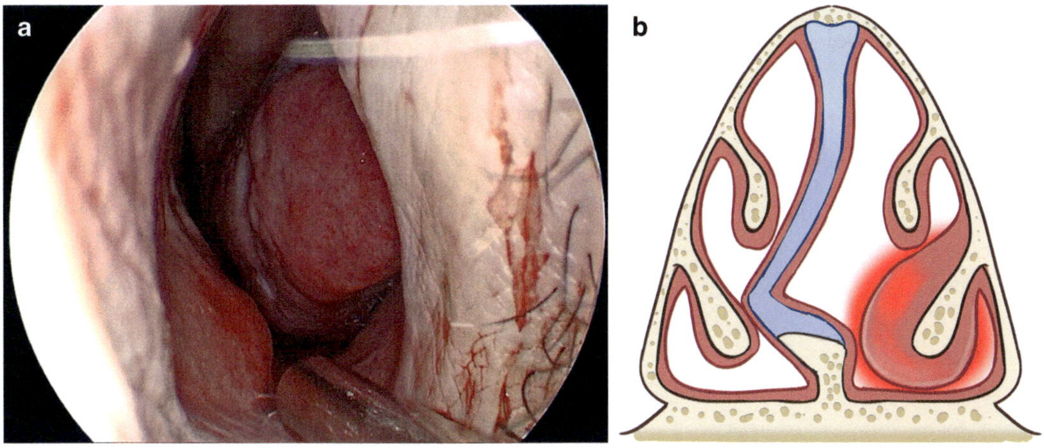

Fig. 16.3 The endoscopic view of the nasal cavity showing hypetrophy of the inferior turbinate (**a**). A cross-sectional diagram of the nasal passage showing a deviation of the septal cartilage to the right side and compensatory hypetrophy of the inferior turbinate on the left side (**b**)

nose by endoscopy before surgery. In addition, I prefer to perform any intervention on the turbinates at this stage, before I start rhinoplasty. I have seen many cases where it can bleed and lengthen the operation time unnecessarily. Therefore, if these interventions are performed at the beginning, simple cotonoids placed in the nasal airways can be very effective in stopping these bleedings.

The middle portion is usually hypertrophied together with the anterior or posterior portion (Fig. 16.3a, b). Sometimes a spine or deviated cartilage can be buried in the inferior turbinate, splitting it into two parts. This can also be the reason for hypertrophy. Another surprising finding was the observation of hypertrophy of the inferior turbinate just behind the deviated portion of the nasal septum, obstructing the nasal airway. Therefore, it is highly recommended to examine the nasal passages using an endoscope at the end of surgery to determine if there is a problem at the posterior portion of the nose and if there are any bleeders. This is the best time to solve these kinds of problems, which can easily be missed during surgery.

The reduction of inferior turbinates can be performed using different surgical techniques, including thermal coagulation, total or partial inferior turbinectomy, turbinoplasty, lateral outfracture, submucosal resection, chemocoagulation, laser surgery, cryosurgery, vidian neurectomy, coblation, and high-intensity focused ultrasound [2, 3].

Inferior turbinate reduction can be performed using various techniques.

16.4.1 Radiofrequency

This is by far the most popular method used in recent years. Radiofrequency energy, applied by a needle-like tip, creates hyperthermic submucosal necrosis with less damage to the surrounding tissue, especially to the mucosa (Figs. 16.4 and 16.5). It is a safe and quick procedure during rhinoplasty, which is completed in 1–2 min. Healing ends with volume reduction due to wound contraction and fibrosis of the submucosa. The submucosal nerve fibers are damaged during the procedure, causing denervation and hyporeactivity of the turbinate mucosa [4].

It can be done through one entry point or multiple entry points on the inferior turbinate, depending on the specifications of the tip of the instrument and the gadget used. I have been using this technique for almost 20 years, and I am very satisfied with the results. It is applied submucosally after penetrating the tip into the head of the inferior turbinate. I find it more practical to address the anterior, middle, and posterior

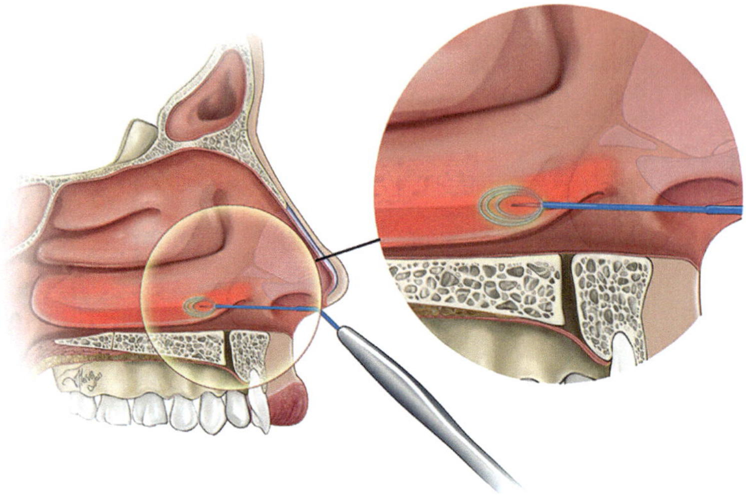

Fig. 16.4 Radiofrequency energy is applied by a needle-like tip, creating hyperthermic submucosal necrosis with less damage to the surrounding tissue

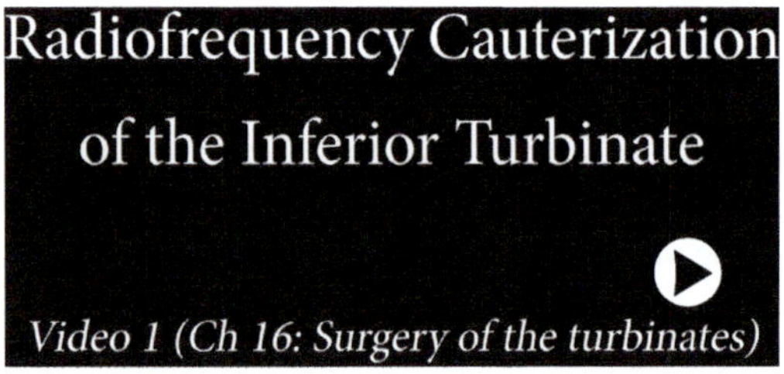

Fig. 16.5 Radiofrequency cauterization of the inferior turbinate (▶ https://doi.org/10.1007/000-dzs)

portions separately through three or more entry points.

What types of instruments are used to apply this technique? There are models that can be used with eye control, and these models are relatively cheaper. I have been using this gadget for 20 years. It is possible to change the intensity and time of exposure. It is applied until blanching and devolumization are seen. What happens when the needle electrode is inserted into the turbinate submucosally? The needle electrode causes a rapid local temperature rise, to a range of 50–90 °C, within seconds to minutes, resulting in thermal injury and irreversible tissue destruction. When the 100 °C threshold is reached, boiling at the electrode–tissue interface results in tissue coagulum adhering to and insulating the electrode, and there is an abrupt drop in current density; tissue heating ceases, as do lesion formation and tissue damage [4].

In recent years, electrosurgical devices developed for needle ablation, i.e., thermal ablation, have incorporated thermistors or other sensors in the electrode to monitor local tissue temperature to prevent tissue near the electrode from attaining 100 °C. The sensor automatically shuts off the current, which determines the maximum lesion size [5]. I have been using these sophisticated radiofrequency generators that allow radiofrequency ablation via impedance feedback and autostop. These machines are more precise and safe, but they are also more costly.

16.4.2 Electrocautery

Electrocautery can be used in linear surface electrocautery, bipolar electrocautery, and submucous diathermy. I have tried all these techniques from 1989 to today. When I started my residency, I had to use submucosal diathermy because a team from my department had designed a gadget for submucosal diathermy after working on animals and humans with good results. I was always scared of touching the bone and pressing the pedal for longer than needed. However, I witnessed patients in my department with excessive crusting lasting 4–8 weeks, as well as bone necrosis and sequestration. This is why I also abandoned this method.

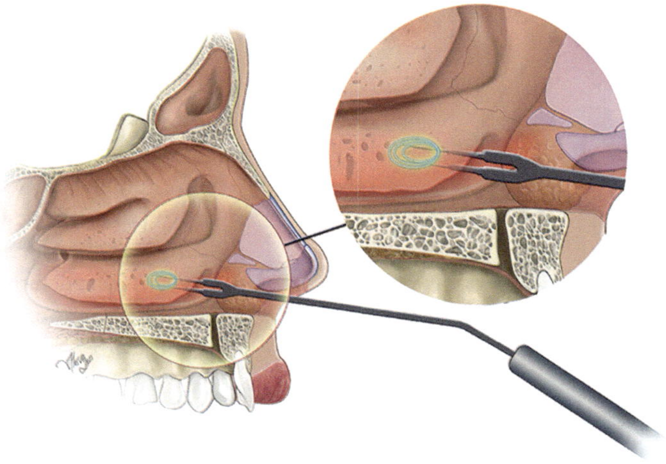

Fig. 16.6 Bipolar electrocautery is a cheap and effective method, using a fork-like tip connected to any cautery gadget available in the operating theater

I have almost never used linear surface electrocautery routinely because this is a technique that directly damages the mucosa and mucociliary action.

In rare instances, I used traditional bipolar electrocautery with bayonet pincettes submucosally. I have also used it in a few cases with polypoid degeneration and hypertrophy of the tail of the inferior turbinate. In these cases, the tail could look like polypoid tissue connected to the turbinate with a pedicle. Using a bipolar cautery to cauterize this pedicle and then resecting it is a good technique that I still use. In recent years, I have been using bipolar cautery tips designed for inferior turbinates. They are very cheap compared to expensive cautery machines, and they can easily be coupled to any electrosurgery machine in the OR (Figs. 16.6 and 16.7). Therefore, if the radiofrequency gadget does not function well on a given day, this is my second choice in the OR.

16.4.3 Coblation

The term coblation is derived from "Controlled ablation." This procedure involves a non-heat-driven process of soft tissue dissolution using bipolar radiofrequency energy under a conductive medium such as normal saline. Coblation devices work at temperatures of 40–70 °C; thermal penetration is minimal; the effect on target tissue is gentle removal and dissolution, and collateral damage to the surrounding tissue is minimal. Conventional electrosurgical devices work at temperatures of 400–600 °C; thermal penetration is deep; the effect on target tissue is rapid heating, charring, burning, and cutting; and the effect on surrounding tissue is inadvertent charring and/or burning [4]. I have tried this gadget in a certain number of cases. I can easily say that it is really tissue-friendly with satisfactory results, but it took a much longer time to use this method on patients compared with traditional electrosurgical methods.

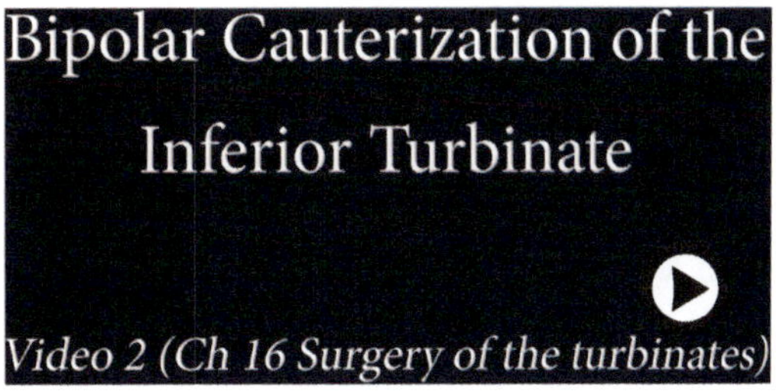

Fig. 16.7 Bipolar cauterization of the inferior turbinate (▶ https://doi.org/10.1007/000-dzr)

16.4.4 Outfracturing of the Inferior Turbinate

Using a blunt elevator to displace the turbinate laterally is a technique with minimal morbidity (Fig. 16.8). Improvement in the nasal airway can

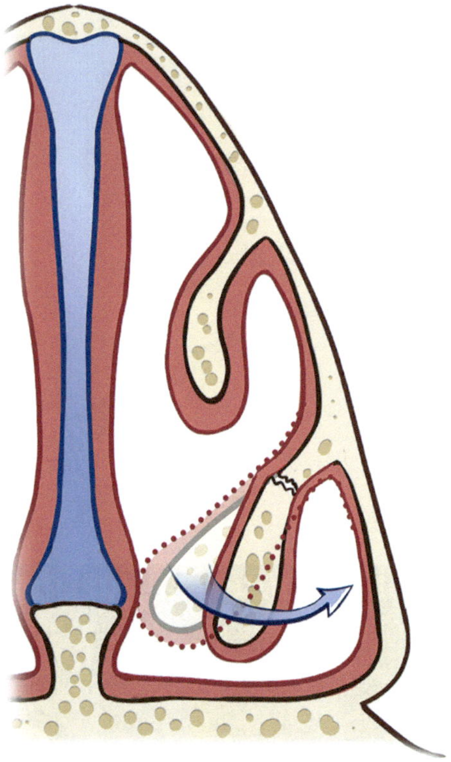

Fig. 16.8 Outfracture of the inferior turbinate can be done by using a blunt elevator to displace the turbinate laterally

be transient. In fact, it seems that it is effective in the patients I use because I usually keep the Doyle splints for a week, which can splint the fractured turbinate in place for a week, although I did not do a study on it. There are studies showing its efficacy, whereas there are authors who have published against its usage. The technique also does not address the underlying pathology of hypertrophied turbinate mucosa. Turbinate outfracture, therefore, is often performed concomitantly with another procedure [2].

16.4.5 Submucous Resection

It was first described by Spielberg in 1924 [6]. After a small incision at the anterior part of the turbinate, the submucosal erectile tissue and/or inferior turbinate bone were removed, leaving the overlying mucosa intact (Fig. 16.9). By maintaining the mucosal flaps, normal mucosal function is preserved, thereby reducing the likelihood of complications, such as crusting and atrophic rhinitis. Only minimal crusting is typically observed along the incision site. Another reported advantage of this method is the very low incidence of

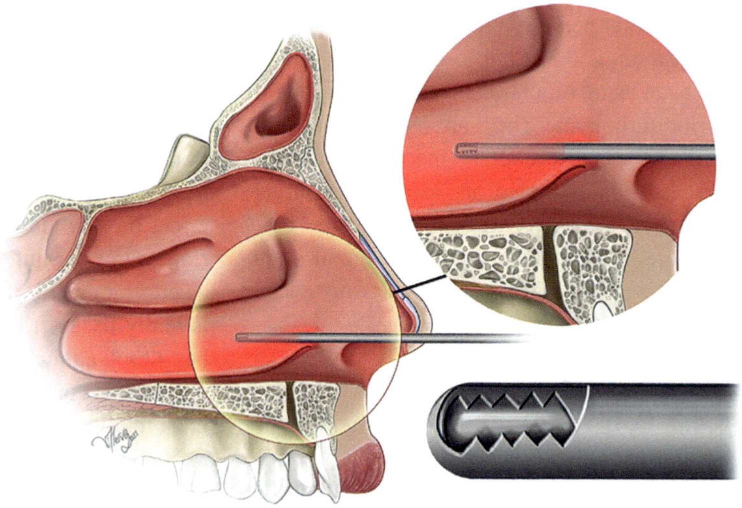

Fig. 16.9 Submucous resection of the inferior turbinate is realized after a small incision at its anterior part. The submucosal erectile tissue and/or inferior turbinate bone can be removed using forceps, microdebrider, or piezotome

postoperative bleeding [7]. The effectiveness of traditional submucous resection is even more pronounced in cases of conchal bone hypertrophy. The primary disadvantages of traditional submucous resection are the potential for mucosal shredding in inexperienced hands and the need for nasal packing postoperatively [8].

This surgery can be performed with traditional surgical instruments, such as through-cut forceps or Takahashi forceps, if bone is intended to be removed. Piezoelectric instruments can also be very helpful because they work only on bone and not on soft tissue. When erectile soft tissue resection is desired, microdebriders are more favorable than traditional forceps because of ease and predictability of application [9].

16.4.6 Turbinoplasty

The term inferior turbinoplasty was introduced by Mabry in 1982 [8]. In this technique, a local injection using 1% lidocaine with 1:100,000 epinephrine is applied first. I dilute this mixture with an equal amount of saline to inject more and facilitate hydrodissection of the mucosa and submucosal tissues away from the turbinate bone. The inferior turbinate is then fractured medially using a Freer or Joseph elevator. A deep incision is made at the anterior margin of the inferior turbinate, reaching the conchal bone. A Freer elevator is then employed to elevate the soft tissue and mucosa off the medial surface of the conchal bone. At this point, I would like to use Heyman scissors vertically by placing one jaw in the lower portion of the pocket and the other jaw in the nose, matching the lower margin of the inferior turbinate, to make a long cut until the posterior end of the turbinate. The second cut is performed with the same Kaplan bone-cutting scissors, with one jaw between the conchal bone and the elevated flap and the other jaw below and lateral to the turbinate attachment. The scissors are closed and advanced to completely resect the conchal bone from its attachment to the lateral nasal wall. The remaining posterior attachment of the resected bone and mucosa can be resected under endoscopic control using bipolar cautery and endoscopic scissors. The remaining flap of the turbinate is rolled upon itself from medial to lateral to form a neo-turbinate with two opposing internal raw surfaces and an external mucosal-lined surface (Fig. 16.10). Packing is then carried out in whatever manner is desired. I used this technique a lot in the past and was very happy with the result because it is a very efficient technique for reducing the volume and size of the inferior turbinate while maintaining most of the medial mucosa. However, I only had one case of severe bleeding in which the patient needed to be hospitalized for a week, and that event discouraged me from using this technique more often.

When the resection of bone and parenchyma is restricted to the anterior part of the turbinate, it is called as "anterior turbinoplasty" [2]. An L-shaped incision is made at the anterior portion of the turbinate, and the lateral portion of the mucosa and bone is resected. Therefore, it is a partial turbinoplasty addressing the anterior portion of the turbinate (Fig. 16.11).

Schmelzer [10] reported the use of partial inferior turbinoplasty. In this method, two separate incisions are made that join in the center of the concha. A wedge-shaped piece of the turbinate is then removed, and the margins of the resulting defect are brought together (Fig. 16.12).

In turbinoplasty, all mucosal functions are preserved, and there is a very low incidence of postoperative bleeding and crusting.

16.4.7 Turbinectomy

Partial turbinectomy was described in 1882 [11], and total turbinectomy was first reported in 1895 [12]. Technically, they are both easy techniques. After medialization of the inferior turbinate by a Freer elevator, Heymann scissors are used. If the cut is done at the middle of the turbinate, this is called partial (Fig. 16.13), and if the scissors are placed at the lateral attachment of the turbinate and cut, it is called total turbinectomy (Fig. 16.14). Total turbinectomy is not compatible with the

a

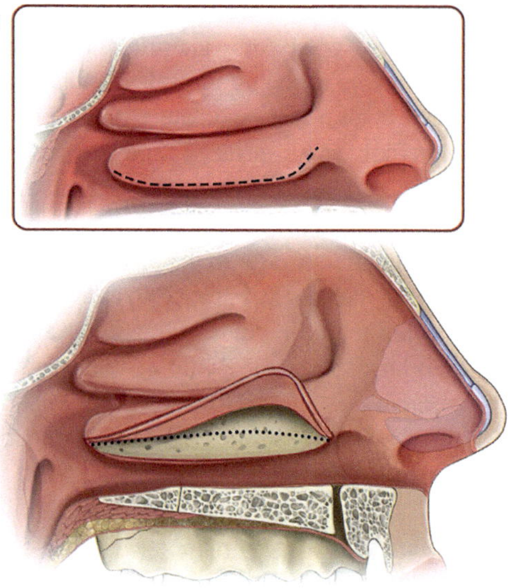

b

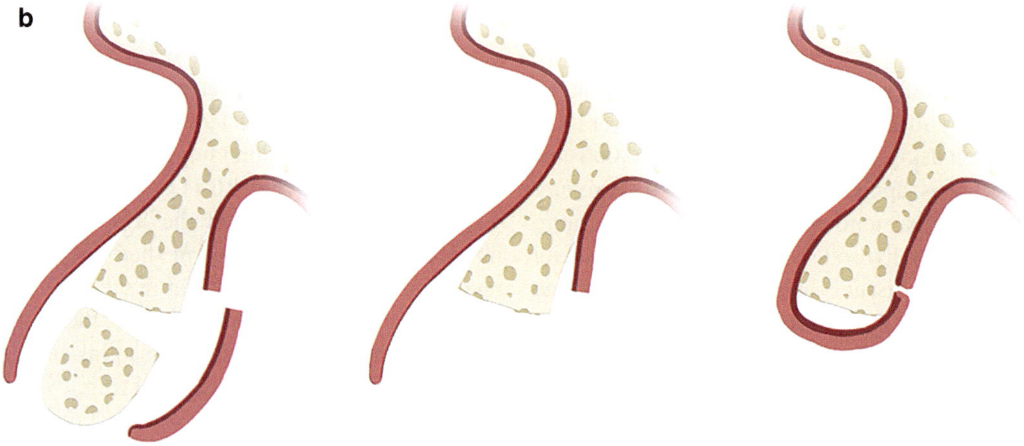

Fig. 16.10 Turbinoplasty starts with a deep incision made at the anterior margin of the inferior turbinate. The mucosa and soft tissues are dissected away from the medial surface of the conchal bone using a Freer elevator. The lower half of the inferior turbinate is cut and resected (**a**). The medial flap of the turbinate is rolled upon itself from medial to lateral (**b**)

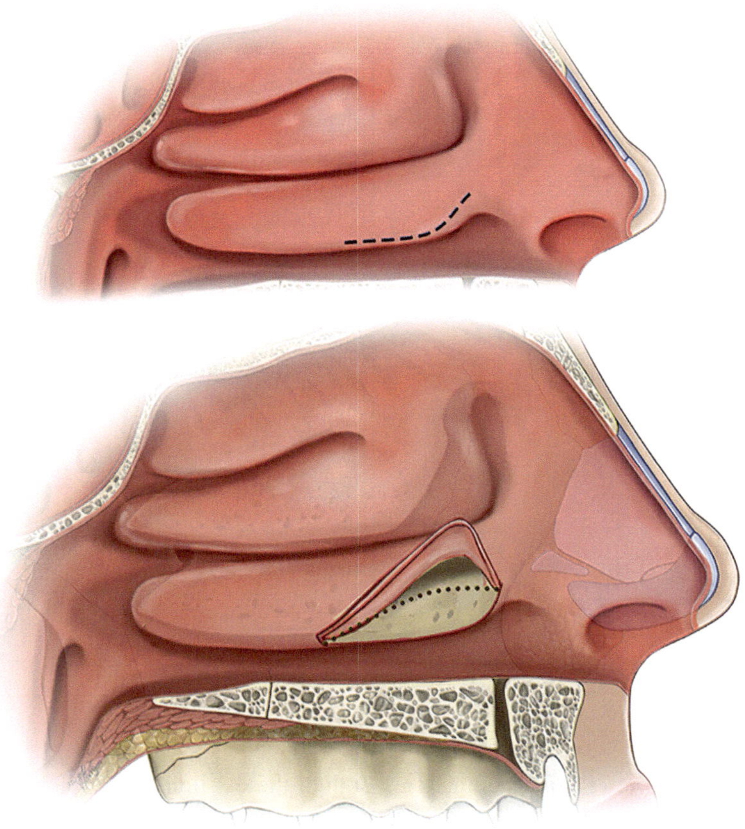

Fig. 16.11 In anterior turbinoplasty, an L-shaped incision is made at the anterior portion of the turbinate, and the lateral portion of the mucosa and bone is resected

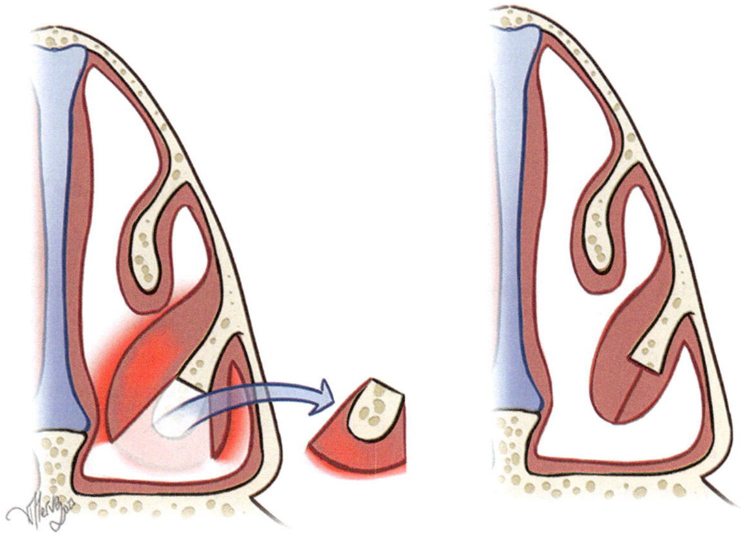

Fig. 16.12 Partial inferior turbinoplasty comprises two separate incisions joining in the center of the concha. A wedge-shaped piece of the turbinate is then removed, and the margins of the resulting defect are brought together

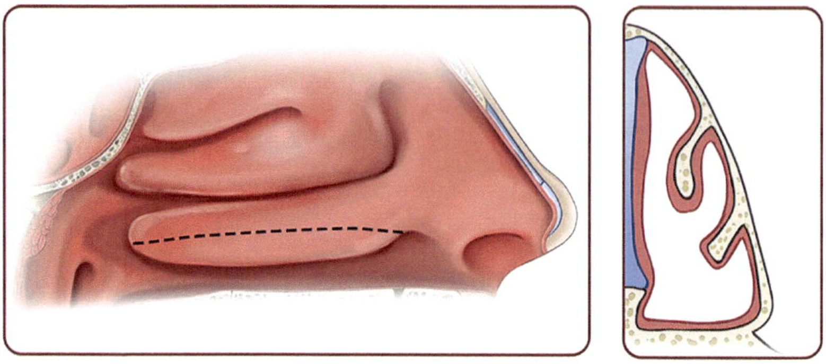

Fig. 16.13 In turbinectomy, the lower half of the inferior turbinate is simply cut with Heymann scissors and resected

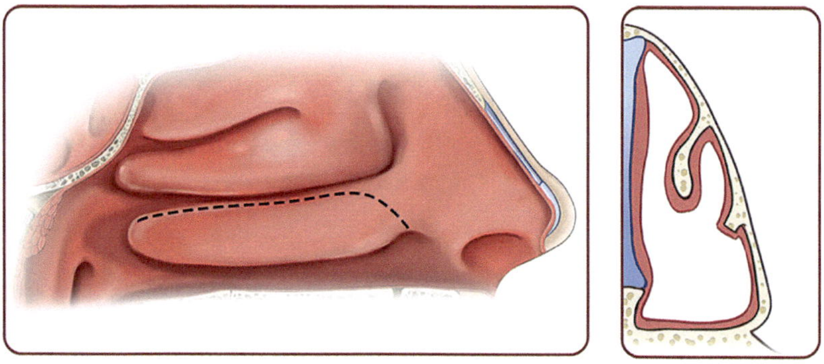

Fig. 16.14 Total turbinectomy means resecting the entire inferior turbinate

goal of "preservation of function." Both of these techniques are irreversible.

First, it is against the aerodynamics of the nasal airway. There must be resistance in the nasal cavities to obtain turbulence and pressure differences, so that the air can flow faster and more consistently. Second, it can create postoperative hemorrhage, crusting, and atrophic rhinitis. Therefore, I think that rhinoplasty surgeons should consider these two procedures as historical techniques.

16.4.8 Ultrasound Treatment

High-intensity focused ultrasound (HIFU) is a new noninvasive treatment modality that focuses an ultrasound beam on the target tissue in the body and generates high energy, which selectively and rapidly causes coagulation necrosis of the target tissue without damaging adjacent or superficial tissues. HIFU turbinoplasty showed no complications, such as bleeding or scar formation. Histological examinations revealed decreased glandular structure and increased fibrosis. It has been described that HIFU can be as effective as coblation for treating inferior turbinate hypertrophy [3].

HIFU can be an effective and safe noninvasive alternative to current surgical modalities for inferior turbinate hypertrophy.

16.4.9 Other Treatment Modalities

Different lasers have been described to be used for inferior turbinate resection [13, 14]. Although they were effective in turbinate reduction, they were never widely used because the equipment was expensive and required additional expertise, training, and safety precautions.

Cryosurgery was introduced by Ozenberger in 1970 [15]. This method involves freezing the turbinate under local anesthesia with a cryoprobe that uses nitrous oxide or liquid nitrogen as a cooling agent. It was abandoned because the amount of volume reduction was hard to predict, and the long-term results were disappointing.

16.5 Surgery of the Middle Turbinate

If we look at the issue from a rhinologist's perspective, middle turbinate anatomy and management is a crucial issue because it is one of the key anatomic structures in functional endoscopic sinus surgery. However, the middle turbinate is very rarely a matter of concern for the rhinoplasty surgeon because it does not cause any problems during or after rhinoplasty.

The major problem for a rhinoplasty surgeon can be the existence of a concha bullosa (Fig. 16.15), which is aeration of the middle turbinate. It is reported to be present in 34% of the population on at least one side. There is a strong association between the presence of a concha bullosa and contralateral deviation of the nasal septum. However, the necessity to perform surgical intervention is very rarely needed. Throughout all these years, I had to deal with concha bullosa in very severely crooked noses.

What is the best way to address concha bullosa [16]? After decongestion of the nasal mucosa using pledgets soaked in lidocaine and adrenaline, the incision site is injected with lidocaine and adrenaline. I also like using bipolar cautery to cauterize the incision tract to reduce bleeding during the intervention. Then, I use a #15 blade to make a deep incision in the anterior–inferior end of the middle turbinate. It is usually easy to penetrate through the tough bone of the concha bullosa and keep cutting up and down. Heymann scissors are very effective for further cutting the concha bullosa. I have been using a loupe and/or endoscope for this surgery. A freer or suction elevator can be helpful to detach the cut lateral

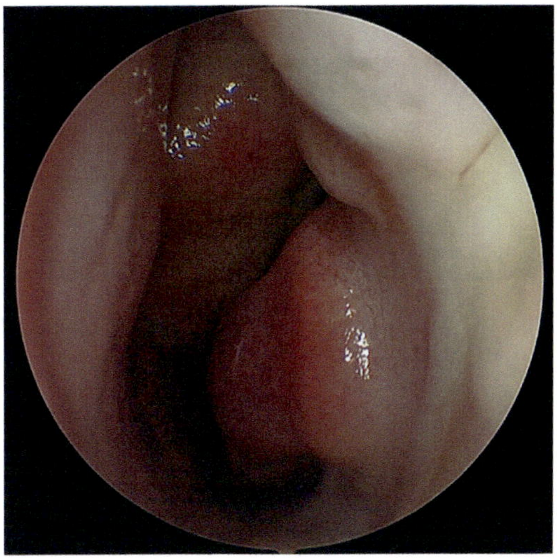

Fig. 16.15 Concha bullosa, endoscopic view

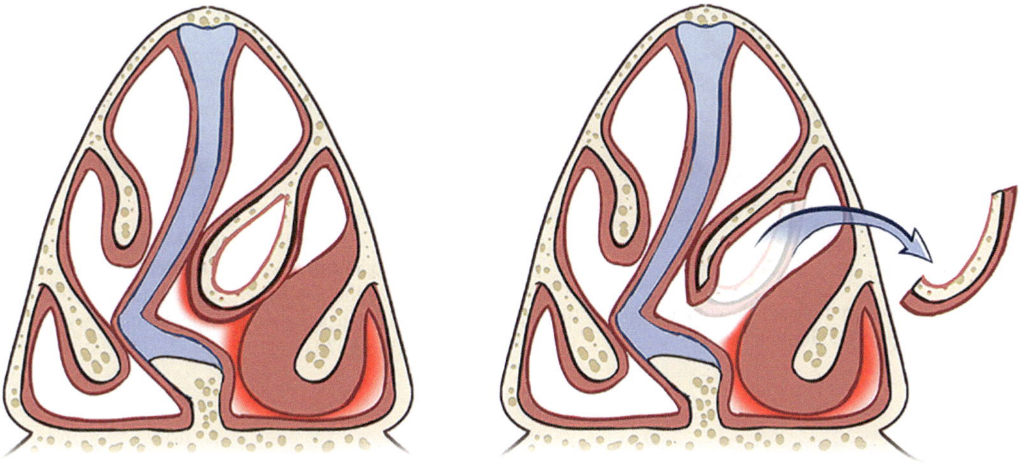

Fig. 16.16 Concha bullosaplasty is simply resecting the lateral lamella of it

portion of the concha bullosa and identify the holding parts (Fig. 16.16). Endoscopic scissors are then used to cut the remaining portions to resect the lateral lamella of the concha bullosa (Fig. 16.17). Cotton pledgets are inserted to stop bleeding if there is any. Then, the bleeders are inspected and cauterized. An absorbable packing is placed in the middle meatus. It must be kept in mind that nasty bleeding can happen after this surgery in the postoperative period. Therefore, the surgeon should take all the measures to identify and stop all the bleeders during surgery.

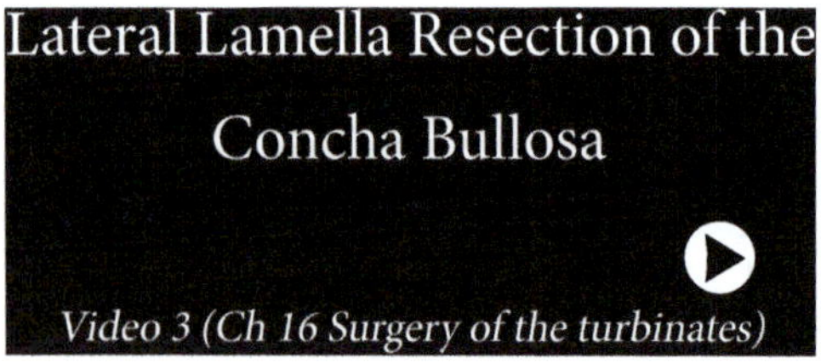

Fig. 16.17 Concha bullosaplasty (▶ https://doi.org/10.1007/000-dzt)

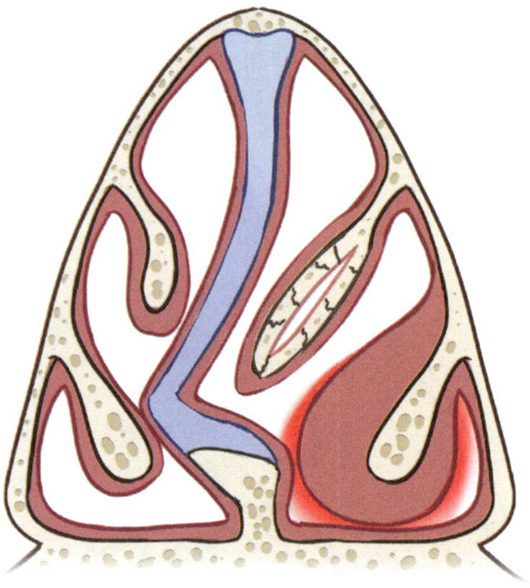

Fig. 16.18 Concha bullosa can be managed by crushing it with the help of Takahashi forceps

A second treatment option for concha bullosa is crushing it using forceps, such as Takahashi forceps (Fig. 16.18). This is a less bloody and easier intervention, but lateral lamella excision is more successful in my experience.

To sum up, there are many alternatives in the management of inferior and middle turbinate problems. Every surgeon has a certain way after experiencing some of the methods mentioned in this chapter. All of these methods have advantages and disadvantages. So, the choice will depend on the surgeon's expertise.

References

1. Lang J. Clinical anatomy of the nose, nasal cavity, and paranasal sinuses. 1st ed. George Thieme Verlag; 1989.
2. Hol MK, Huizing EH. Treatment of inferior turbinate pathology: a review and critical evaluation of the different techniques. Rhinology. 2000;38:157–66.
3. Kim HG, Kim DS, Choi YS, Lee ES, Yoo HJ, Kim DY. High-intensity focused ultrasound therapy versus coblation for the treatment of inferior turbinate hypertrophy: a clinical trial. Clin Exp Otorhinolaryngol. 2023;16:141–7.
4. Li KK, Powell NB, Riley RW, et al. Radiofrequency volumetric tissue reduction for the treatment of turbinate hypertrophy: a pilot study. Otolaryngol Head Neck Surg. 1998;119:569–73.
5. Smith TL, Smith JM. Electrosurgery in otolaryngology-head and neck surgery: principles, advances, and complications. Laryngoscope. 2001;111:769–80.
6. Elwany S, Harrison R. Inferior turbinectomy: comparison of four techniques. J Laryngol Otol. 1990;104:206–9.
7. Jackson LE, Koch R, James MD. Controversies in the management of inferior turbinate hypertrophy: a comprehensive review. Plast Reconstr Surg. 1999;103:300–12.
8. Mabry RL. Inferior turbinoplasty: patient selection, technique, and long-term consequences. Otolaryngol Head Neck Surg. 1988;98:60–6.
9. Chen YL, Tan CT, Huang HM. Long-term efficacy of microdebrider-assisted inferior turbinoplasty with lateralization for hypertrophic inferior turbinates in patients with perennial allergic rhinitis. Laryngoscope. 2008;118:1270–4.

10. Schmelzer B, Katz S, Vidts G. Long-term efficacy of our surgical approach to turbinate hypertrophy. Am J Rhinol. 1999;13:357–61.
11. Jarvis WMC. Removal of hypertrophied turbinated tissue by écrasement with the cold wire. Arch Laryngol. 1882;3:105–11.
12. Jones M. Turbinal hypertrophy. Lancet. 1895;2:895.
13. Lenz H, Eichler J, Knof J, Salk J, Schafer G. Endonasal Ar+-laser beam guide system and first clinical application in vasomotor rhinitis. Laryngol Rhinol Otol (Stuttgart). 1977;56:749.
14. Mittelman H. CO2-laser turbinectomies for chronic, obstructive rhinitis. Lasers Surg Med. 1982;2:29–36.
15. Ozenberger JM. Cryosurgery in chronic rhinitis. Laryngoscope. 1970;80:723–34.
16. Stammberger H. Endoscopic endonasal surgery—concepts in treatment of recurring rhinosinusitis. Part II. Surgical technique. Otolaryngol Head Neck Surg. 1986;94:147–56.

17 Packing and Splinting for Septal Surgery

17.1 Introduction

One of the most controversial issues in septoplasty and rhinoplasty is the use of packing and splints. In this chapter, I want to share my experience on this issue since 1987. When I first started septal surgery as submucous resection in 1988, sterile dry gauze strips or petroleum-impregnated gauze strips were the only options available to prevent postoperative bleeding and hematoma. I used to insert 5–6 gauze strips of 8–10 cm in length into each nasal passage. I later learned to use splints cut from used X-ray films. I learned to use sterile gauze strips in glove fingers. Then, the Merocel sponges came to the market, which was a revolutionary event for all of us. In the 1990s, I started using quilting sutures without any packing. Silicone splints were later introduced and became very popular. Recently, more technologically high-end products, such as self-dissolving materials in the nose, have become available.

17.2 Packs

17.2.1 Gauze Strips

The use of linen strips inside the nose dates back to Egyptian times, meaning they have been in use for thousands of years [1]. The use of gauze strips for epistaxis was the first thing I learned when I started residency. They are relatively practical and very cheap. I have a great deal of experience using this kind of packing after septoplasty and for epistaxis. You can see in drawings from earlier textbooks the application of a long gauze in the nose (Fig. 17.1). In our department, they were cut into 10-cm-long strips of gauze. I used to apply 5–6 pieces to each nasal passage. However, they were occlusive and very discomfortable for the patient, even though they were kept in place for 2 days. The major difficulty was in sleeping and eating for the patients during this time. An additional discomfort for the patient was during the removal of the gauze strips. Because they

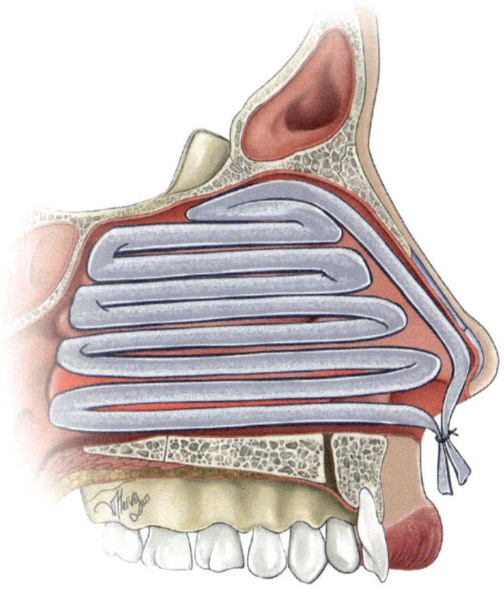

Fig. 17.1 Gauze strips were described as being used in cases of epistaxis and septal surgery

© The Author(s), under exclusive license to Springer Nature Switzerland AG 2025
F. Apaydın, *Septal Surgery Challenges in Rhinoplasty*,
https://doi.org/10.1007/978-3-031-74734-2_17

tended to swell and stick to the mucosa of the nose, their removal was extremely painful. I used to apply an oily drop into the nasal passages to soften the gauze strips and ease their removal. Besides, they could cause lacerations of the nasal mucosa ending with synechias.

17.2.2 Glove Finger

I learned about this method from my German colleagues when I was working in Tübingen as a researcher in 1993. I liked the idea very much because I was filling a glove finger with gauze strips and tying it. They were easy to apply and very easy to remove in seconds, which was extraordinary progress for me and my patients. I could not use them for a long time because Merocel® came to the market at that time.

17.2.3 Merocel

Merocel (Medtronic Xomed Inc., FL, USA) is a compressed, dehydrated sponge composed of hydroxylated polyvinyl acetate [2]. After insertion, it requires rehydration with normal saline to achieve its optimal size within the nasal cavity and compress the bleeding vessels. When it comes in contact with blood, it is decompressed (Fig. 17.2). When it became available, it was a revolutionary contribution for surgeons who had been using gauze packing since Egyptian times. When compared to gauze strips, they were more comfortable for the patients, and removal was quick, although painful. It was presented in two forms: 8 cm and 10 cm. The longer one could reach the nasopharynx to prevent posterior bleeding; however, they were more discomfortable for the patient. I used them for a long time until I started using quilting sutures and silicone splints. Currently, I do not use them at all after septoplasty or rhinoplasty. However, they are always in my office in case of severe bleeding, which I have not experienced during the last 15 years.

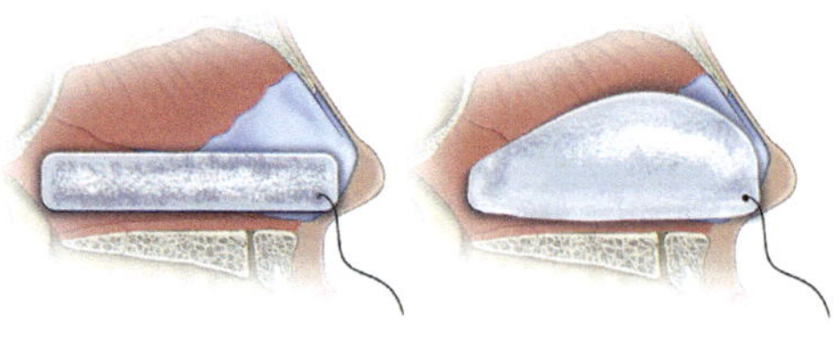

Fig. 17.2 Merocel is a compressed, dehydrated sponge composed of hydroxylated polyvinyl acetate, which decompresses inside the nose after insertion

Merocel with an airway was also brought to us to overcome some problems created by Merocel. They were quite helpful to the patients. When the patients were recovering from anesthesia, they did not feel a blocked nose, and they could breathe through their noses for some time after surgery.

Merocel caused all the problems created by gauze packs, except that it caused less discomfort for the patients than gauze packs, especially during removal. It was reported to be used in a glove finger, something which I never tried [3].

17.2.4 Absorbable Packs

I have been using absorbable products as an adjunct during or after rhinoplasty and septoplasty since 1989. I used three products all over these years, and I want to share my experience with them.

Gelfoam (Pharmacia & Upjohn Company, New York, NY, USA) is absorbable gelatin in the form of a sterile compressed sponge. It is intended for application to bleeding surfaces as a hemostatic agent. It is a water-insoluble, off-white, nonelastic, porous, pliable product prepared from purified porcine skin [4]. My chairman used to use it in tympanoplasties, and we started using it for epistaxis control and during the follow-up of septoplasty during my residency. Although it was not good enough to apply pressure on the nasal walls, it was good enough to stop bleeding and dissolved by itself in 2 weeks. After using it for almost 15 years, the supplier stopped marketing it.

Spongostan (Ferrosan, Copenhagen, Denmark) is an absorbable hemostatic gelatin sponge made from purified pork skin gelatin [5] (Fig. 17.3). It can be applied to the bleeding site,

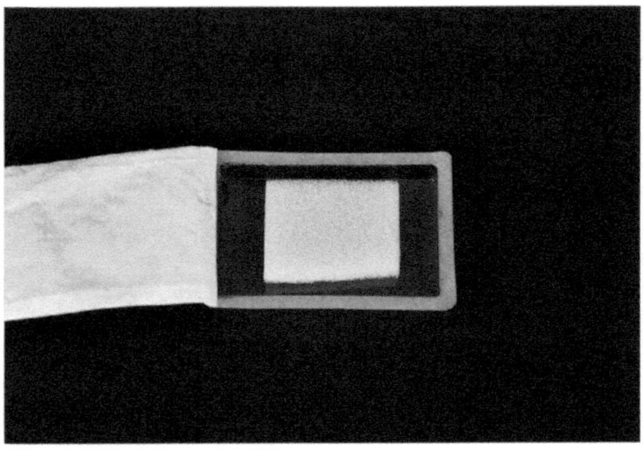

Fig. 17.3 Spongostan is an absorbable hemostatic gelatin sponge made from purified pork skin gelatin

cut in the form of a nasal pack like Gelfoam. I have been using this product for more than 20 years with great enthusiasm. In cases of concha bullosa, when the lateral lamella is resected, there is a tendency to bleed. In these situations, I fill the middle meatus with Spongostan strips. If the tail of the inferior turbinate needs resection, which is very rare in my practice, or a turbinoplasty is applied, I use Spongostan strips mixed with antibiotic ointment.

Surgicel (Johnson & Johnson) is an oxidized regenerated cellulose that has been used clinically since 1960 [6]. It absorbs water and swells to provide tamponade at the bleeding sites. I use it in rare conditions. At the end of rhinoplasty, if I feel that there may be some oozing from the needle insertion sites or due to a laceration in the nasal mucosa, I would like to cover these places with Surgicel strips. The advantage of it is that it is thin like a paper and does not add bulk to the nose like Spongostan. Sometimes, I place it under the internal valve area to help the mucoperichondrium stabilize because silicone splints cannot always reach those areas. There are more products available on the market, but I will not go into detail because I do not have experience with them [7].

17.3 Splints

I used splints cut from X-ray films in a very limited number of patients, and I have little experience with them [8]. However, I have been using Doyle silicone splints with an airway, which was presented in 1977 by Doyle et al. The original form was two splints connected to each other by a silicone band touching the columella [9, 10]. Silicone splints are my favorite splinting option (Fig. 17.4). There are three main types: plain silicone splints (without airway), silicone splints with airway, and silicone splints with airway and sponge.

I have been using the plain silicone splint after the management of septal perforations, where I can leave them in place for 2–3 weeks. They are very well tolerated by patients, and they work quite well while epithelization can continue under the silicone without any problems. When I used grafts to cover the tympanic perforations, silicone sheets were my workhorse for similar reasons. I have been using these splints after opening large synechiae as well.

Silicone splints with an airway are my favorite choice when I need a splint after finishing rhinoplasty or septoplasty. The splints are covered with a thin layer of antibiotic ointment and inserted into the nasal passages. They are fixated to the caudal septum using one mattress suture with 3-0 silk. All these years, I kept them for 1–7 days and learned the behavior of patients with these splints. At the moment, I keep them for 6 days, and for me, this is the optimal time. Why not 2, it is 6? Because I observed that the maximum swelling in the nose occurs during the first 4–5 days. In cases where I use a quilting suture, this period lasts even longer, and the patients cannot breathe through their noses for 2–3 weeks. However, if this faster swelling time is overcome with silicone splints in the nose and they are removed 6 days after surgery, patients can often start breathing through the nose immediately after splint removal. Therefore, patients usually tolerate silicone splints with an airway quite well.

There are additional advantages of silicone splints with an airway. When the inferior turbinate is outfractured, the splint can keep them in a lateralized position for almost a week, so the chance of remedialization is decreased. In cases of crooked noses where splinting of the nasal septum is realized, the splints are helpful for further

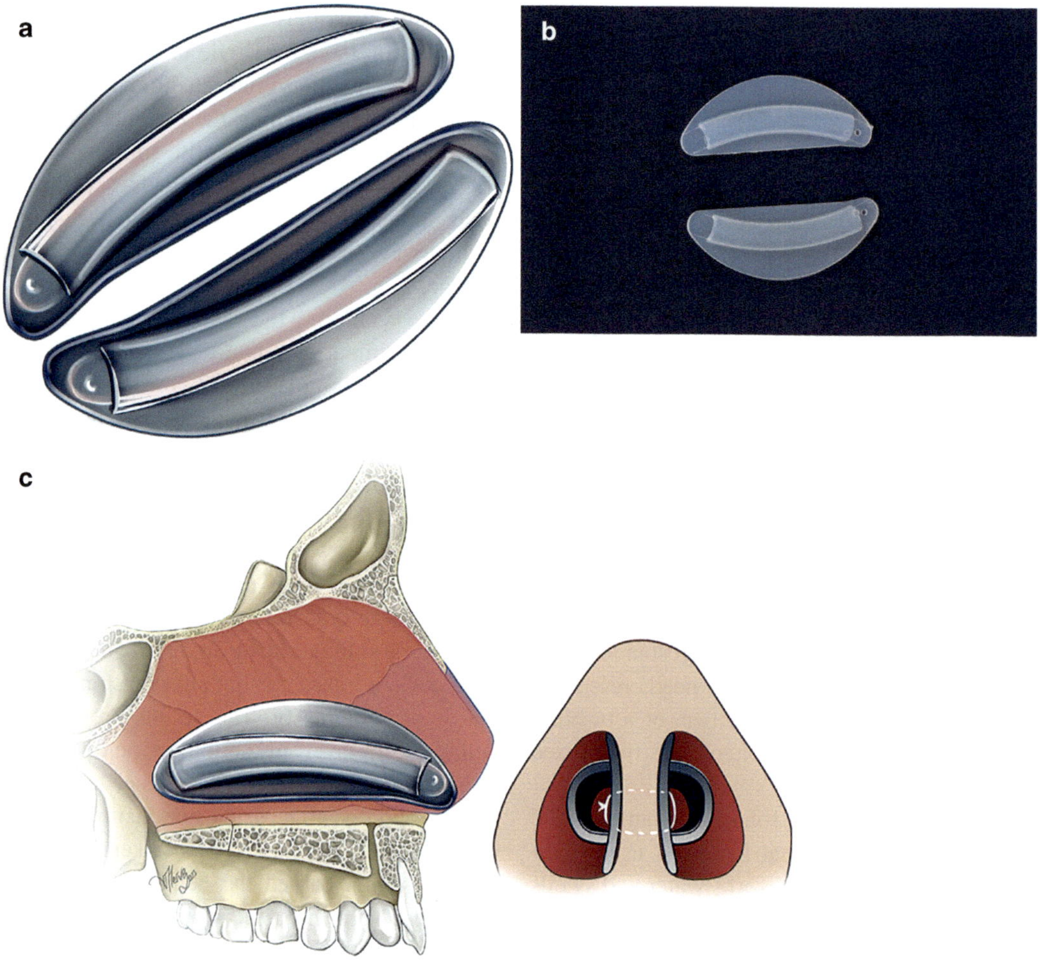

Fig. 17.4 Doyle silicone splints are my favorite packing material if needed as seen as an illustration (**a**) and in the picture (**b**). They are sutured to each other after being inserted into the nasal airways (**c**). They can stay inside from 2 to 7 days

stabilization of the reconstructed nasal septum. In cases where lateral crural repositioning is performed, these splints act as support to prevent hematoma formation under the lateral crura.

What are the drawbacks of these splints? The presence of a foreign body in the nose can cause discomfort, sneezing, and mucus discharge from the nose. In the first few days after surgery, because of the swelling, the patients can express a feeling of fullness around the nose. The anterior margins of the splints can irritate the nostril sils and very rarely create a wound there. The patient is asked to apply Bacitracin for 10–14 days routinely, and this treatment accelerates the healing of these wounds. Of course, the most stressful issue for the patient is the fear of silicone removal. There is a widespread belief in society that the removal of nasal packing is very painful, and patients can even faint during removal.

17.4 Transseptal Quilting Suture

I have been using transseptal quilting sutures for septoplasty since 1993 and for rhinoplasty since 1999 [11]. At the end of surgery, cotonoids soaked in 1% lidocaine with 1:100,000 adrenaline are inserted into the nose to decongest the mucosa. A 4-0 Vicryl Rapide (polyglactin 910; Ethicon) on a 13-mm Keith needle makes it eas-

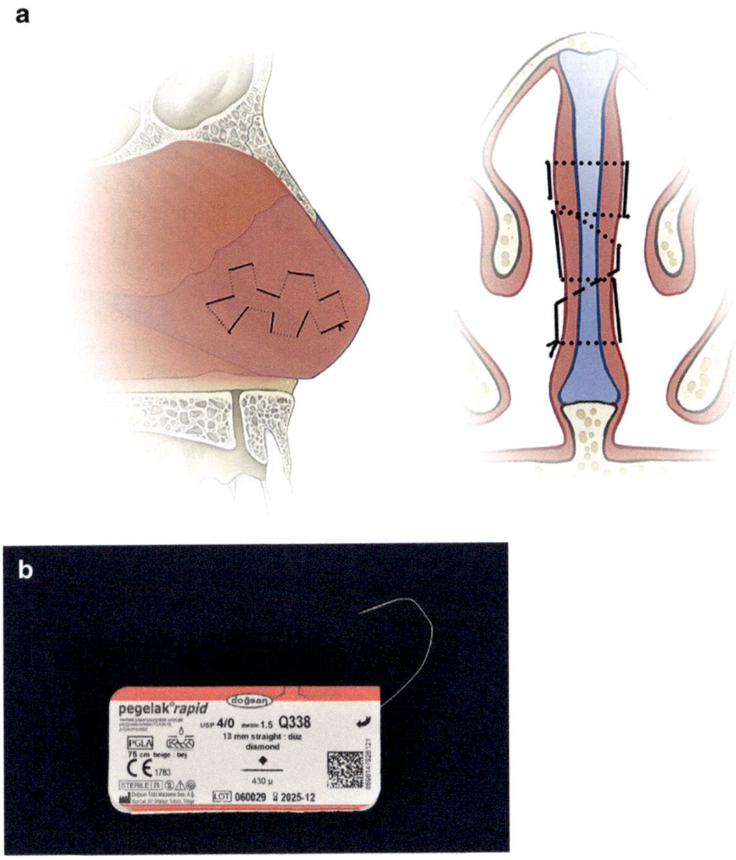

Fig. 17.5 Transseptal quilting suture is an elegant way to avoid packing. The illustrations show in two planes the zigzag pattern of suturing to close the dead space between the mucoperichondrial flaps (**a**). I like using 4-0 Vicryl Rapide on a 13 mm Keith needle (**b**)

ier to manipulate and suture inside the nose (Fig. 17.5). I have also used Vicryl for this purpose, but because it stayed longer, the patients felt a bad smell, and I saw crust formation around these sutures. So, I stopped using Vicryl in the nose for quilting.

How many sutures should we place, and how far should we go back? The idea is to close the dead space to prevent hematoma formation in the nose. So, I try to pass as much suture as possible at 4–5 mm apart from each other, starting from the anterior and then going back. The main reason I start anteriorly is that I would like to close the dead space, especially in Cottle zones 1–3, since these areas are more prone to septal hematoma formation. I usually go in a zigzag formation posteriorly. It is much easier to pass sutures up to 3 cm, but then it becomes more difficult. In addition, it is more difficult to pass sutures at the bony septum zone because the needle cannot pass through the bone. In cases of deviations reaching the bone, when the mucoperichondrium is dissected here, and if some of the bony septum is intact, I prefer to stop suturing at this point and insert silicone splints. If the bony septum is intact, quilting sutures are sufficient, and there is no need for splints.

I do not touch the nasal septum at all in less than 5% of my patients where the septal hump is resected, spreader flaps are used, and the resected cartilage can be used as a columellar strut. If the septal surgery is only confined to the cartilaginous dorsum, I prefer using transseptal quilting sutures. However, if the septal surgery is extended to the bony septum or a complex reconstruction of the nasal septum is performed, I like using silicone Doyle splints. If additional turbinate surgery is conducted, absorbable packs are used.

References

1. Elsberg CA. The Edwin Smith Surgical Papyrus: and the diagnosis and treatment of injuries to the skull and spine 5000 years ago. Ann Med Hist. 1931;3:271–9.
2. Weber R, Keerl R, Hochapfel F, Draf W, Toffel PH. Packing in endonasal surgery. Am J Otolaryngol. 2001;22:306–20.
3. Seyhan T. A comfortable and practical nasal packing method: tied Merocel in clear glove finger impregnated with lidocaine-prilocaine cream. Plast Reconstr Surg. 2010;125:111e–2e.
4. Anderson RL. Gelfoam packing after dacryocystorhinostomy. Arch Ophthalmol. 1977;95:520.
5. Cho KS, Park CH, Hong SL, Kim MJ, Kim JY, Kim YW, Koo SK, Roh HJ. Comparative analysis of Cutanplast and Spongostan nasal packing after endoscopic sinus surgery: a prospective, randomized, multicenter study. Eur Arch Otorrinolaringol. 2015;272:1699–705.
6. Gabay M. Absorbable hemostatic agents. Am J Health Syst Pharm. 2006;63:1244–53.
7. Massey CJ, Singh A. Advances in absorbable biomaterials and nasal packing. Otolaryngol Clin N Am. 2017;50:545–63.
8. Salinger S, Cohen BM. Surgery of the difficult septum. AMA Arch Otolaryngol. 1955;61:419–21.
9. Doyle DE, House LF, Hall WP. Description of a new device: an intranasal airway/splint. Laryngoscope. 1977;87:608–12.
10. Lau J, Elhassan HA, Singh N. History of intranasal splints. J Laryngol Otol. 2018;132:198–201.
11. Sessions RB. Membrane approximation by continuous mattress sutures following septoplasty. Laryngoscope. 1984;94:702–3.

18 Postoperative Follow-Up and Care After Rhinoplasty

18.1 Introduction

The patient–surgeon relationship moves to a new stage just after the surgery. The patient feels more vulnerable and scared after surgery because they face two important issues that they never have to face in their normal life routine: anesthesia and surgery. Therefore, the surgeon should prepare the patient by informing them about these two situations beforehand. However, even though all operations performed under general anesthesia create a comfortable environment for both the patient and the surgeon, the effect on the patient is very variable. Regardless of this situation, surgeons should always provide the best possible care just after surgery to the patient, family members, and/or friends. The surgeon should inform the patient about the course of the postoperative period and repeat the postoperative instructions (Table 18.1). These instructions should be given to the patient in written form. Besides, they should exist on your website or social media accounts as video instructions, if possible

© The Author(s), under exclusive license to Springer Nature Switzerland AG 2025
F. Apaydın, *Septal Surgery Challenges in Rhinoplasty*,
https://doi.org/10.1007/978-3-031-74734-2_18

Table 18.1 List of things to do by the patient after rhinoplasty

1.	Sleep with the head of the bed elevated or use two to three pillows. Do not move your head to the sides more than 45°. If you do more, the fractured fragments of the nose can move and result in unwanted distortion of the nose. Please follow this rule for at least 8 weeks until told otherwise. You can use a traveler pillow while sleeping because it prevents you from making a complete turn of your head to both sides.
2.	Keep your head elevated while leaning on the floor to prevent nose bleeding.
3.	Do not consume scalding drinks because the vapor coming from the drinks can increase nasal congestion and bleeding.
4.	Do not blow your nose until instructed. Wipe or dab the nose gently with Kleenex if necessary. You can clean the secretions and crusts in the nose gently by wiping with hydrogen peroxide and Bacitracin ointment.
5.	You will have a gauze drip pad placed beneath your nose. Change this pad when it is wet for the first 2–3 days following surgery.
6.	Use cold gels or ice packs over the nose and around the eyes and cheeks. Do not place ice packs directly on your skin. Please place a gauze or linen napkin between the applied areas and the cold gel.
7.	The nasal cast will remain in place for approximately 1 week and will be removed by the doctor. Please do not disturb it and keep it dry.
8.	Brush teeth gently with a soft toothbrush only. Avoid manipulation of the upper lip to keep the nose at rest.
9.	Avoid foods that require prolonged chewing. Please use less salt for at least 1 month after surgery.
10.	Rest for at least 1 week. Avoid athletic and sexual activities for 2 weeks.
11.	You may wash your face carefully, avoiding the cast. Take a shower, bypassing your head or tub baths, until the cast is removed. Go to a hairdresser for 1 week who can wash your hair without touching the cast unless you have someone who can do it for you. Do not get the nasal dressings wet.
12.	Avoid excessive or prolonged telephone conversations and social activities for at least 10–14 days.
13.	Avoid smiling, grinning, and excessive facial movements for 1 week.
14.	Wear clothing that fastens in front or back for 1 week. Avoid slipover sweaters, T-shirts, and turtlenecks.
15.	Avoid sun or sun lamps for 6 weeks after surgery because heat may cause swelling of the nose.
16.	Do not swim for at least 1 month. You may easily be confronted with some kind of trauma during swimming.
17.	Your face will be swollen within 3–4 days after surgery. The swelling usually subsides within 2–3 weeks. The whole swelling usually disappears within 12–18 months.
18.	You may have bruising around the eyes within 1–2 weeks after surgery. It is usually gone after 10 days. If it persists longer, camouflage with makeup can be applied.
19.	Take only medications prescribed by your doctor.
20.	Do not wear regular glasses or sunglasses that rest on the bridge of the nose for at least 8 weeks. Please use the thermoplastic cast removed from your nose for an additional 7 weeks if you wish to wear glasses or a mask.
21.	You can wear contact lenses 2–3 days after surgery.
22.	When the cast and tape are removed, the nasal skin can be gently cleaned with soaps and moisturizers. You should avoid applying pressure on your nose and clean it like a fragile ceramic for 8 weeks.

18.2 Immediate Postoperative Period (First 24 h, Table 18.2, Fig. 18.1)

The first few hours after surgery are the most critical for the patient because of surgical site pain, nausea, and vomiting. I usually administer an analgesic such as acetaminophen and/or a nonsteroidal anti-inflammatory drug such as diclofenac, along with an antiemetic agent such as ondansetron, usually half an hour before the patient recovers from anesthesia. In fact, anesthesiologists know much better than surgeons about the possible effects and side effects of the drugs used for anesthesiology during surgery. Therefore, it is highly critical to have close cooperation with them and ask for their help during the first 24 h.

18.2.1 Pain and Discomfort

I am a firm believer in preemptive analgesia to prevent breakthrough pain. The patient receives IV/IM acetaminophen during the first 12–24 h in the hospital. I like to prescribe a nonsteroidal anti-inflammatory drug such as diclofenac for 3–5 days after surgery. I would also like to inform the patient that a fullness or discomfort around the nose can occur because of the existence of

Table 18.2 List of complaints during the first 24 h and procedures performed during the first week

Postoperative period				
Immediate postoperative period (24 h)				
Pain	[ ] None	[ ] Mild	[ ] Moderate	[ ] Severe
Discomfort	[ ] None	[ ] Mild	[ ] Moderate	[ ] Severe
Nausea	[ ] None	[ ] Mild	[ ] Moderate	[ ] Severe
Vomiting	[ ] None	[ ] Mild	[ ] Moderate	[ ] Severe
Additional remarks				
Early postoperative period (24 h to 1 month)				
Suture removal				
Columellar	[ ] Days			
Alar base reduction	[ ] Days			
Intranasal	[ ] Days			
Auricular	[ ] Days			
Chest	[ ] Days			
Other	[ ] Days			
Nasal packing removal	[ ] Days			
Nasal cast removal	[ ] Days			
Intranasal splint removal	[ ] Days			

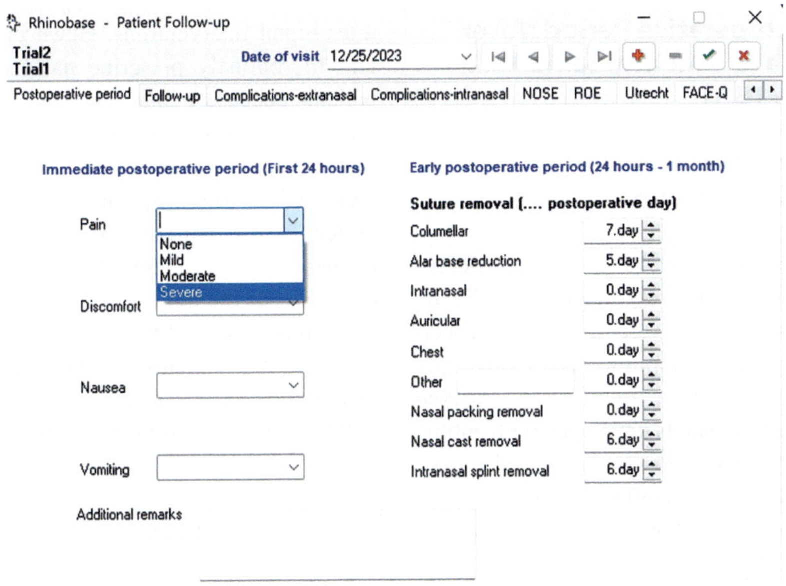

Fig. 18.1 The image shows a patient follow-up interface for postoperative care in a software named Rhinobase. The screen is divided into sections for the immediate postoperative period and early postoperative period. The immediate section includes dropdowns for selecting pain levels, with options ranging from "None" to "Severe," and fields for discomfort, nausea, vomiting, and additional remarks. The early postoperative section lists suture removal timelines for various areas, such as columellar and alar base reduction, with specified days for each. The date of visit is set to 12/25/2023

Doyle splints if they are used. It is very rare for patients to need a second analgesic or an opioid-type analgesic. In my opinion, the key factor in pain management is to prepare the patient preoperatively for pain after surgery and then provide close care after surgery.

18.2.2 Nausea and Vomiting

The anesthetist is asked to administer ondansetron half an hour before the end of the surgery so that it can be effective after recovery. I do not like to add corticosteroids with ondansetron to treat nausea. In my personal experience, I did not find any difference between the use of ondansetron and a combination of corticosteroid and ondansetron. The patient is allowed to drink water for 2 h and soup 4 h after recovery from anesthesia. However, it should also be noted that the patient can feel nausea and vomit as a reaction to anesthetic agents for 1–2 days.

18.3 Postoperative Period (After 24 h to 1 Month, Table 18.2, Fig. 18.1)

18.3.1 Decongestants: Antihistamines

Decongestants are available as topical or systemic agents. They are very helpful for relieving nasal congestion. However, in addition to congestion, allergy-like symptoms such as sneezing, pruritus, and rhinorrhea are usually observed. Therefore, decongestants developed with antihistamines are the way to go to relieve nasal congestion and the allergic symptom complex.

The primary effect of antihistamines is to diminish pruritus, sneezing, and rhinorrhea. The preferred antihistamines are loratadine, acrivastine, cetirizine, and fexofenadine. These preparations are reported to have no cardiotoxic side effects and are generally considered nonsedating at normal doses [1].

The best systematic agent as a decongestant is pseudoephedrine. The most common side effect of these agents is cardiovascular stimulation, such as blood pressure elevation, tachycardia, palpitations, and even arrhythmias. The central nervous system can be stimulated, and anxiety and insomnia can be observed in these patients. Therefore, systemic decongestants should be administered cautiously and in reduced doses in patients with hypertension, atherosclerotic coronary artery disease, and hyperthyroidism, and in those with urinary retention [2, 3].

As a topical decongestant, I routinely administer oxymetazoline after surgery unless there are splints in the nose for 5 days, three times a day. If there are Doyle nasal splints, an oxymetazoline spray is applied after splint removal for 5 days.

18.3.2 Nasal Saline

Topical nasal saline can be used for nasal douches after rhinoplasty. I used hypertonic nasal saline irrigation after septoplasty starting from my residency years. Hypertonic saline is more powerful than normal saline in reducing mucosal swelling after septal interventions. However, I am reluctant to routinely prescribe nasal saline to my patients because I cannot be sure how well they will apply it. The main reason is that I am scared that they could mobilize the osteotomized fragments of the bony pyramid during irrigation. I prefer that the patients clean their nostrils with oxygen peroxide or Bacitracin ointment applied on Q-tips. If the patient insists, then I explain in detail how it should be used. One of the biggest mistakes that patients can make is reading the instructions on the bottle and using nasal saline with too much pressure inside the nose.

18.3.3 Antibiotics

There is no consensus among surgeons on the use of antibiotics after rhinoplasty. I have been using Amoxicillin/clavulanate postoperatively for 1 week for three decades. I did not see any serious side effects except for a few in the form of allergic reactions and diarrhea.

Toriumi et al. recently reported that the use of antibiotic soaks and irrigation reduced infection rates after rhinoplasty, particularly in secondary rhinoplasty. It is suggested to use them in patients undergoing rhinoplasty, particularly those with a history of extensive revision, trauma, filler, prior infection, or underlying disease processes [4].

A meta-analysis investigating the value of preventive antibiotics in rhinoplasty was published in 2019. These results suggest that the use of preventive antibiotic therapy in rhinoplasty is not recommended [5]. However, this is a hot topic that we have been discussing with the most prominent surgeons in our meetings. I know from personal communications that many of them use antibiotics for their patients after rhinoplasty.

18.3.4 Steroid Use

I have not been using steroids perioperatively for any of my patients over the years. I tried in some patients but did not see any significant difference. A meta-analysis of this subject was performed in 2016. It was stated that there was high-quality evidence that a single dose of systemic perioperative corticosteroids reduced edema and ecchymosis on day 1. However, there was no significant change on day 7. It was also stated that the addition of a postoperative oral steroid course did not change the results. It was concluded that perioperative steroid treatment remains an option for patients undergoing rhinoplasty to reduce short-term soft tissue side effects [6].

18.3.5 Packing

I prefer using silicone Doyle splints if any procedure is performed at the bony septum or a major reconstruction of the L-strut framework is performed in a crooked nose. I usually remove them on the sixth postoperative day. I do not apply any packing if the intervention is made only on the septal cartilage and the dead space can be closed by quilting sutures. I have provided detailed information in the previous chapter on why I did not remove them earlier.

18.3.6 Cold Application

When the patient comes out of the OR, the nurses start cold application on and around the nose immediately. It is applied for 4–6 h on the operation day. Then, it is applied three times a day for 2 h for 3 days. The edema is the greatest for the first 3–4 days after surgery. Then, they start to migrate to the cheeks and down the face. Ideally, patients should continue cold application as long as possible during the first week, but it is not very easy because of staying in bed during that time.

As the source of the cold, I prefer using gels kept in the refrigerator. They are flexible, can be molded to fit on the midface, and can remain cold for 5–15 min. The cheaper ones are covered with nylon, and gauze must be kept on the skin to prevent skin damage from direct application of cold. There are more expensive types of gels covered by fabric instead of nylon, which do not necessitate the use of any additional gauze on the face. Some surgeons ask nurses to put ice cubes in their surgical gloves and use them. I do not find them as effective as gel packs. Some machines connected to facial masks can help the patient adjust the temperature on the face. Although this method seems to be the best for me, it is much more expensive for the patient.

18.3.7 Cast Removal

I have been using thermoplastic casts for 24 years without any complaints from patients or complications. When I was a resident, the traditional plaster of Paris was the standard application for a rhinoplasty cast. My chairman was so obsessive about trying to immobilize the entire nose, and the cast was so big that it extended to the forehead and cheeks, and then a surgical dressing was used all around the face. The patient looked like a mummy after rhinoplasty for a week. My mentor, Eugene Tardy, used to put a Denver splint as a cast. Having used three of these methods during the last three decades, I like thermoplastic casting the most. First, it is much easier to customize the thermoplastic cast for each patient after rhinoplasty. Second, it maintains its shape well and applies the same pressure because of its elasticity during the first week after rhinoplasty. The nose starts swelling immediately after surgery, the swelling reaches its peak during the first 3–4 days, and then starts subsiding incrementally in 4–7 days. The plaster of Paris and Denver splints are deformed during the swelling period and then stay bigger than the nose without applying any pressure on it. Third, it is much better tolerated by the patient in daily life. Fourth, I give the cast back to the patient to keep using it in case of putting on glasses or wearing masks for an additional 7 weeks. It gives relief to the patient and me as the surgeon because the cast can prevent any kind of trauma caused by the glasses and masks.

How long do I keep the cast in place? When I returned from Chicago 24 years ago, I tended to keep the cast in place for 5 days, as I had learned from my mentor, Dr. Dean Toriumi. Over time, I realized that the swelling could persist on the fifth day in my patients, and it would be better to remove it on the sixth or seventh day. I keep the cast for 10 days in crooked noses or in preservation rhinoplasty cases, thinking that the patients need longer stability of the nose. In my conversations with my colleagues, I learned that some of them tended to keep the cast for 2 weeks. I never tried it because I observed some skin reactions in 5–10 days, especially in patients with thick, oily skin.

How do I remove the cast from the patient? I used to pour Detachol on the cast and tape, an adhesive remover that I liked very much. Unfortunately, this solution does not exist in Türkiye, and it was not always easy to find. I started pouring alcohol for some time, but some of the patients felt discomfort, mainly because of the alcohol's irritation on the damaged skin. Then I changed to baby lotion, which is used on babies to prevent diaper rash. It is useful to moisturize and nourish the damaged skin due to trauma from the tape and cast. Besides, it has antiseptic properties.

18.3.8 Taping

I like using taping for one more week after cast removal. In my opinion, it is often a neglected and underrated part of rhinoplasty. Surgeons tend to leave this part to their residents, fellows, or nurse practitioners. I saw in one of my cases that the tape was about to cause partial skin necrosis of the columellar flap. I learned from this case that the surface of the tape should always touch the skin evenly. It should not be applied too tightly, keeping in mind that the nose will swell. As mentioned above, when the cast is removed within a week, the tape is removed as well. I always apply taping for one more week after cast removal. I learned from my colleagues in the Middle East that they were using taping for at least a month and even longer, up to 6 months. The main reason for this application is to decrease the edema of the thick skin, especially at the supratip area.

Ozucer et al. reported in a randomized study that 2 weeks of postoperative taping was sufficient for thin skin patients, whereas it should be for 4 weeks in patients with thick skin to decrease postoperative swelling, especially at the supratip area [7]. I do not like patients to apply taping by themselves for two reasons: (1) I do not trust them that they can apply taping properly. (2) The removal of tapes by the patient can cause more trauma to the nose.

18.3.9 Sutures

I have been using endonasal and external rhinoplasty approaches for almost 30 years. There was a time when I used 6-0 Prolene (polypropylene; Ethicon) sutures for closing the inverted-V incision. When a patient of mine left my office because of her fear of stitch removal in 2006, I switched to absorbable sutures for all kinds of wound closures in rhinoplasty, except wedge excision and revision rhinoplasty cases. I have been using Vicryl Rapide 6-0 for inverted-V closure since 2006. I also tried Monocryl recently, thinking that it could create fewer reactions because of its monofilament structure. Surprisingly, I did not observe a major difference between the two in terms of wound healing and scar formation. Marginal incisions, hemitransfixion incisions, quilting sutures, and chest incisions for rib harvest are closed with absorbable sutures. Therefore, I rarely remove stitches. I always ask the patient to cover the suture lines with Bacitracin ointment for 2 weeks.

On a special note, I have been using 4-0 Vicryl Rapide on a 13-mm Keith needle for quilting sutures for almost 30 years. I have started using Vicryl sutures before. However, it caused crusting and a bad smell because it was absorbed in 6–8 weeks. Therefore, I never use Vicryl sutures for closing the dead space inside the nose.

18.4 Follow-Up

I have a statement that I tell my fellows and residents: "Until you operate on a patient, you have the power. After rhinoplasty, the roles change, and the patient has the power." Because rhinoplasty is a psychosurgery, you should always take care of your patient after surgery and act like a psychologist in addition to being a surgeon. Experienced surgeons know that this is not an easy task. I know of surgeons who wanted to quit facial plastic surgery because of the heavy pressure coming from the patients after surgery. Therefore, please never abandon your patient and try to stay calm and not get angry.

My rhinoplasty cases leave the hospital if I operate on them in the morning and stay in the hospital if I operate on them in the afternoon. I always see them before being discharged and speak about the instructions at home. On postoperative days 1 and 2, I always call to determine how they are. The next visit is usually 6–7 days after surgery in my office, where the cast and splints are removed. Taping is applied in the office after cast removal.

The patient comes for a routine visit 2 weeks after surgery for tape removal. If the patient is from a distant place, she/he is said to take a shower where the tapes come off easily. The bruising usually subsides within 2 weeks. The patient is examined one more time to see if there are any crusting, bleeding sites, discharge, dryness, or swelling in the nose (Fig. 18.2, Table 18.3).

The third visit is 6 weeks after surgery. The patient is questioned about the airway and esthetic appearance even though the nose is still swollen. The following visits are on the 12th week, 6th month, and 1 year after surgery. During these visits, the nose is examined to determine if there are any external or intranasal complications (Figs. 18.3 and 18.4; Tables 18.4 and 18.5). The patient is given a SCHNOS questionnaire in the sixth month and 1 year after surgery (Fig. 18.5). At the end of 1 year, if the patient has functional

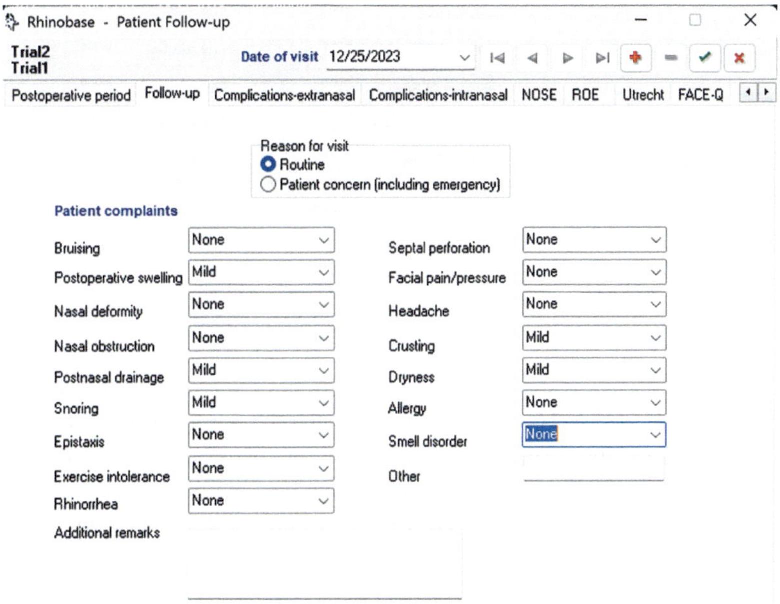

Fig. 18.2 The possible complaints that a rhinoplasty patient can have in the follow-up period are listed in this screenshot

Table 18.3 List of complaints that can be reported by the patient during the follow-up period

Patient complaints				
Reason for the visit	[ ] Routine	[ ] Patient concern		
Bruising	[ ] None	[ ] Mild	[ ] Moderate	[ ] Severe
Postoperative swelling	[ ] None	[ ] Mild	[ ] Moderate	[ ] Severe
Nasal deformity	[ ] None	[ ] Mild	[ ] Moderate	[ ] Severe
Nasal obstruction	[ ] None	[ ] Mild	[ ] Moderate	[ ] Severe
Postnasal drainage	[ ] None	[ ] Mild	[ ] Moderate	[ ] Severe
Snoring	[ ] None	[ ] Mild	[ ] Moderate	[ ] Severe
Epistaxis	[ ] None	[ ] Mild	[ ] Moderate	[ ] Severe
Exercise intolerance	[ ] None	[ ] Mild	[ ] Moderate	[ ] Severe
Rhinorrhea	[ ] None	[ ] Mild	[ ] Moderate	[ ] Severe
Septal perforation	[ ] None	[ ] Mild	[ ] Moderate	[ ] Severe
Facial pain/pressure	[ ] None	[ ] Mild	[ ] Moderate	[ ] Severe
Headache	[ ] None	[ ] Mild	[ ] Moderate	[ ] Severe
Crusting	[ ] None	[ ] Mild	[ ] Moderate	[ ] Severe
Dryness	[ ] None	[ ] Mild	[ ] Moderate	[ ] Severe
Allergy	[ ] None	[ ] Mild	[ ] Moderate	[ ] Severe
Smell disorder	[ ] None	[ ] Mild	[ ] Moderate	[ ] Severe
Additional remarks				

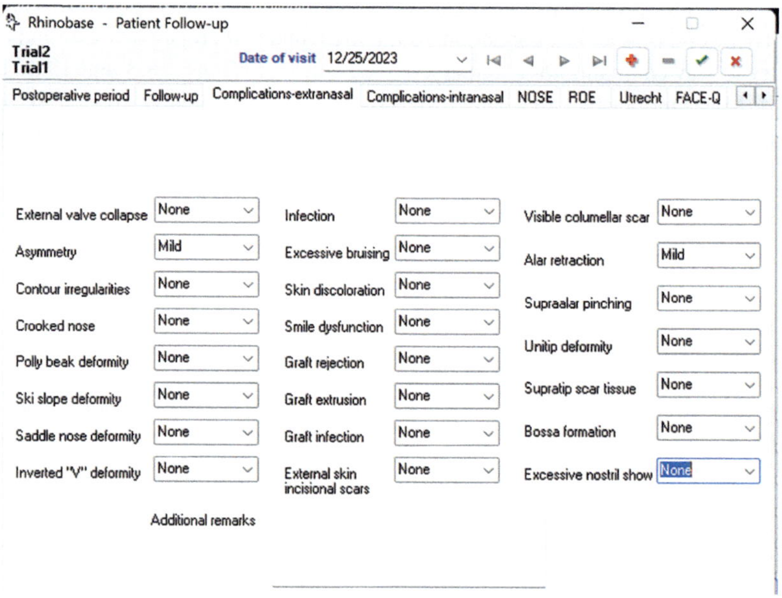

Fig. 18.3 Extranasal complications after rhinoplasty are listed here

or esthetic concerns, they are discussed with the patient after detailed intranasal and extranasal examination. If the concerns of the patient have a basis, the pros and cons of revision rhinoplasty are discussed with the patient. All the tables and screenshots presented in this chapter are from Rhinobase, a special software that we have been using since 2000. It is a database program that allows surgeons to enter all kinds of data before, during and after surgery in a systematic way [8].

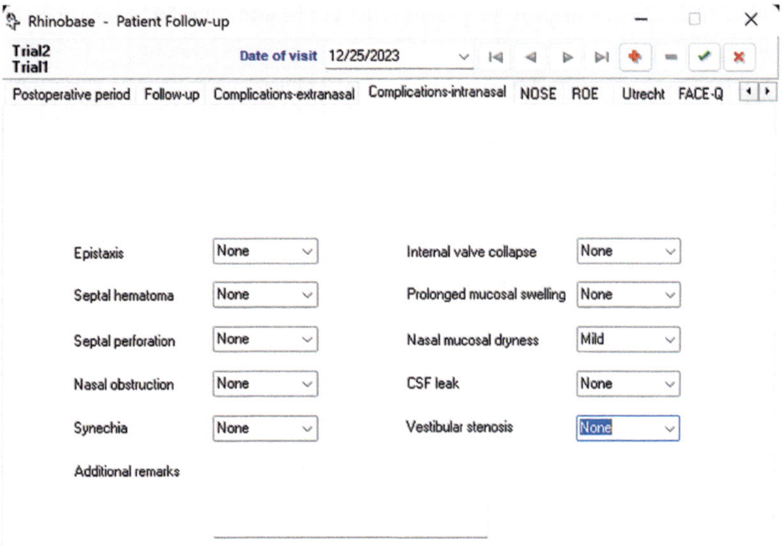

Fig. 18.4 This screenshot from Rhinobase shows the possible intranasal complications after rhinoplasty

Table 18.4 List of extranasal complications that can be seen in the follow-up period

Extranasal complications				
External valve collapse	[ ] None	[ ] Mild	[ ] Moderate	[ ] Severe
Asymmetry	[ ] None	[ ] Mild	[ ] Moderate	[ ] Severe
Contour irregularities	[ ] None	[ ] Mild	[ ] Moderate	[ ] Severe
Crooked nose	[ ] None	[ ] Mild	[ ] Moderate	[ ] Severe
Polly beak deformity	[ ] None	[ ] Mild	[ ] Moderate	[ ] Severe
Saddle nose deformity	[ ] None	[ ] Mild	[ ] Moderate	[ ] Severe
Inverted V deformity	[ ] None	[ ] Mild	[ ] Moderate	[ ] Severe
Infection	[ ] None	[ ] Mild	[ ] Moderate	[ ] Severe
Excessive bruising	[ ] None	[ ] Mild	[ ] Moderate	[ ] Severe
Skin discoloration	[ ] None	[ ] Mild	[ ] Moderate	[ ] Severe
Smile dysfunction	[ ] None	[ ] Mild	[ ] Moderate	[ ] Severe
Graft rejection	[ ] None	[ ] Mild	[ ] Moderate	[ ] Severe
Graft extrusion	[ ] None	[ ] Mild	[ ] Moderate	[ ] Severe
Graft infection	[ ] None	[ ] Mild	[ ] Moderate	[ ] Severe
External skin incisional scar	[ ] None	[ ] Mild	[ ] Moderate	[ ] Severe
Visible columellar scar	[ ] None	[ ] Mild	[ ] Moderate	[ ] Severe
Alar retraction	[ ] None	[ ] Mild	[ ] Moderate	[ ] Severe
Supraalar pinching	[ ] None	[ ] Mild	[ ] Moderate	[ ] Severe
Unitip deformity	[ ] None	[ ] Mild	[ ] Moderate	[ ] Severe
Supratip scar tissue	[ ] None	[ ] Mild	[ ] Moderate	[ ] Severe
Bossa formation	[ ] None	[ ] Mild	[ ] Moderate	[ ] Severe
Excessive nostril show	[ ] None	[ ] Mild	[ ] Moderate	[ ] Severe
Additional remarks				

Table 18.5 List of intranasal complications that can be seen in the follow-up period

Intranasal complications				
Epistaxis	[ ] None	[ ] Mild	[ ] Moderate	[ ] Severe
Septal hematoma	[ ] None	[ ] Mild	[ ] Moderate	[ ] Severe
Septal perforation	[ ] None	[ ] Mild	[ ] Moderate	[ ] Severe
Nasal obstruction	[ ] None	[ ] Mild	[ ] Moderate	[ ] Severe
Synechia	[ ] None	[ ] Mild	[ ] Moderate	[ ] Severe
Internal valve collapse	[ ] None	[ ] Mild	[ ] Moderate	[ ] Severe
Prolonged mucosal swelling	[ ] None	[ ] Mild	[ ] Moderate	[ ] Severe
Nasal mucosal dryness	[ ] None	[ ] Mild	[ ] Moderate	[ ] Severe
CSF leak	[ ] None	[ ] Mild	[ ] Moderate	[ ] Severe
Vestibular stenosis	[ ] None	[ ] Mild	[ ] Moderate	[ ] Severe
Additional remarks				

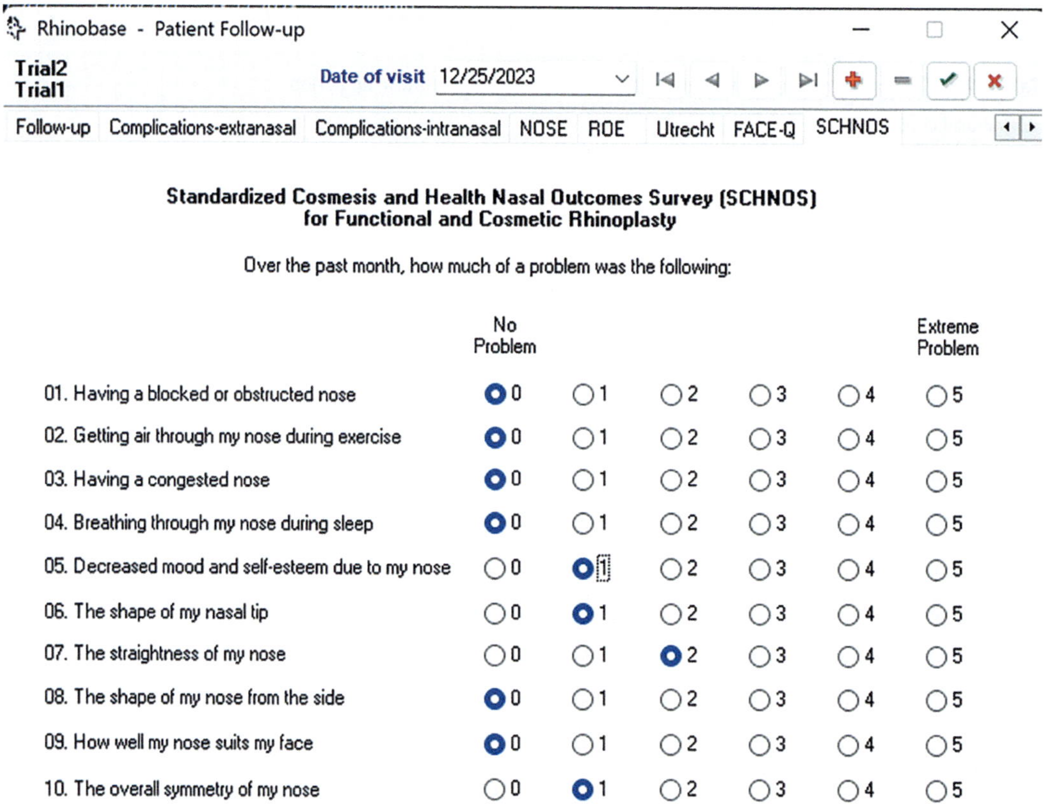

Fig. 18.5 It is important to follow the rhinoplasty patients by using patient-reported outcome measures to assess the functional, psychological, and esthetic status at a particular point in time

The patient's care after surgery is a very important time when the patient should never feel abandoned. Because this is the time when nothing is done surgically, but the surgeon should show his/her role as a good psychologist.

References

1. Hindmarch I, Shamsi Z. Antihistamines: models to assess sedative properties, assessment of sedation, safety and other side-effects. Clin Exp Allergy. 1999;29(Suppl 3):133–42.
2. Beck RA, Mercano DL, Seguin SM, Andrade WP, Cushner HM. Cardiovascular effects of pseudoephedrine in medically controlled hypertensive patients. Arch Intern Med. 1992;152:1242–5.
3. Kroenke K, Omori DM, Simmons JO, Wood DR, Meier NJ. The safety of phenylpropanolamine in patients with stable hypertension. Ann Intern Med. 1989;111:1043–4.
4. Toriumi DM, Kowalczyk DM, Cristel RT, Caniglia AJ, Curran N, Lombard R, Kerolus JL. Evaluation of postoperative infection rates in 3084 rhinoplasty cases using antibiotic soaks and/or irrigations. Facial Plast Surg Aesthet Med. 2021;23:368–74.
5. Nuyen B, Kandathil CK, Laimi K, Rudy SF, Most SP, Saltychev M. Evaluation of antibiotic prophylaxis in rhinoplasty: a systematic review and meta-analysis. JAMA Facial Plast Surg. 2019;21:12–7.
6. Coroneos CJ, Voineskos SH, Cook DJ, Farrokyar F, Thoma A. Perioperative corticosteroids reduce short-term edema and ecchymosis in rhinoplasty: a meta-analysis. Aesthet Surg J. 2016;36:136–46.
7. Ozucer B, Yildirim YS, Veyseller B, Tugrul S, Eren SB, Aksoy F, Uysal O, Ozturan O. Effect of postrhinoplasty taping on postoperative edema and nasal draping: a randomized clinical trial. JAMA Facial Plast Surg. 2016;18:157–63.
8. Apaydin F, Akyildiz S, Hecht DA, Toriumi DM. Rhinobase: a comprehensive database, facial analysis, and picture-archiving software for rhinoplasty. Arch Facial Plast Surg. 2009;11:209–11.

19 Lamb Head as a Training Model for Septorhinoplasty

19.1 Introduction

There is no doubt that fresh frozen cadavers are the gold standard in teaching septoplasty and rhinoplasty. However, reaching cadavers for surgical training has become very difficult and expensive recently worldwide. Therefore, teachers are always in search of a good method to help trainees practice septoplasty and rhinoplasty. To my knowledge, apart from silicone models of the face and nose, there is not a good alternative as a training model for trainees to exercise the surgical steps of septoplasty and rhinoplasty.

In 2009, I was invited by Ranko Mladina from Zagreb to lecture on rhinoplasty and participate in a lamb head dissection course. He developed a lamb head model for sinus surgery [1] and asked me if I wanted to try it for rhinoplasty. I was quite amazed with the specifications of the model at that time, but I must admit that due to lack of experience and only using it once discouraged me from using it later. In 2019, one of my fellows asked me if there was a good model for practicing all the techniques he was learning. At that time, the lamb head came to mind, and I decided to work on it in a systematic way to see if it would be an ideal model for my residents and fellows to practice before they start operating on patients.

We conducted two studies with my fellows using the lamb head as a model with great success from 2019 to 2022 [2, 3]. In the first one, a systematic dissection plan was applied to 21 lamb heads, which then became our routine dissection plan. It is very easy to reach lamb heads in Türkiye because they are sold in the butchers for a reasonable price, because they are a delicacy in Turkish cuisine. However, these lamb heads are without skin, and they can be used easily to practice most of the surgical steps. However, I advise you to use heads with skin for dissection (Fig. 19.1). Therefore, it needs to be ordered from the butcher in advance. They come fresh frozen with intact skin. One night before the dissection, the heads should be kept at room temperature for defrosting. While writing the articles, we found that Brazilian colleagues have already published an article using lamb head as a model for training rhinoplasty [4].

Supplementary Information The online version contains supplementary material available at https://doi.org/10.1007/978-3-031-74734-2_19. The videos can be accessed individually by clicking the DOI link in the accompanying figure caption or by scanning this link with the SN More Media App.

© The Author(s), under exclusive license to Springer Nature Switzerland AG 2025

F. Apaydın, *Septal Surgery Challenges in Rhinoplasty*,
https://doi.org/10.1007/978-3-031-74734-2_19

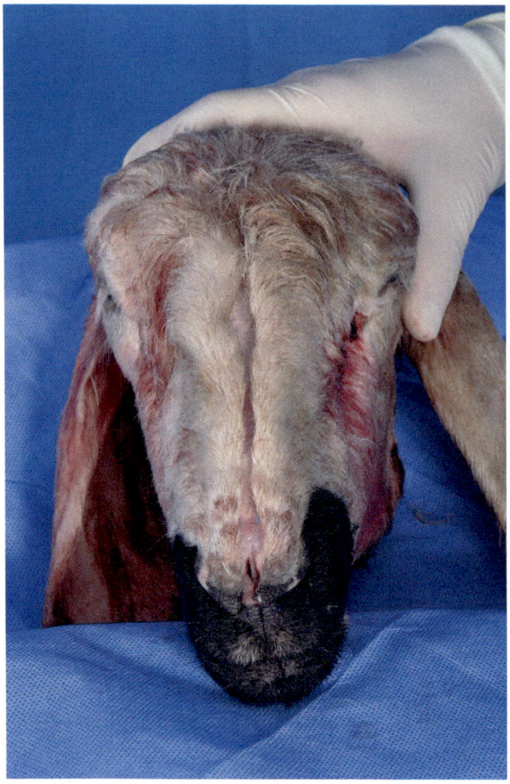

Fig. 19.1 Lamb head with skin. A gloved hand holds the head of a sheep, which is positioned on a blue surgical drape

Table 19.1 Dissection plan for structural rhinoplasty on lamb head

1. Preparation of the lamb head
2. Preparation of the surgical setting
3. Injection of the tip and dorsum
4. Columellar incision
5. Tip exposure
6. Dorsum exposure
7. Dissection of the skin and cutting it in the midline
8. Elevation of perichondrial and periosteal flaps
9. Caudal septum exposure
10. Bilateral elevation of mucoperichondrial flaps
11. Separate the upper lateral cartilages from septum
12. Cartilaginous hump removal
13. Application of spreader flaps
14. Bony hump removal (Rubin osteotome and Piezotome)
15. Osteotomies
    (a) Medial
    (b) Transverse
    (c) Lateral
16. Septal cartilage harvest
17. Carve grafts
    (a) Spreader graft: First suture these at the level and then under the level of the dorsal margin
    (b) Tip onlay graft
    (c) Shield graft
    (d) Articulated rim graft
    (e) Septal extension graft
18. Application of spreader grafts
19. Apply septal extension graft
20. Cephalic trim
21. Apply suture techniques
    (a) Domal suture
    (b) Hemitransdomal suture
    (c) Cranial tip suture
    (d) Dome equalizing suture
    (e) Tongue-in-groove suture
22. Use tip grafts
    (a) Tip onlay graft
    (b) Shield graft
    (c) Articulated rim graft
23. Camouflage
    (a) Diced cartilage
    (b) Cartilage chips
    (c) Cartilage dust

19.2 Dissection for Structural Rhinoplasty Techniques

The lamb head dissection can be performed anywhere, which is a big advantage for the trainee. A table with a comfortable chair is recommended. The trainee should carry a headlight, standard surgical gown, and gloves. Caving headlights are a cheaper solution to use during a dissection session. A basic rhinoplasty operation set should be present on the table. Prof. Mladina has designed a special holder for the lamb head; however, we have been using surgical drapes to hold the head in position, which work fine.

Our first task was to standardize the surgical steps of structural rhinoplasty in lamb heads (Table 19.1). The procedure begins with the injection of the incision lines and dissection planes. An inverted "V" and marginal incisions are performed using the No. 15 blade. The columella and medial crura are too short in lamb heads, and utmost care should be taken to complete the incisions. The tip and dorsum are exposed after dissecting the soft tissue envelope. The average anteroposterior length of the lateral crura was 17.8 mm, and the average cephalocaudal length was 11.6 mm in lamb heads in our study. It is approximately 22 × 12 mm in Caucasians, as I have measured it many times

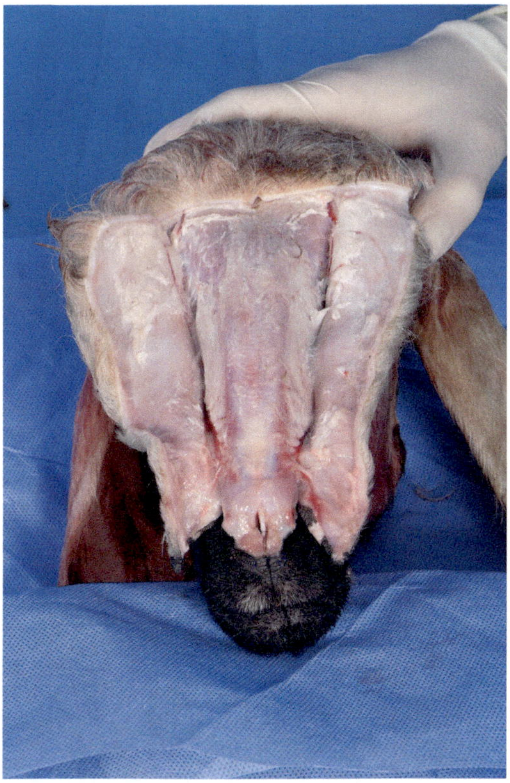

Fig. 19.2 After inverted-V incision, the dorsum is elevated, and the skin over the dorsum is cut in the midline to expose the whole dorsum

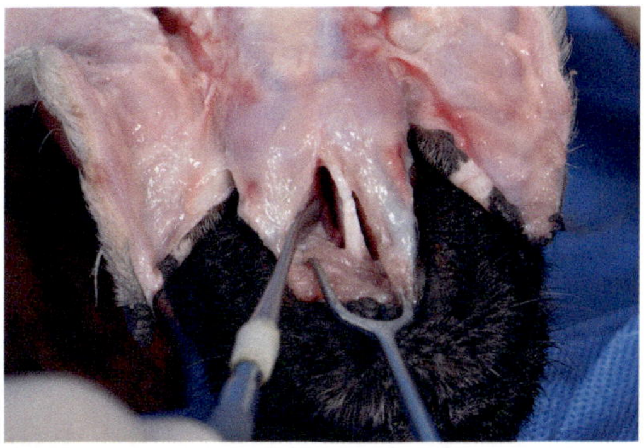

Fig. 19.3 The caudal septum is reached after dividing the soft tissues in the midline. The lamb has no medial crura. Mucoperichondrial flaps are elevated on both sides

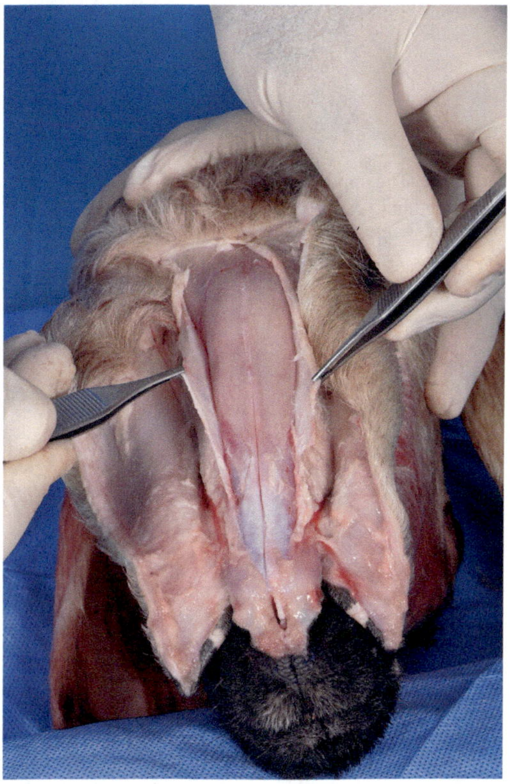

Fig. 19.4 Perichondrio-periosteal flap elevated on the nasal dorsum

during my surgeries. The average interdomal distance was found to be 8.1 mm, and the average domal width was 3.7 mm [2].

The dorsal skin was cut vertically at the midline to the level of the nasion for better exposure (Fig. 19.2). Perichondrial and periosteal flaps are elevated after a midline incision on the osseocartilaginous dorsum (Fig. 19.3).

The average length of the upper lateral cartilages was 31.1 mm at the lateral margin and 21.2 mm at the midline. The average length of the nasal bones was 63.9 mm, and the width was 16 mm. The nasal bones are much larger than those in human specimens. Therefore, the trainee can practice osteotomies for a longer time on a bigger surface (Fig. 19.4).

The average dimension of the harvested septal cartilage was 45 × 20 mm without removing the bony dorsum. However, it is best to wait for cartilage harvest after bony hump removal because it is possible to obtain a larger cartilage graft [2].

The caudal septum is exposed after dissecting the short medial crura in the midline, followed by elevation of bilateral mucoperichondrial flaps.

The upper lateral cartilage is cut away from the septal cartilage (Figs. 19.5 and 19.6). Septal humpectomy of 3–4 mm is performed using a scalpel (Fig. 19.7). The spreader flaps are created to reconstruct the middle vault at the lower half of the dorsum (Fig. 19.8). It is recommended to use two to three mattress sutures.

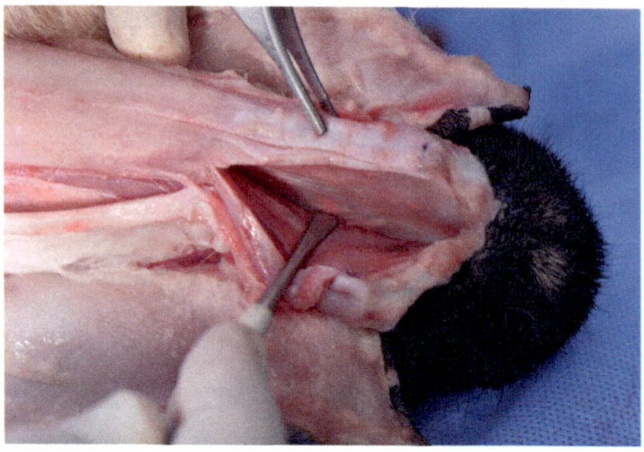

Fig. 19.5 The upper lateral cartilage is cut away from the nasal septum to expose the nasal septum

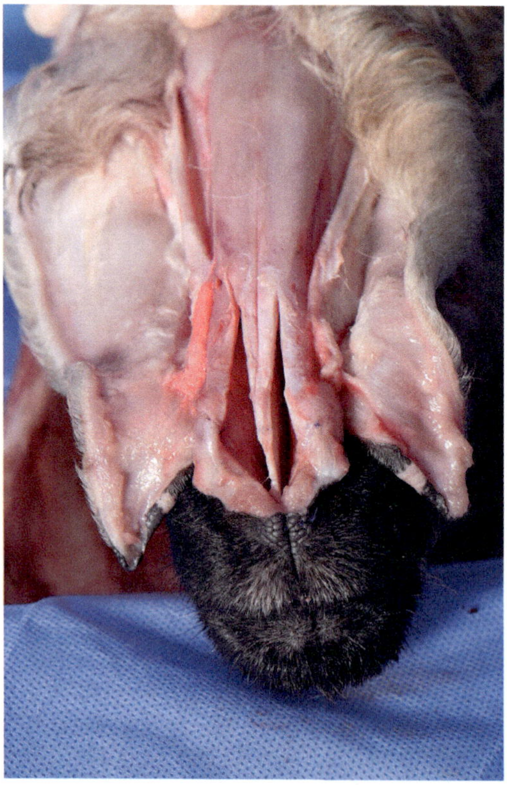

Fig. 19.6 Both upper lateral cartilages are cut away from the nasal septum

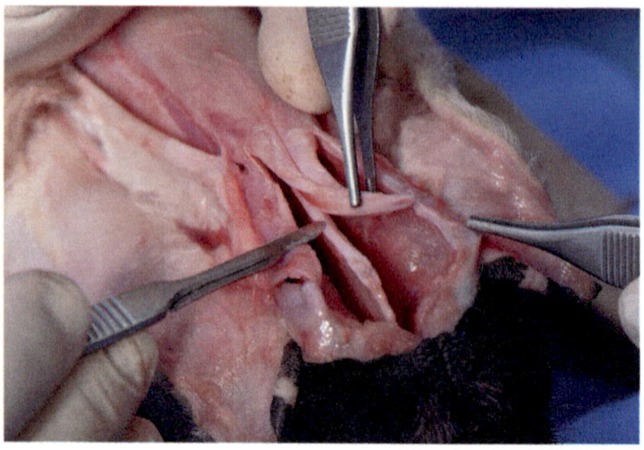

Fig. 19.7 Cartilaginous hump is resected

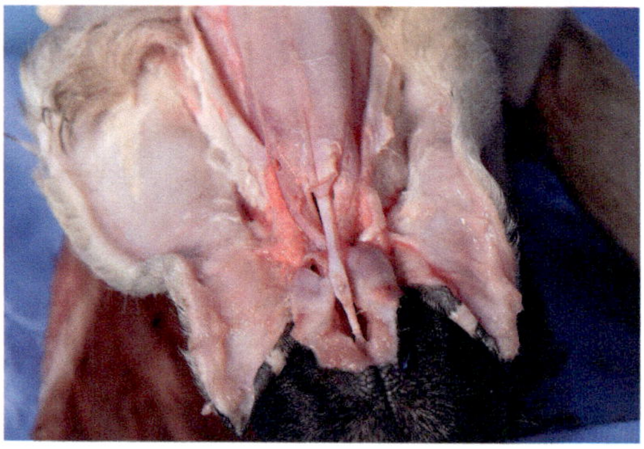

Fig. 19.8 Spreader flaps are sutured in the midline to reconstruct the middle vault

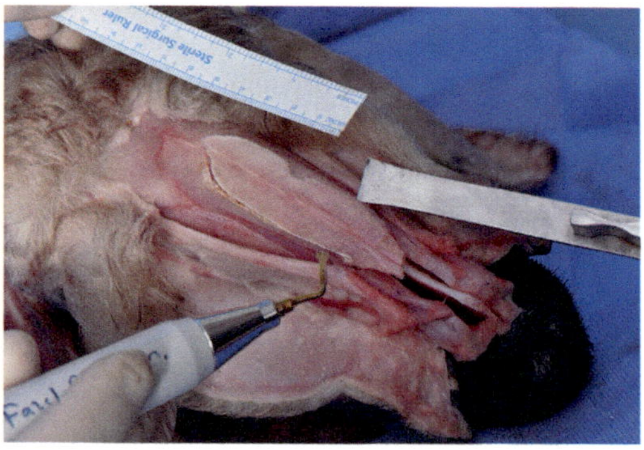

Fig. 19.9 Bony hump is resected by using Piezotome and Rubin osteotome. Since the nasal bones are much longer and bigger than in humans, this is a great model for trainees to learn the behavior of Piezotome and handheld instruments such as Rubin osteotome

The bony hump can be removed using different instruments to compare their efficacy, such as the Rubin osteotome, rasps, piezo, and/or burr (Fig. 19.9). Thus, the surgeon can have a clear

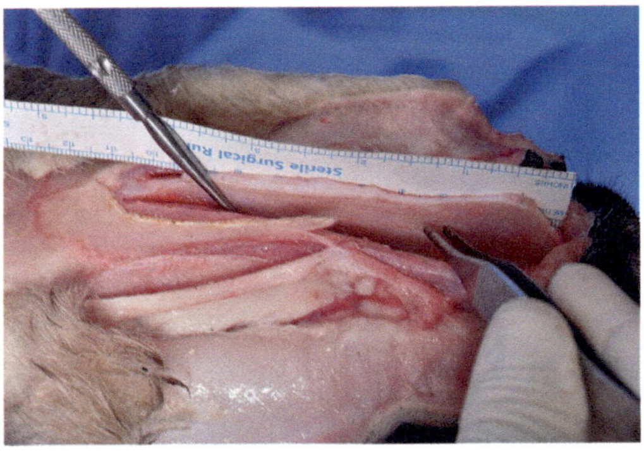

Fig. 19.10 After humpectomy, the nasal septum is exposed entirely. In lamb heads, the nasal septum can reach up to 12 cm in length

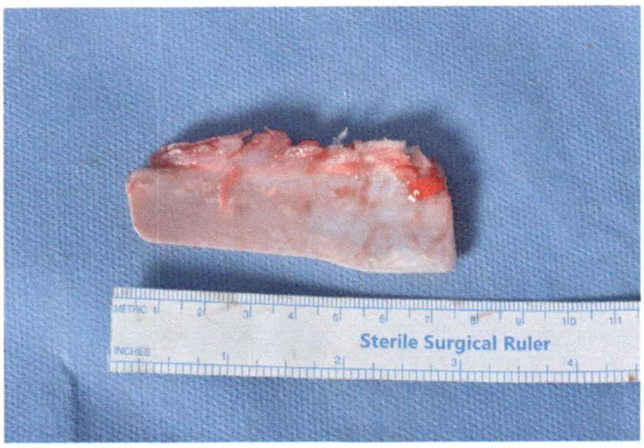

Fig. 19.11 The septal cartilage is harvested, and it is almost 8 cm after leaving the L-strut framework in place

understanding of how these instruments work on the bony pyramid. It is better to harvest the septal cartilage at this stage, leaving an 8–10 mm L-strut in place (Fig. 19.10). The cartilage obtained can be as long as 10 cm and 2 cm in height (Fig. 19.11). From this large piece of cartilage, it is possible to carve spreader grafts, tip onlay grafts, lateral crural onlay grafts, shield grafts, articulated rim grafts, and septal extension grafts (Fig. 19.12).

The spreader grafts are sutured to both sides of the dorsal septum (Fig. 19.13). The spreader grafts can be sutured at the upper margin of the dorsal segment of the nasal cartilage and/or 1–2 mm below the upper margin. By doing so, the effect of both methods can be observed by the surgeon. It is suggested to keep the spreader grafts long enough so that the caudal portions can exceed the anterior septal angle by 3–4 mm. Upper lateral cartilages are sutured to the spreader grafts and septum to reconstruct the middle vault (Fig. 19.14). A caudal septal extension graft can be sutured to the caudal portions of the spreader grafts. The septal extension graft is fixed to the caudal portion of the nasal septum using simple and figure-of-eight sutures. In addition, supportive grafts can be experienced at this stage to further fix the septal extension graft (Fig. 19.15). Another technique to try is suturing the septal extension graft to overlap on the caudal septum to determine its effectiveness.

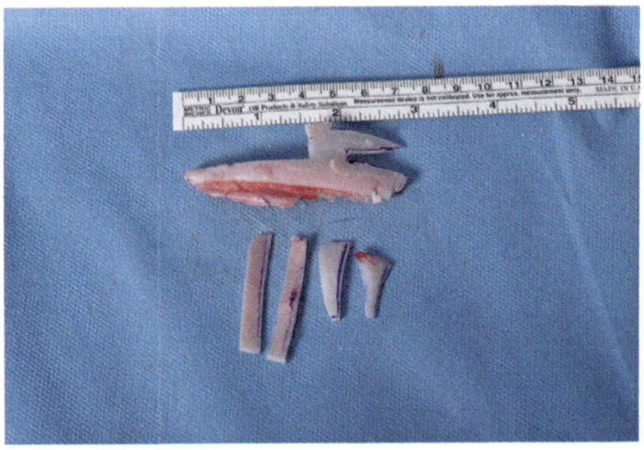

Fig. 19.12 Two spreader grafts, a septal extension graft, and a shield graft are sculpted from the harvested cartilage

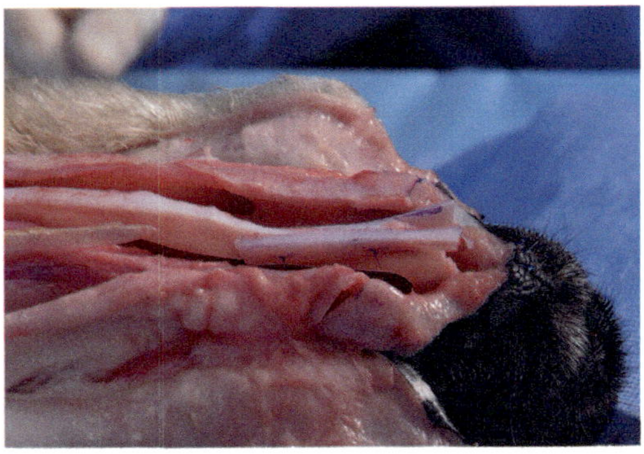

Fig. 19.13 Two spreader grafts are sutured to the dorsal septum

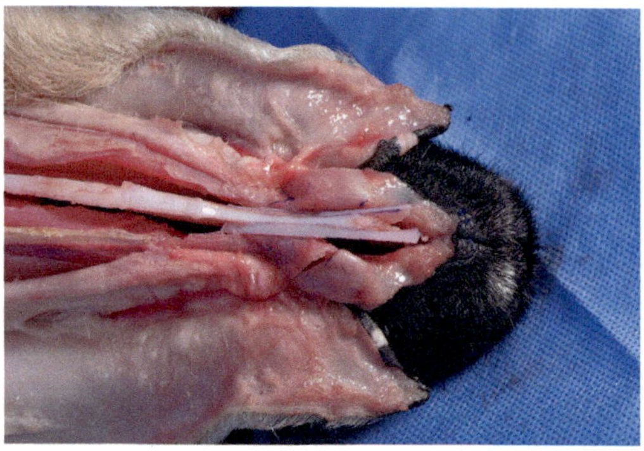

Fig. 19.14 Upper lateral cartilages are sutured to the spreader grafts and septum to reconstruct the middle vault

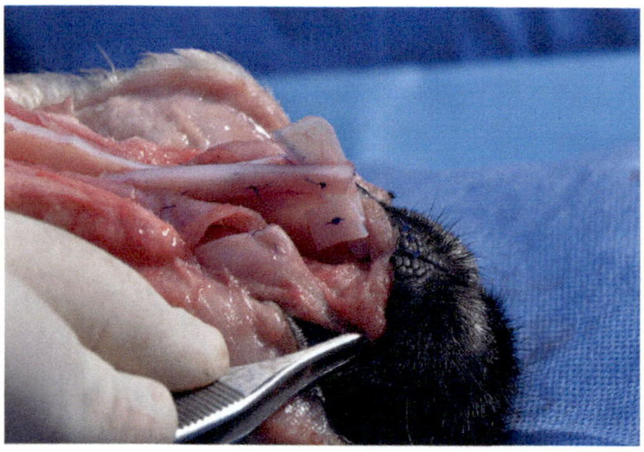

Fig. 19.15 Septal extension graft is fixed in place by suturing it to the spreader grafts and supporting septal graft

Tip surgery starts with a cephalic trim. The lateral crura is shorter and thinner in lambs. Therefore, lateral crural turn-in-flap is not easy to perform. Lateral crural steal of 2–3 mm is performed bilaterally. Dome sutures, such as traditional domal suture, high domal, hemitransdomal, and cranial tip suture, should be exercised (Fig. 19.16). Dome equalizing sutures are applied to shape the tip. The tongue-in-groove technique is used to fixate the tip in the midline on the caudal septal extension graft. At this stage, various grafts, such as shield grafts, tip grafts, articulated alar rim grafts, and dorsal onlay grafts, can be easily exercised (Fig. 19.17).

Medial, transverse, and lateral osteotomies are performed using osteotomes and/or a piezo device (Figs. 19.18 and 19.19a). The surgeon can have a clear understanding of how different osteotomy techniques and instruments work on bone. Percutaneous osteotomies can be performed before dissecting the skin on the bony pyramid

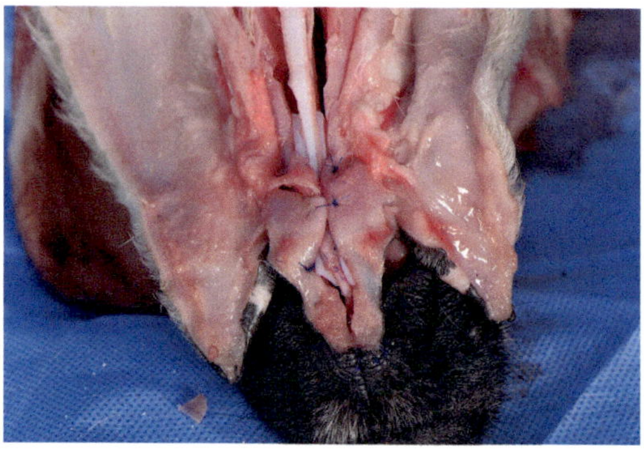

Fig. 19.16 Right-sided domal suture, right-sided cephalic trim, and dome equalization suture are performed

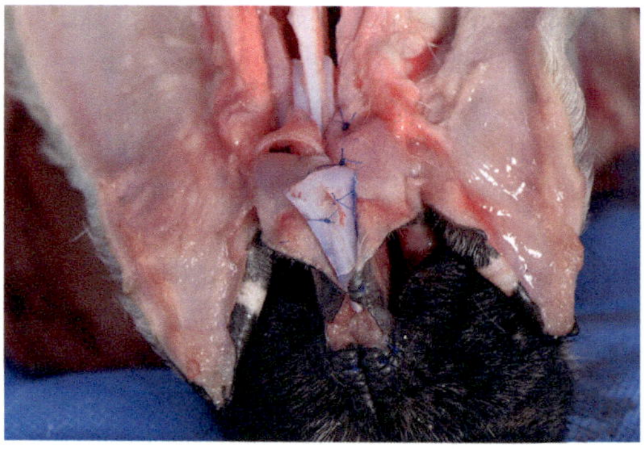

Fig. 19.17 Shield graft is sutured on the tip

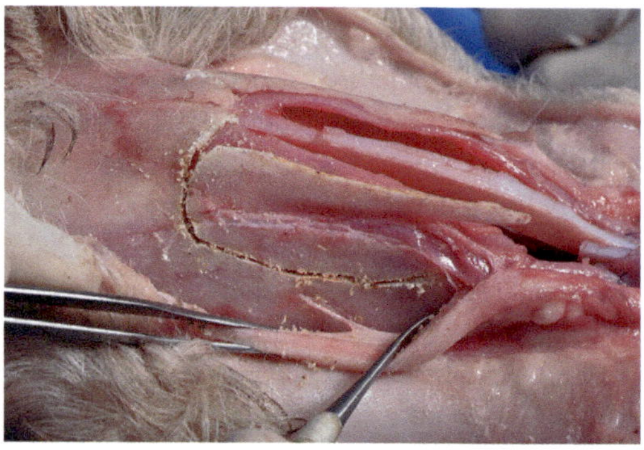

Fig. 19.18 Transverse, and lateral osteotomies are performed using Piezo on the right side

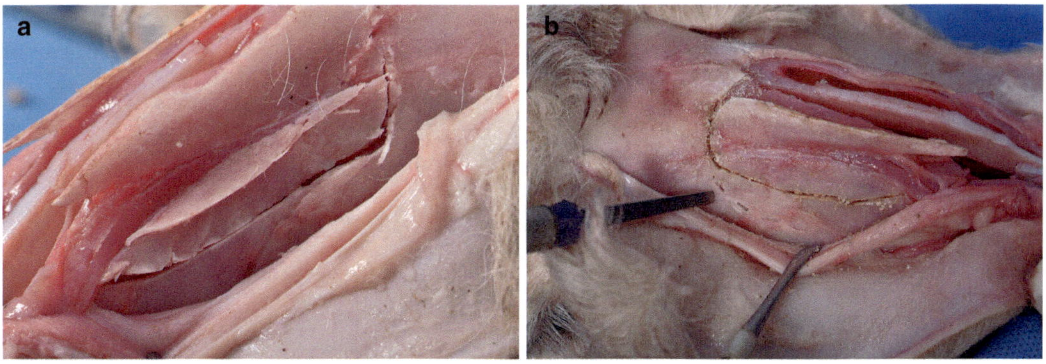

Fig. 19.19 Transverse, intermediate, and lateral osteotomies are performed using a handheld osteotome on the left side (**a**). Perforating osteotomies are performed on the right side to mimic percutaneous osteotomies (**b**)

(Fig. 19.19b). Its effect can later be evaluated after skin dissection. I heard that many colleagues were reluctant to use Piezo because they were not willing to use it in humans before they understood how it worked. This is the best model to work with Piezo and to understand how it works with different tips and different bone thicknesses.

19.3 Dissection for Preservation Rhinoplasty Techniques

Preservation rhinoplasty techniques have become popular in recent years. Surgeons who would like to learn and try these techniques will need to work on cadavers. I decided to use the lamb head if it could be a good model for learning preservation rhinoplasty techniques. If a lamb head with skin is used, the first 9 steps for structural rhinoplasty are the same. However, if the surgeon intends to perform a dissection for preservation techniques, the lamb heads can be directly bought from the butcher because the skin is not needed. It is advised to start working on the bony pyramid first (Table 19.2; Figs. 19.20 and 19.21). Lateral osteotomies are performed perpendicular to the face to facilitate the push-down of the bony pyramid (Fig. 19.22). Then, lateral wedge resections are performed as in the let-down procedure. The trainee can use osteotomes, a piezo, or a burr to work on the bony pyramid. Then, the bony-cartilaginous skeleton and part of the maxilla on the right side are resected to fully expose the

Table 19.2 Dissection plan for preservation rhinoplasty

1.	Preparation of the lamb head
2.	Preparation of the surgical setting
3.	Injection of the tip and dorsum
4.	Columellar incision
5.	Tip exposure
6.	Dorsum exposure
7.	Dissection of the skin and cutting it in the midline
8.	Elevation of perichondrial and periosteal flaps
9.	Caudal septum exposure
10.	Lateral osteotomy on the right side
11.	Wedge resection on the left side (let down)
12.	Resection of the bony-cartilaginous skeleton and part of the maxilla on the right side to fully expose the nasal septum
13.	Dissection and resection of right-sided mucosa of the nasal septum
14.	Planning different strip techniques on the long septal cartilage
15.	Low strip (caudal one-third of the nasal septum)
16.	High strip (middle one-third of the nasal septum)
17.	Intermediate strip (cephalic one-third of the nasal septum)

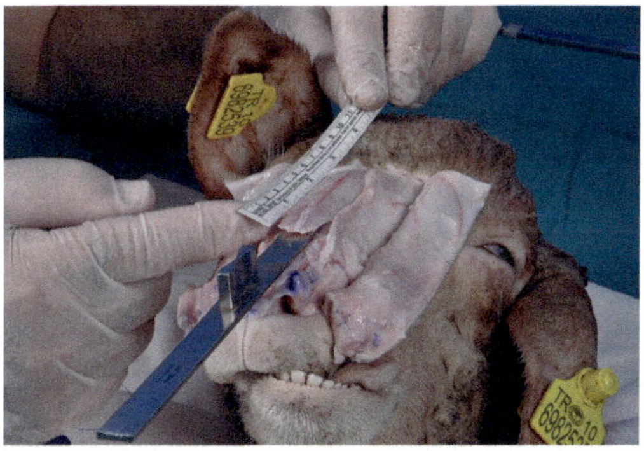

Fig. 19.20 Bony hump removal by Rubin osteotome and/or Piezotome. The bony dorsum is three times longer than in humans

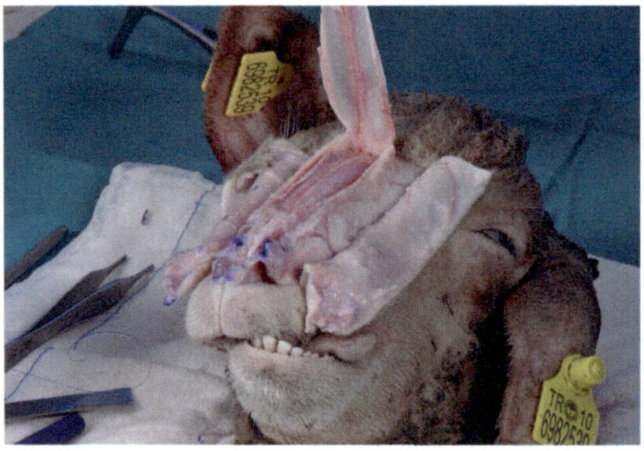

Fig. 19.21 When the bony hump is removed, the cartilaginous and soft tissue structures under it should stay intact

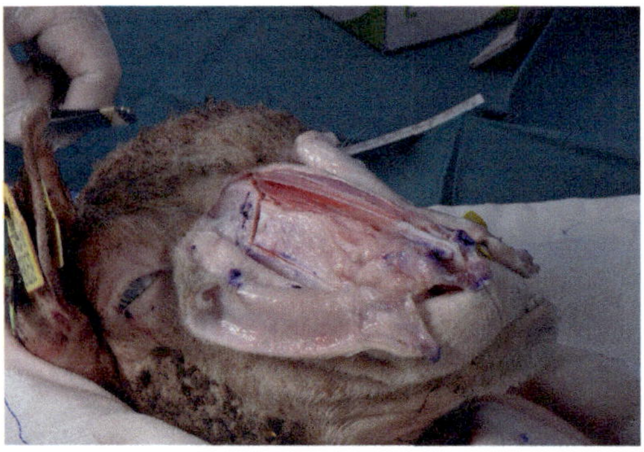

Fig. 19.22 Lateral and transverse osteotomies on the right side

nasal septum (Fig. 19.23). The mucosa of the nasal septum on the right side is dissected and then resected to expose the entire cartilage. The length of the nasal septum was found to be 11.5 cm in width and 4.1 cm in height in our previous studies. The ethmoid did not exist in lamb heads. We also learned during our previous studies that a satisfactory profile could not be obtained without removing the long bony cap in lambs. The advantage of the long septal cartilage is that the surgeon can perform two or three techniques on the same head (Fig. 19.24). It is best to start with high strip [5], and intermediate techniques such as the Tetris technique [6] (Figs. 19.25 and 19.26), and/or modified subdorsal Cottle tech-

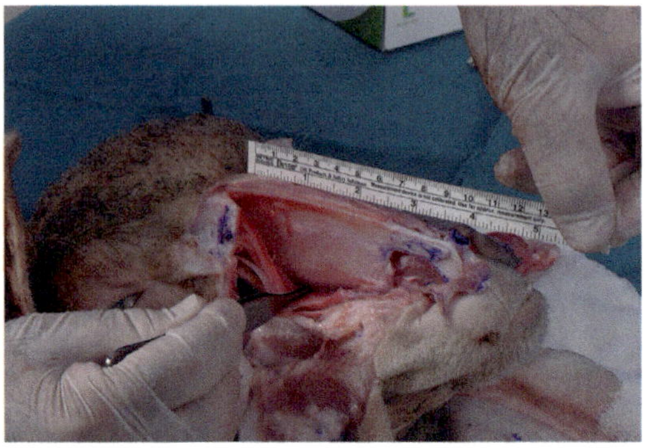

Fig. 19.23 Resection of the bony-cartilaginous skeleton and part of the maxilla on the right side to fully expose the nasal septum, and the mucosa of the nasal septum is dissected

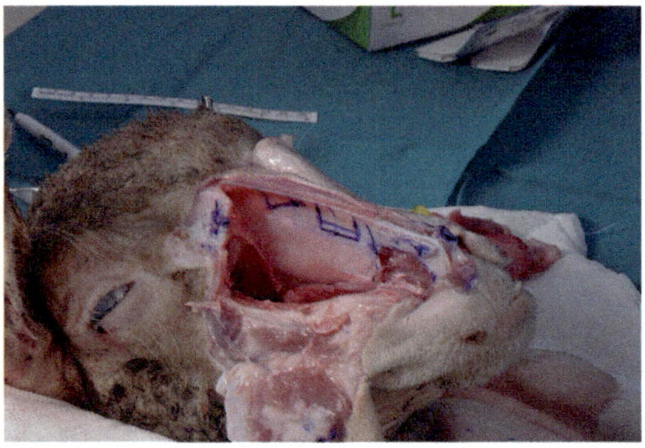

Fig. 19.24 Planning different strip techniques on the septal cartilage can be done because of very long nasal septal cartilage. Tetris and Z-flap markings are already done on the septal cartilage

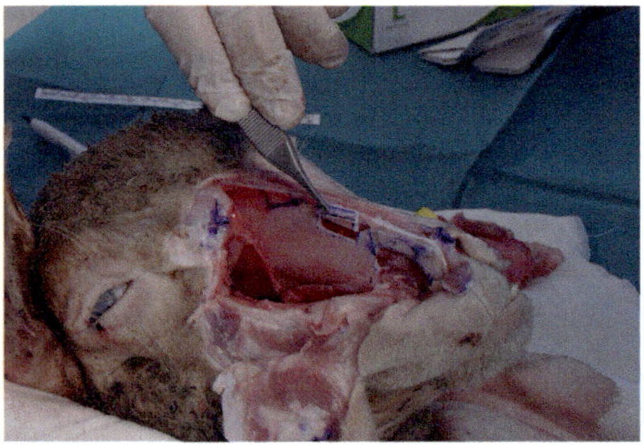

Fig. 19.25 In the Tetris type, a rectangular piece of cartilage is removed to lower the nasal dorsum

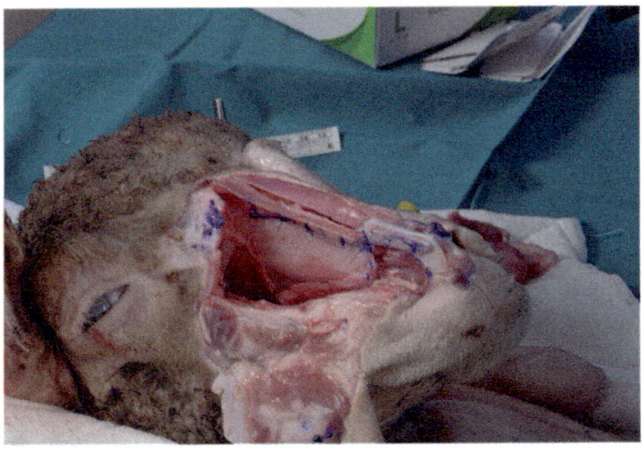

Fig. 19.26 The nasal dorsum is lowered by using Tetris and Z-flap methods

nique [7] (Fig. 19.28) and their variations, such as overlapping the cartilage instead of resecting. The low strip can be attempted after suturing the high strip and intermediate technique cuts [8] (Figs. 19.27 and 19.29).

I have been using lamb head to teach rhinoplasty and septoplasty to residents and course participants. Until now, I had the opportunity to perform lamb head dissections for rhinoplasty in Turkey, Colombia, and Peru. I am organizing courses for my residents in my university department. I am pretty sure that either I and/or my fellows will continue using lamb head dissections.

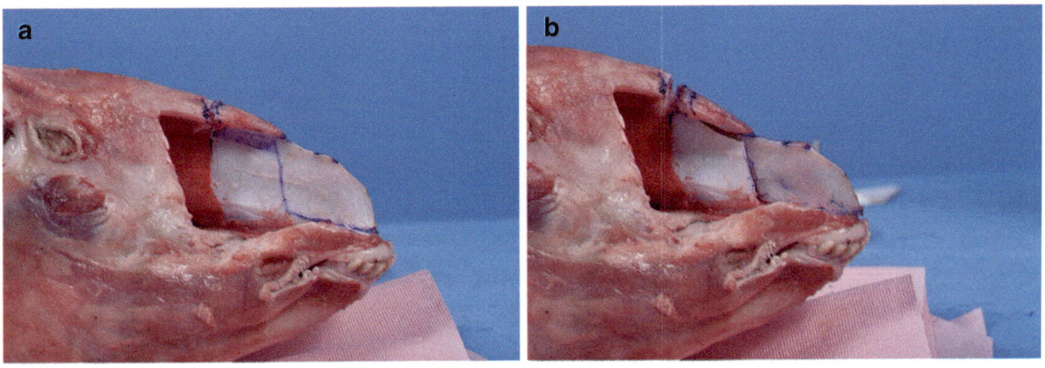

Fig. 19.27 The nasal dorsum is lowered by using Cottle type of low strip procedure

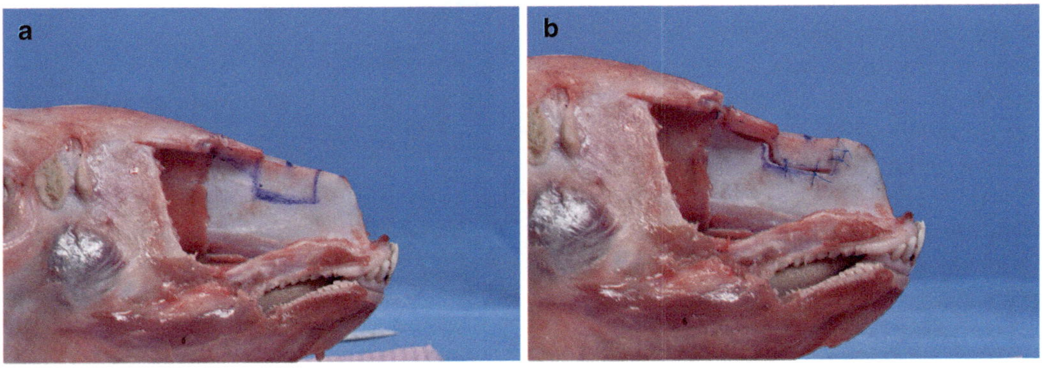

Fig. 19.28 The resection area of the is marked first (**a**), and then a strip of cartilage is resected and the cartilaginous flap is sutured to the nasal septum

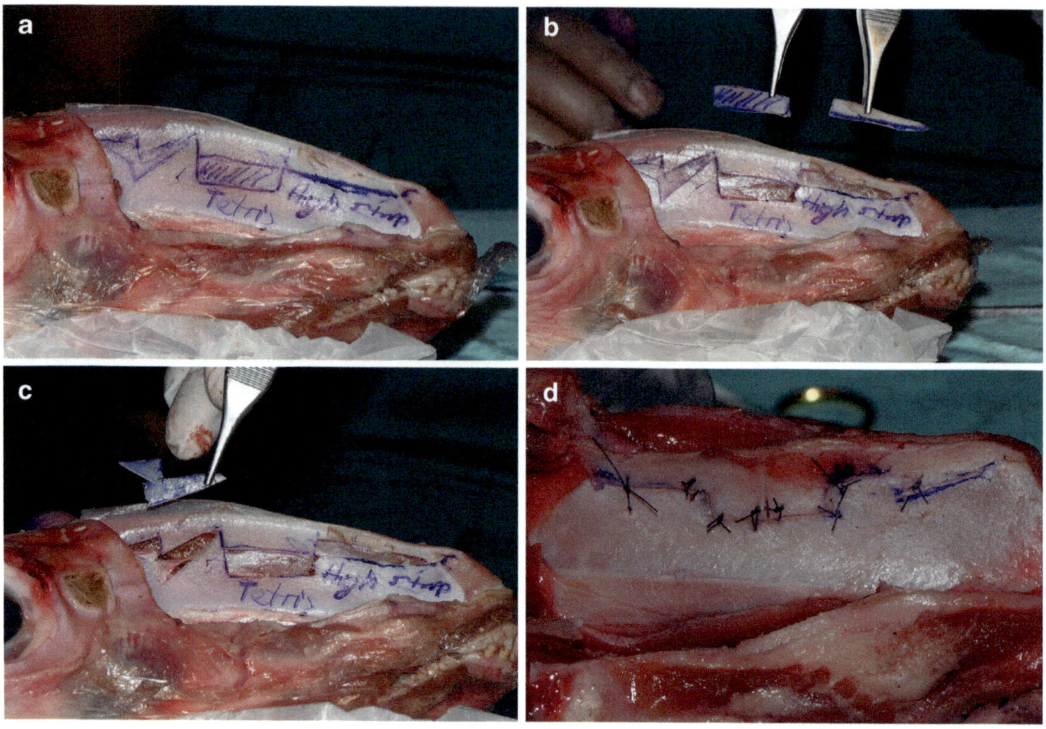

Fig. 19.29 The high strip, intermediate techniques of Tetris, and Z-flap can be planned on the same specimen (**a**). Cartilage resections are performed to bring the nasal dorsum down (**b, c**). The edges of the cartilage are sutured, and the effects of these three techniques can be compared on one specimen (**d**)

I also try to encourage my colleagues all over the world to start cadaver dissection courses with lamb head and then pass to human cadaver dissection. I have been teaching rhinoplasty to my colleagues on human cadavers for more than 20 years. If trainees start working on an entire lamb head, they have a chance to practice all the steps of rhinoplasty alone. When they pass to the human cadaver head, they feel more accustomed to working on soft tissues and bone, even though they dissect only one side of the head.

All the steps presented for structural rhinoplasty can be clearly seen in the demonstration video attached in this chapter (Fig. 19.30).

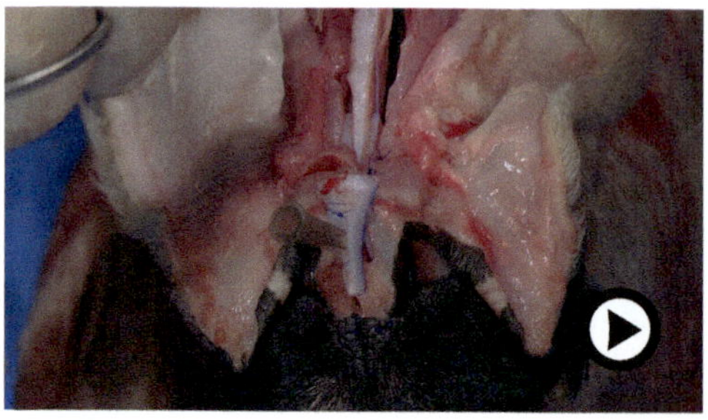

Fig. 19.30 A lamb head dissection is performed as an ex vivo animal model for septorhinoplasty training (▶ https://doi.org/10.1007/000-dzv)

In short, the lamb head is a very useful and cheap model to train on rhinoplasty and septoplasty. A surgeon can practice all surgical maneuvers of structural and preservation rhinoplasty. It can be practiced anywhere without the need for a special setting like an anatomy lab.

References

1. Mladina R, Vuković K, Štern Padovan R, Skitarelić N. An animal model for endoscopic endonasal surgery and dacryocystorhinostomy training: uses and limitations of the lamb's head. J Laryngol Otol. 2011;125:696–700.
2. Apaydin F, Saghir M, Garcia RFFP, Daoud M, Jaber A. Lamb head as a training model for septoplasty and rhinoplasty. Facial Plast Surg. 2022;38:525–9.
3. Erol O, Soto-Galindo GA, Apaydin F. Biomechanics of septal L-strut on lamb head models. Facial Plast Surg. 2022;38:518–24.
4. Dini GM, Gonella HA, Fregadolli L, Nunes B, Gozzano R. Training rhinoseptoplasty, sinusectomy, and turbinectomy in an animal model. Plast Reconstr Surg. 2012;130:224e–6e.
5. Saban Y, Daniel RK, Polselli R, Trapasso M, Palhazi P. Dorsal preservation: the push down technique reassessed. Aesthet Surg J. 2018;38:117–31.
6. Neves JC, Arancibia Tagle D, Dewes W, Ferraz M. The segmental preservation rhinoplasty: the split tetris concept. Facial Plast Surg. 2021;37:36–44.
7. Kovacevic M, Buttler E, Haack S, Riedel F, Veit JA. Dorsal preservation septorhinoplasty [in German]. HNO. 2021;69:817–27.
8. Cottle MH, Loring RM. Corrective surgery of the external nasal pyramid and the nasal septum for restoration of normal physiology. Ill Med J. 1946;90:119–35.

Index

© The Editor(s) (if applicable) and The Author(s), under exclusive license to Springer Nature Switzerland AG 2025
F. Apaydin, *Septal Surgery Challenges in Rhinoplasty*,
https://doi.org/10.1007/978-3-031-74734-2

GPSR Compliance

The European Union's (EU) General Product Safety Regulation (GPSR) is a set of rules that requires consumer products to be safe and our obligations to ensure this.

If you have any concerns about our products, you can contact us on ProductSafety@springernature.com

In case Publisher is established outside the EU, the EU authorized representative is:

Springer Nature Customer Service Center GmbH
Europaplatz 3
69115 Heidelberg, Germany

Batch number: 10732801

Printed by Printforce, the Netherlands